Property o
FAU School
Social Wo

MW00666886

20198284

SOCIAL WORK PRACTICE WITH CHILDREN

Clinical Practice with Children, Adolescents, and Families
(formerly Social Work Practice with Children and Families)

Nancy Boyd Webb, *Series Editor*

www.guilford.com/CPCAF

This series presents a broad range of topics relevant for today's social workers, psychologists, counselors, and other professionals who work with children, adolescents, and families. Designed for practical use, volumes feature specific discussions on assessment, interventions, therapeutic roadblocks, the therapeutic relationship, and professional and value issues, illuminated by numerous case examples.

Social Work Practice with Children, Fourth Edition
NANCY BOYD WEBB

Play Therapy with Children and Adolescents in Crisis, Fourth Edition
NANCY BOYD WEBB, EDITOR

Group Work with Adolescents, Third Edition: Principles and Practice
ANDREW MALEKOFF

Working with Adolescents: A Guide for Practitioners
JULIE ANNE LASER AND NICOLE NICOTERA

Child Development, Third Edition: A Practitioner's Guide
DOUGLAS DAVIES

Helping Bereaved Children, Third Edition: A Handbook for Practitioners
NANCY BOYD WEBB, EDITOR

Social Work in Schools: Principles and Practice
LINDA OPENSHAW

Working with Traumatized Youth in Child Welfare
NANCY BOYD WEBB, EDITOR

Mass Trauma and Violence: Helping Families and Children Cope
NANCY BOYD WEBB, EDITOR

Culturally Competent Practice with Immigrant and Refugee Children and Families
ROWENA FONG, EDITOR

Complex Adoption and Assisted Reproductive Technology: A Developmental Approach to Clinical Practice
VIVIAN B. SHAPIRO, JANET R. SHAPIRO, AND ISABEL H. PARET

SOCIAL WORK PRACTICE WITH CHILDREN

FOURTH EDITION

Nancy Boyd Webb

Foreword by Luis H. Zayas

THE GUILFORD PRESS
New York London

Copyright © 2019 The Guilford Press
A Division of Guilford Publications, Inc.
370 Seventh Avenue, Suite 1200, New York, NY 10001
www.guilford.com

All rights reserved

Except as indicated, no part of this book may be reproduced, translated, stored in a retrieval system, or transmitted, in any form or by any means, electronic, mechanical, photocopying, microfilming, recording, or otherwise, without written permission from the publisher.

Printed in the United States of America

This book is printed on acid-free paper.

Last digit is print number: 9 8 7 6 5 4 3 2 1

LIMITED DUPLICATION LICENSE

These materials are intended for use only by qualified professionals.

The publisher grants to individual purchasers of this book nonassignable permission to reproduce all materials for which permission is specifically granted in a footnote. This license is limited to you, the individual purchaser, for personal use or use with clients. This license does not grant the right to reproduce these materials for resale, redistribution, electronic display, or any other purposes (including but not limited to books, pamphlets, articles, video- or audiotapes, blogs, file-sharing sites, Internet or intranet sites, and handouts or slides for lectures, workshops, or webinars, whether or not a fee is charged). Permission to reproduce these materials for these and any other purposes must be obtained in writing from the Permissions Department of Guilford Publications.

The author has checked with sources believed to be reliable in her efforts to provide information that is complete and generally in accord with the standards of practice that are accepted at the time of publication. However, in view of the possibility of human error or changes in behavioral, mental health, or medical sciences, neither the author, nor the editors and publisher, nor any other party who has been involved in the preparation or publication of this work warrants that the information contained herein is in every respect accurate or complete, and they are not responsible for any errors or omissions or the results obtained from the use of such information. Readers are encouraged to confirm the information contained in this book with other sources.

Library of Congress Cataloging-in-Publication Data

Names: Webb, Nancy Boyd, author.
Title: Social work practice with children, fourth edition / Nancy Boyd Webb ; foreword by Luis H. Zayas.
Description: Fourth edition. | New York, NY : The Guilford Press, 2019. | Series: Clinical practice with children, adolescents, and families | Revised edition of the author's Social work practice with children, c2011. | Includes bibliographical references and index.
Identifiers: LCCN 2018042395 | ISBN 9781462537556 (hardback : alk. paper)
Subjects: LCSH: Social work with children. | BISAC: SOCIAL SCIENCE / Social Work. | PSYCHOLOGY / Psychotherapy / Child & Adolescent. | MEDICAL / Psychiatry / Child & Adolescent. | PSYCHOLOGY / Psychotherapy / Couples & Family.
Classification: LCC HV713 .W39 2018 | DDC 362.7/253—dc23
LC record available at *https://lccn.loc.gov/2018042395*

About the Author

Nancy Boyd Webb, DSW, LICSW, RPT-S, is a leading authority on play therapy with children who have experienced loss and traumatic bereavement. She is University Distinguished Professor Emerita of Social Work in the Graduate School of Social Service at Fordham University, where she held an endowed Chair in Child Welfare Studies, founded the Post-Master's Certificate Program in Child and Adolescent Therapy, and taught clinical practice for 30 years. She has published numerous books on child therapy, trauma, and bereavement, including *Helping Bereaved Children, Third Edition*, and *Play Therapy with Children and Adolescents in Crisis, Fourth Edition.* Dr. Webb is an active supervisor, consultant, and trainer who presents frequently at conferences in the United States and internationally. She is a recipient of honors including the Day-Garrett Award from the Smith College School for Social Work, the Clinical Practice Award from the Association for Death Education and Counseling, and the designation of Distinguished Scholar by the National Academies of Practice in Social Work.

Foreword

Being a professional social worker who treats children and adolescents in any field of practice (e.g., child welfare, mental health, schools, juvenile justice) calls for clinicians to be watchful of the contemporary social, cultural, economic, and political changes and of the scientific and professional advances that are happening around us and our young clients. In fact, this need to monitor the world that our clients and their families are experiencing brings me back to an exhortation I heard often from clinical supervisors: "If you are practicing today the way you did yesterday, you are stagnating." Like other advice I give supervisees, this is one that I return to. It makes clear that to keep up with our clients, we have to change what we do and how we do it. It reminds us that we must be attentive to the forces affecting us and refresh our practice regularly.

Nancy Boyd Webb has been alert to the world around her. She has been so since the first edition of this book and her other writings. She is a disciplined and deeply empathic writer and therapist. Webb is a keen observer of a child's world and doesn't get distracted by fads in, say, child rearing, or trendy therapies. And she is attentive to how social work practice must change. One thing you can always count on is that Webb refreshes her thinking, her practice, and her writings. But she also keeps in mind tried-and-true principles of human behavior from the foundations of attachment and bonding, psychological and social individuation, the arc of human development, and the universality of loss, grief, and mourning. The fourth edition of *Social Work Practice with Children* reflects the author's integration of the traditional and the new.

Refreshing our practice means integrating the contemporary knowledge with the solid, age-old pillars of practice (e.g., "getting in our client's shoes"; listening actively; reflecting and reframing). These skills have to take into consideration the many contemporary issues that practitioners have to integrate. From Webb's book and my own thinking, I alight on three major issues of our day: social–cultural forces, technological changes, and scientific advancement.

Social and cultural forces are readily seen in such places as the United States and other developed countries, where the greatest changes are being brought by one of the largest streams of migrations in recorded history. Refugees, asylum seekers, and immigrants move in search of security, safety, and prosperity. These newcomers carry with them a host of reasons for their moves, such as poverty, persecution, natural disasters, wars and violence, or social instability. And in their proverbial rucksacks, these newcomers bring their suffering and their need for help to social workers, making for a complex and totally modern interaction. Social workers in receiving countries must adapt their practice to this reality; staying tied to the practice of the past will fail the newest clients. There are many other social and cultural changes in the world that children and their families must grapple with, from new and different definitions of gender identity and gender expression to the unease parents feel about whom they can trust with their children and whom they cannot trust. No parent today can obscure (change to avoid) the violence in the world. Children see and hear about killings with bombs, cars and trucks, and any other weapon in the name of religion. On any given day, children see news on television or the Internet about mass shootings, such as those in schools, workplaces, temples of worship, and celebrations. When it happens to other children, such as happened at Sandy Hook Elementary School in the state of Connecticut, it becomes much more real, as the victims were children like themselves and teachers like the ones they engage with every day.

Technology—its impact and its utility—is the second transformative issue for humankind. In a world that didn't have the communications technology of today, much of the news of tragedies would trickle in, as it did perhaps a hundred years ago. But technology now brings it to us rapidly. Laptop computers, tablets, and mobile phones are ubiquitous and are making life easier in many ways. Telemedicine can bring patients and doctors together from remote parts. Now child clients can have more regular and immediate access to their social workers. The therapeutic alliance has found new ways to be sustained and strengthened through technology. The transitional objects that clients in the past relied on can now be in the palms of their hands. A child feeling alone, bereft of help, misunderstood, or confused can reach the therapist and summon the therapist's image or words, thereby invoking the soothing aspect of the therapeutic relationship. To change and move ahead our practice, contemporary social work practitioners need to know how to use the tools of technology therapeutically, judiciously, and ethically.

Neuroscience and the increasing knowledge of the brain is the third major factor in our lives and in improving our practice. Keeping our practice fresh and relevant means actively pursuing learning and understanding the neurobiology of behavior, to understand who we are and why we do what we do. This isn't to say that we discard tried-and-true knowledge of, say, human behavior and principles of practice. We know full well that emotional attachments and dynamics of human interaction, much of them stemming from both family patterns and deep psychic forces (e.g., fear and envy, humiliation, self-worth), are what make us human after hundreds of thousands of years of evolution. Similarly, knowing how to engage clients and sustain therapeutic relationships are bread-and-butter practice skills. It's these kinds of issues that do not change. Yet the neurosciences can reveal mysteries associated with, for example, the nature of early attachment relationships. Inevitably, we will work with severely traumatized children suffering from posttraumatic stress disorder and other responses to trauma. Comprehending that the neurobiology of trauma involves deep links with brain growth and such things as emotional regulation, problem solving, cognition, and other executive functions that help us manage in our world is important for the practitioner. Scientific knowledge from biology, psychology, and the neurosciences is helping the modern practitioner. We might say that we are at a place in history in which neuroscience can help us resolve the centuries-long debate of nature versus nurture.

Webb emphasizes the impact that deteriorating social conditions have on children's health and well-being. From family dysfunction to rampant drug use and family and community violence, children become frightened and feel very vulnerable. Modern practitioners need to keep up with understanding the *long-term effects* on children who are exposed to different forms of family dysfunction, such as domestic violence, abuse and neglect, substance use, and parental absence and/or abandonment. Reactive disorders in the form of externalizing or internalizing behaviors or reactive attachment problems are not uncommon. As children forge their identities, social workers must acknowledge with the child the changing norms about gender identity. Social work practice must take into account how this may affect children's beliefs and their own experiences.

Refreshing our practice involves drawing on evidence-based research that can guide our selections of interventions with children. The modern practitioner cannot simply pluck "off the shelf" the easiest or most accessible evidence-based intervention. The practitioner has to know *how* to evaluate the science and make informed choices. Practicing culturally competent social work involves understanding our clients and adapting our practices to their needs. Webb's list reminds us to consider carefully at what level we should intervene on behalf of our child clients. Should it be solely the child? The family? The school? Parents' social networks? The list is as complex as are the lives of our clients. Webb points us toward how to make the decisions.

In helping us be better social workers with children (and all our clients), Webb doesn't lose sight of us, the practitioners. Just as she sees the suffering of children, she also sees what can happen to the modern clinician working with such difficult cases. In this book, Webb reminds us of the importance of self-care to avoid being traumatized and burned out by our work. Self-care is an individual choice, of course, but Webb suggests that we appreciate the healing effects of mindfulness in self-caring.

As I stated at the outset, Nancy Boyd Webb has been alert to the world around her. Her scholarship has always kept in mind how the changes in that world will affect our practice with children and families. For decades, I have been impressed with her writings. Her books guided my own practice with children and adolescents decades ago. My respect for her authenticity as a teacher and clinician grew when we were colleagues on the same faculty of social work. With the publication of the fourth edition of *Social Work Practice with Children*, my admiration has only grown more. I trust the next generation of social workers will feel similarly as it learns from Nancy Boyd Webb.

Luis H. Zayas, PhD
Dean and Robert Lee Sutherland Chair in Mental Health and Social Policy,
Steve Hicks School of Social Work, and
Professor of Psychiatry, Dell Medical School,
The University of Texas at Austin

Preface

When I completed the third edition of this book in 2011, I believed that it would serve as a guide for practitioners for many years. It has done so, but the increasingly complex crises, traumas, and stresses confronting families during the second decade of the 21st century have required greatly enhanced understanding and skills on the part of helping professionals. This fourth edition seeks to increase practitioners' knowledge about the impact of multiple and intense stressors in children's lives, while also presenting a range of effective helping approaches to assist them. The focus remains on the numerous problems that may interfere with children's development, including the helpful and/or harmful influences of family, peers, and others in their lives.

The everyday environment of many children today is toxic rather than beneficial. Children may live in a family in which one or both parents are addicted to alcohol or other substances, they may be victims of or witnesses to bullying at school, and some may suffer from poor nutrition and/or personal health issues. Children need to grow up in a loving home where the adults cherish and value them, so that a positive attachment relationship develops, which then serves as a buffer when the child encounters negative treatment from peers or others. Too often, when parents use substances, they ignore their children, who then must learn to take care of themselves. Children may witness interpersonal violence in the family, which also may be directed at them, leaving them feeling helpless and confused. Sadly, this is not a new situation, but we have learned more about the consequences of early neglect and trauma on the young child's brain and his or her future development. This topic is discussed in this edition, together with some approaches to helping the families and children who are struggling with the aftereffects of poor parenting and the absence of positive attachments.

As in previous editions, this book is divided into four major sections. Part I presents the ecological framework for understanding children in the context of their environments and the challenges for practitioners who are committed to this helping effort. Part II reviews the process of helping children, utilizing the case of a homeless girl over three chapters that focus on the necessary steps in any helping effort. Part III deals with the different methods of helping children, beginning with methods to help the family help their child, and also includes chapters describing play therapy with the individual child, group work, and school-based collaboration. Part IV devotes separate chapters to children in special circumstances, such as in divorcing families, in families affected by illness and death, and in substance-using families. One chapter focuses on the interpersonal violence of bullying, and another chapter, new to this volume, focuses on helping children who are immigrants and refugees.

Although the format of this volume is similar to earlier editions, much new content is included in the various chapters, such as helping families deal with young children who present with gender identity issues, and new treatment approaches such as cognitive-behavioral trauma-focused therapy, mindfulness, and parent–child interaction therapy. The assessment chapter now considers the updated fifth edition of the *Diagnostic and Statistical Manual of Mental Disorders* (DSM-5) as part of the diagnostic process, together with a discussion of the effects of early trauma on parent–child attachment. The importance of therapist self-care practice is emphasized throughout. Case illustrations demonstrate details about the helping process.

This book can be used as a text for undergraduate- or graduate-level social work courses. Each chapter ends with Discussion Questions and suggestions for possible role-play exercises. These are intended to encourage class discussion of the content in each chapter. It is essential that social workers receive specialized training focused on the child's individual needs, apart from those of the family. Although it is always incumbent on a practitioner working with a child to involve the family, it is seldom sufficient to focus on family work alone, without some sessions devoted to helping the child individually, based on his or her developmental level. Family therapy involves a lot of talking, and this puts the young child at a disadvantage; examples in this book demonstrate how to involve family members in playing with their child under a therapist's guidance to help them deepen their relationship and resolve some family issues.

My hope is that this book will make social workers more eager and confident about working one on one, using play therapy with a child client, thereby helping to resolve problems before they intensify and become more resistant to intervention. Social workers can have a pivotal role in turning a child's life around, and this not only is a gift to the child and the family, but is also both personally and professionally gratifying for the worker.

Acknowledgments

Each book has its own history, even one with three previous editions. Unique to this fourth edition is that I am now retired from Fordham University and no longer have the benefits of a secretarial staff and research assistants to help with many of the details that accompany any publication. Fortunately, Jane Keislar, Senior Assistant Editor at The Guilford Press, has very successfully filled this role. I am grateful to her and to Jim Nageotte, Senior Editor at Guilford, for their steady support and helpful suggestions, as well as to Jeannie Tang, Senior Production Editor at Guilford.

This book represents my evolution and work with children and families during the past 35 years. All the case material has been disguised to protect client confidentiality, except in instances in which this privilege was previously waived. A few cases are composites of children and families based on numerous past cases. In most instances, clients (including children, whenever possible) gave their written permission. The profession owes a tremendous debt of gratitude to these parents and children, who permitted the use of their personal situations to benefit future social workers and other practitioners in their efforts to help children and families.

I continue to feel very grateful to the filmmaker Kathryn Hunt, whose documentary film *No Place Like Home* (1992) portrayed the case of Barbie and her family that serves as the basis for Chapters 3, 4, and 5. Kathryn helped me locate Barbie for both the second and third editions of this book, when she gave her permission for me to write about her experiences. Neither Kathryn nor I have had any recent contact with Barbie, who now would be in her 30s. Because of the very positive feedback about this case from instructors who have used it in teaching over the years, I have preserved the case without alteration in all editions of this book. I sincerely hope that professionals who work with homeless families and educators who teach about families in economic duress will continue to benefit from this true-life case example. I thank Barbie most sincerely for her willingness to permit me to describe her life as a 10-year-old. Her openness in this regard means that countless others will learn from her experiences.

The first edition of this volume inaugurated Guilford's Social Work Practice with Children and Families series. Since 1996, 10 additional titles have been published in the series (now titled Clinical Practice with Children, Adolescents, and Families), several in three editions. I want to acknowledge the commitment made by this commercial publishing house to the issues confronting social work practice. I continue to be grateful for Seymour Weingarten's endorsement of this venture that connects Guilford to cutting-edge issues in social work education and practice in the 21st century.

Several social work educators and practitioners have offered useful consultation regarding specific chapters in this edition that correspond to their own areas of expertise. Dr. Linda Openshaw of the University of Texas provided invaluable consultation and assistance for Chapter 9, on school-based interventions. Dr. Lala Straussner's writings about substance-using families provided a helpful foundation for Chapter 13, as did the clinical examples provided by Madeline Zevon of Westchester County. I am very grateful to them for their expertise and generosity in sharing their responses and suggestions.

Other invaluable help came from my granddaughter Sophia Webb, who carefully worked to integrate numerous updates into the Appendices. We all know that the devil is in the details, and these people worked diligently to produce a final product of which we all are proud. Once again, my husband, Kempton, has provided concrete assistance and psychological support during this process. His steady optimism and respect for the value of my work is consistent and inspirational. As our family has increased since the previous edition to include four grandchildren, my lifelong commitment to children and their basic rights has taken on special meaning.

Contents

Part II. The Process of Helping Children: A Running Case Illustration of a Child in a Single-Parent Homeless Family

Part III. Different Methods of Helping Children

Appendices

Purchasers of this book can download and print enlarged versions of select materials at *www.guilford.com/webb-forms* for personal use or use with clients only (see copyright page for details).

List of Figures, Tables, and Cases

FIGURES

TABLES

CASES

PART I

AN ECOLOGICAL–DEVELOPMENTAL FRAMEWORK FOR HELPING CHILDREN

CHAPTER 1

The Challenge of Meeting Children's Needs in the Context of Difficult Family and Community Environments

Babies are born dependent on others to meet their physical, psychological/emotional, and cognitive/intellectual needs. A committed caregiver and/or an entire family typically devotes much time and energy to nurturing the baby and helping him or her grow and develop. Ideally, this caretaking process results in the formation of a two-way attachment relationship that serves as the template through which the growing infant experiences the world and learns to relate to others. In the best of all possible worlds, a family feels great happiness anticipating the birth of a child. When prepared emotionally, physically, and financially, most families can deal with the mixture of pleasure and stress associated with raising a child. However, unpredictable circumstances related to the home situation, the baby's health, the family's economic and psychological state, and the community and neighborhood in which the family lives can cause the birth experience and the child's early years to be shrouded with worry and concern. Unforeseen challenges may set in motion a chain of reactions when parents are not prepared to deal with the inevitable responsibilities associated with raising their new baby or when their personal situation changes, as following the death of a family member or a deployment into the military. When parents cannot care for their baby, relatives may do so, and when the extended family is unavailable, the child welfare system may step in. Society therefore maintains a vested interest in ensuring that families meet the needs of their children.

Social workers assist families and children, either through small-scale direct interventions or on a larger scale by helping communities establish and maintain essential services. This book presents different methods of helping children within their families, in schools, and in community settings. Whereas much of the focus here is on micro-level clinical practice with children and their families, the ecological perspective that guides such interventions always evaluates and considers the surrounding physical, economic, and political environments that may facilitate or hinder helping efforts.

THE SOCIAL CONTEXT OF CHILDREN'S LIVES

Children's basic needs include nurturance, responsiveness, predictability, support, and guidance from caretakers (Garbarino, Stott, & Associates, 1989; Garbarino, 1992). Fulfilling these needs requires at least one caring adult who will take the responsibility of being an active presence in the child's life. Over time an attachment relationship develops between the dependent baby and the nurturing caretaker, and this relationship has a crucial role in determining how the child will respond to others in the future. When the child's early relationships are neglectful, abusive, or traumatic, this can result in enduring emotional, behavioral, cognitive, social, and emotional problems later in the child's life (Perry, 2006; Osofsky, 1997).

Statistics from 2016 indicate that approximately 9.2 million poor children in the United States were living in single-parent families, with the majority in single-mother families (Children's Defense Fund, 2016). It is very challenging to balance the economic necessities of earning a living with finding the time to take care of home responsibilities and, in addition, to nurture and develop and maintain a loving relationship with a baby and young child. Although some mothers manage this very well, others do not, and the children may suffer neglect or abuse.

According to the Children's Defense Fund (2016), in 2014 nearly 1 in 11 children lived in extreme poverty (defined as an annual income of less than half the poverty level), and children in single-parent families were more likely to be poor. Black children have the highest poverty rate. Single mothers experience the combined effects of social isolation, economic pressure, and the burden of having sole responsibility for raising a child (Gustafsson, Larson, Nelson, & Gustafsson, 2009; American Psychological Association, 2007). These factors can seriously affect the mothers' ability to form a positive attachment with their babies.

What is the impact on children of living in impoverished environments, which may be characterized by unemployment, pervasive substance abuse, inadequate health care, poor quality child care, and high levels of child abuse and neglect? Numerous studies have found that these socioeconomic disadvantages can contribute to higher incidences of impairment in children's social, behavioral, and academic functioning (Achenbach, Howell, Quay, & Conners, 1991; Achenbach, McConaughy, & Howell, 1987; American Psychological Association, 2007; Brooks-Gunn & Duncan, 1997; Institute of Medicine, 1989; Perry, 2006; Perry & Szalavitz, 2006; Schteingart, Molnar, Klein, Lowe, & Hartmann, 1995; Siegel, 2012). Poverty is a serious social and personal crisis, and interventions to help poor children and families require broad-based efforts to find political and economic remedies, in addition to helping children with their emotional–behavioral difficulties.

However, all children raised in poverty do not develop psychological problems. The ratio of risk and resilience cannot be calculated with certainty, although practitioners should certainly try to reduce risk factors and do whatever possible to stack the deck in favor of the child and family. Sometimes an intervention to help the mother will have trickle-down positive effects on the child. The assessment of risk and resilience factors is discussed more fully as part of the tripartite assessment in Chapter 4.

The *ecological–transactional focus* of this book emphasizes the interacting multisystemic factors that contribute to children's mental, emotional, and behavioral difficulties, including both familial and environmental influences. Developmental factors also play a critical role in how children respond to favorable and stressful events in their lives. However, as previously mentioned, it is important to emphasize that any single element alone is seldom sufficient to lead to emotional problems. It is far more likely that *multiple factors,* both developmental and systemic, will interact to produce problematic behavior in a child (Cicchetti, 2008).

As depicted in Figure 1.1, the complex interplay between children and their social environments makes it essential to consider *simultaneously* a troubled child's biological, temperamental, and developmental status, the surrounding familial cultural context, and his or her physical and social environment. Although political advocacy may be essential for long-term improvement of the insidious effects of poverty, substance abuse/dependence, and violence, immediate supportive assistance must be offered to children and their families who are living in the midst of and trying to cope with these conditions. Children demonstrating troubled and troubling behaviors require prompt, direct services, even when these are provided in less than ideal social environments.

THE CASE OF JACOB, AGE 10, AND DAMIEN, AGE 14

The following account is taken from a front-page article in *The New York Times* (Wilkerson, 1994). As when I prepared the second and third editions of this book, I wondered whether this case would seem out of date for this fourth edition over 20 years later. Sadly, it is not; the situation of urban children who live in high-crime, drug-infested neighborhoods is as bad as ever, and this case could just as easily appear in our local newspapers today.

Presenting Problem Situation

Damien, age 14, and Jacob, age 10, were arrested for armed robbery in the shooting death of a pregnant woman who refused to hand over money she had withdrawn from an automated teller machine. Jacob gave the go-ahead signal

FIGURE 1.1. Interactive influences of child, family, and environment.

Nuclear and Extended Family and Culture	Social and Physical Environment
Ethnicity	Peers
Values and Beliefs	School
Family Lifestyle	Housing
Structure and Boundaries	Neighborhood/Community
Socioeconomic Status	Recreational Resources
Role Expectations	Hazards
Religion	

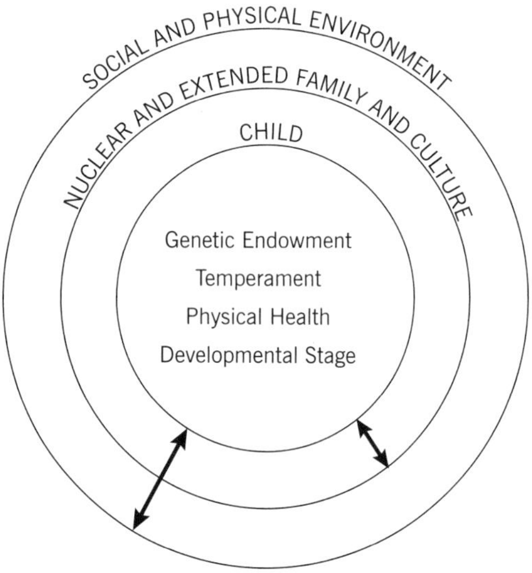

for the robbery, and Damien, a drug dealer who was trying to obtain money to pay drug debts, carried out the shooting. Damien pleaded guilty to second-degree murder, and both boys received the maximum sentence for juveniles—remaining in state custody until the age of 21.

Family Information

Both boys were born to mothers on welfare, each of whom had first given birth at age 14. Damien's father had abandoned his family, and Jacob's father was shot to death in a bar fight when the boy was 4 or 5 years old. Both boys grew up in an atmosphere of physical abuse; Jacob's father used to beat his mother, and Damien said that he ran away from home because his mother beat him. Both boys lived in crack houses, and Jacob's mother had a history of alcohol and crack dependence.

Jacob was the youngest of eight children, in a family in which he saw relatives and friends use guns to settle disputes. He saw his sister shot in the face when he was 4 or 5. Another sister introduced him to marijuana when he was

9. His mother did not appear for Jacob's first court hearing on the armed robbery charge, and when she subsequently came to testify, she was intoxicated and could not remember Jacob's birthday.

Damien dropped out of school after the seventh grade and went to live with a teenage older brother who was a drug dealer and who initiated him into the drug trade. Damien had earlier been a ward of the court after his mother was accused of beating one of his brothers. He apparently had no contact with his father. Damien took the gun used in the robbery/murder from his brother's house; in preparation for the attack, in Jacob's presence, Damien sharpened the bullets.

Discussion

It is not difficult to identify the familial and social factors that coalesced in the behaviors resulting in this tragic murder. An overview of this case summary reveals the following negative influences and risk factors in the lives of these boys:

Family Disintegration

Female-headed single-parent households
Absent fathers (Jacob's was killed; Damien's abandoned the family)
Youthful runaway behavior (Damien)

Poverty

Both families were supported on welfare

Exposure to Violence and Abuse

Witness to spouse abuse (between parents—Jacob)
Witness to child abuse (parental abuse of sibling—Damien)
Personal experience of child abuse (Damien)
Witness to gunfights within family (Jacob)

Exposure to Substance Abuse

Residence in crack houses
Parental alcohol and crack dependence (Jacob)
Sibling drug dealing (Damien)
Drug abuse/dependence in the neighborhood
Encouragement to use drugs

Jacob's lawyer summarized his young client's situation by stating that "Jake is the product of his environment. He comes from a dysfunctional family. The older neighborhood boys were his heroes. They sold drugs. They had guns. They were his role models. He wanted to be like them" (quoted in Wilkerson, 1994, p. A-14).

Charles Patrick Ewing, a lawyer and forensic psychologist, comments in his book *Kids Who Kill* (1990): "Juvenile killers are not born but made. . . . Virtually all juvenile killers have been significantly influenced in their homicidal behavior by one or more of a handful of known factors: child abuse, poverty, substance abuse, and access to guns" (p. 157). Certainly, these conditions do not *always* produce child killers; many youngsters manage to survive the ravages of noxious familial and social environments without succumbing to antisocial acts. Some even achieve great success, against all odds (Anthony & Cohler, 1987). Nonetheless, when the cards are stacked so heavily against healthy development, as they were for both Jacob and Damien, the outcome in terms of antisocial behavior is understandable. Furthermore, in addition to Ewing's list of factors contributing to homicidal behavior, we should consider the possibility that Jacob may have been born with fetal alcohol syndrome and/or the effects of his mother's crack addiction and that Damien may have suffered head injuries due to the serious and repeated beatings he received. Furthermore, mothers who are drug or alcohol dependent may be unable to respond appropriately to their babies' emotional needs for bonding. Both boys' seeming lack of empathy may be related to insecure or avoidant attachment due to the abuse and neglect they both suffered in the first 2 years of their lives (Karr-Morse & Wiley, 1997; Perry, 1997; Lieberman, 2004; Siegel, 2012). Heide (1999) points out that many abused youth have not experienced bonding with others and consequently they do not develop the values, empathy, and self-concept that fosters the self-control that might inhibit them from killing. The lack of an attachment figure in the first few years of life may cause an inablity to establish stable relationships later in life (Siegel, 2012).

We know nothing about either boy's academic record, such as possible learning or hyperactivity problems, or about any individual areas of strengths or achievement. However, both boys learned to survive in the face of situations that were, at times, life threatening, and they learned to adapt in circumstances that required great perseverance and strength. If only this resilience could have been focused on more positive interests and goals! This case illustrates how the cumulative influence of individual, familial, and social factors can culminate in juvenile criminal behaviors. Even when social and familial factors appear to predominate as causal, however, remediation necessitates intensive work with such youths on an *individual* basis. It is likely that after years of abuse and neglect, youngsters such as Damien and Jacob internalized and then replicated the dysfunctional behavior they witnessed and experienced during their formative years. Rehabilitation would require much more than environmental change to significantly alter such youngsters' sense of personal identity, their sense of self-respect and competence, and their views about future goals for their lives. Few if any prisons have programs that can provide the kind of in-depth treatment these boys would need. In fact, it is more likely that they would learn more antisocial behaviors from emulating other prisoners. Chapter 14 discusses in detail the treatment approaches for children who witness family and community violence.

EMOTIONAL AND BEHAVIORAL PROBLEMS

As stated by Hinshaw (2008), "emotional and behavioral problems in children and adolescents are distressingly prevalent and often lead to serious impairments in such crucial life domains as academic achievement, interpersonal competencies, and independent living skills" (p. 4). According to the U.S. Department of Health and Human Services (1999), about one in five children and adolescents in the United States suffer from some type of mental health problem during the course of a year. The overall precedence rates of childhood problems are estimated to be between 14 and 22% for all children, and "a significant proportion of children do not grow out of their childhood difficulties" (Mash & Dozois, 1996, p. 9).

Typical Problem Syndromes in Children

Professionals who work with children document that psychopathology in children is a relatively common occurrence, with overall estimates of developmental, emotional, and behavioral disorders ranging from 14 to 23% of all children, with more severe forms of mental disturbance occurring in an estimated 8–10% of all children (Brandenburg, Friedman, & Silver, 1990; Boyle et al., 1987; Mash & Dozois, 1996, 2003; Mash & Barkley, 2007, 2014).

Because of the growing focus on an individual's *strengths,* rather than on deficits, many social workers and social work educators have turned away from the "medical model" in which individuals are categorized with various disorders using classifications of the fifth edition of the Diagnostic and Statistical Manual of Mental Disorders (DSM-5; American Psychiatric Association, 2013). However, the fact is that anyone whose work involves children will inevitably encounter some who are showing great difficulty in adjusting and who will benefit from interventions based on a thorough assessment of their problematic behavior. The process of making such biopsychosocial assessments is discussed in Chapter 4. Knowledge about the specific categories of problematic behavior of children is essential for practitioners in their efforts to formulate an assessment and plan the kind of treatment that will be most helpful.

Achenbach and Howell's (1993) formulation of children's typical problems was derived from parent, teacher, and self-report forms of the Child Behavior Checklist (CBCL) administered to a 1989 sample. This grouping of problems was summarized by the *New York Times* (Goleman, 1993) and later adapted by Mash and Dozois (1996, 2003). These problems also appear in DSM-5 under slightly different categories. Over 20 years later, this listing of children's problems continues to serve as a guide for many practitioners who give parents, teachers, and school-age children the checklists to fill out as part of the assessment process. This topic is discussed more fully in Chapter 4, but some of the categories of behavior that are screened on this form include the following: withdrawn and/or depressed behavior, attention difficulties, aggressive behavior, and anxiety.

All of these behaviors worsened over the 13-year period from 1976 to 1989 among the groups of children who were studied by Achenbach, who suggested that multiple factors probably contributed to the widespread increase in children's problems. Among these, he cited children's exposure to violence; reduced time with parents and reduced parental monitoring of children; more families with both parents working; more single-parent families; and fewer community mentors to help children learn adaptive social and emotional skills. These possible contributing factors continue to be very relevant in the first decades of the 21st century, so it is logical to expect that there has been a continuing increase in children's problems.

Children's Emotional Problems and Resilience

In contrast to the poor advice given by some pediatricians, most children do *not* outgrow their difficulties (Mash & Barkley, 2007), and they can benefit from some form of treatment. It is essential for practitioners who are treating children to be knowledgeable about different types of problematic behaviors seen in children and their recommended treatments, especially evidence-based treatments, when these have been reported in the professional literature. However, practitioners must be able to identify not only the child's problematic behaviors but also his or her areas of strength and positive adaptation. We know that different children respond differently, even in the same family. For example, all children in a multiproblem family could be considered at risk of developing problems. This is not a simple equation, however, as a significant proportion of children who are at risk do not develop problems later (Mash & Barkley, 2007). The term "resilience" has been used to describe children who not only survive adversity but also somehow become stronger in the face of it (Davies, 2011). A comprehensive understanding of any child requires that practitioners assess both the child's maladaptive and adaptive responses. The foundation of this assessment rests on knowledge of normal child development and of the many ways children can respond to stressful situations.

Implications for Social Workers

The fact that millions of children are suffering from serious mental health problems means that social workers, teachers, and others will encounter these children in schools, in child welfare institutions, in jails, in foster homes, and on the streets (LeCroy & Ashford, 1992). Their presence is by no means restricted to mental health clinics, as only about half the children who need mental health services receive them. Important decisions about what services to offer and which family members to include and in what settings depend on a careful biopsychosocial assessment that takes account of cultural and other factors. These issues are discussed in Chapters 4 and 5. It is essential that those working with children have basic knowledge about child development (Davies, 2011), cultural variations in child rearing (Webb, 2001; Fong, 2001, 2004), and the various possible deviations from children's usual developmental course to evaluate a presenting problem in a manner that fully considers the inner world of the child, in addition to all relevant external factors. An understanding of the concepts of risk and resilience (Fraser, 1997; Davies, 2011) can help practitioners avoid a narrow and linear view of causality.

AN ECOLOGICAL PERSPECTIVE ON ETIOLOGY

The Need to Consider Multiple Factors

Nothing in life is simple, as we quickly realize when we are attempting to ascribe causality to human behavior. "The task of unraveling causes and determinants of childhood mental disorders is formidable because of the complexity of interactions between biological, psychological, social, and environmental factors" (Institute of Medicine, 1989, paraphrased in Johnson & Friesen, 1993, p. 27). This view of the etiologies of mental and emotional disorders in children and adolescents has been summarized as follows:

> Support for multifactorial or systems understanding of the etiology of mental disorders has been accruing rapidly during the past two decades. Systems views are replacing univariate and stage theory models in all mental health disciplines, including social work, psychiatry, special education, clinical psychology, and others. (Johnson & Friesen, 1993, p. 27)

Of course, social work has a long history of employing extensive psychosocial assessment, as pointed out by Lieberman (1987); the addition of "bio-" to "psychosocial" represents increased awareness of the importance of innate factors (whether genetic or acquired) that can influence how an individual copes with a problem. Growing understanding about the impact on the brain of adverse experiences in early childhood (Siegel, 2012; Applegate & Shapiro, 2005) further supports the influence of biological factors on the developing child.

The idea that a child him- or herself may be an active agent influencing the systems of family, school, and government was first proposed by Bronfenbrenner (1979). It has subsequently been elaborated by many, including Stern (1985) and Siegel (2012) with regard to the infant–mother interaction and in the publications of the Erikson Institute (Garbarino et al., 1989), which stress the mutual influences between children and their physical, social, and cultural contexts. The implications of this dynamic view lead to a more complex understanding of social interactions, which are no longer viewed as unidirectional.

For example, when a highly active, intensely reactive, distractible child is adopted by a low-key, calm mother, she may believe that the child is "hyper" because of her own inability to soothe and quiet the baby. However, temperamental differences between parents and children, whether the children are biological or adopted, attest to the notion of "match" or "goodness of fit" between parent and child as the appropriate unit of attention, rather than the maladaptation of the individual parent or child (Thomas, Chess, & Birch, 1968; Shapiro, Shapiro, & Paret, 2001a). Simplistic, single-cause explanations no longer suffice in a multisystems perspective that considers "the continual, mutually influencing forces of biology, culture, behaviors of significant others, organizational processes, economics, and politics" (Johnson, 1993b, p. 86). If this wider view seems cumbersome and broad, it certainly avoids the previous overemphasis on parental pathology as *the* cause of children's problems. Germain and Gitterman (1987) state that "neither the people served, nor their environments, can be fully understood except in relationship to each other" (p. 493).

The Importance of Cultural Factors

It is also essential that social workers understand their own cultural biases and learn about the culturally based beliefs of their clients regarding role expectations, typical ways of expressing feelings, and patterns of social exchange (Webb, 2001; Fong, 2001, 2004). For example, a male child who has been taught both implicitly and explicitly that being "macho" means "stand up for yourself and don't let anyone get away with insulting you or your family" cannot be criticized for initiating a fistfight with a bully who called him a "wimp" and his sister a "tramp." To label this child "aggressive" misses the child's compelling motivation to defend his family's honor in a culturally sanctioned manner. This situation challenges the school social worker, who may be brought in to devise a creative response that respects the child's cultural identity even as it discourages fighting on the school premises. Different cultures have different beliefs about child behaviors that are acceptable and those that are not. Furthermore, attitudes about accepting help in the form of social or mental health services vary greatly among cultures, and practitioners must be sensitive to the implications of discussing a child's "problem behaviors" with a parent who may feel that the child's behavior reflects directly on the quality of her or his parenting and even on the family's honor (Webb, 2001).

Children and adolescents in immigrant families are often in conflict between two competing sets of values and norms, which may require them to follow one set of behaviors in the family setting and another in the school and community (Huang, 1989; Wu, 2001; Fong, 2001). This situation will require concerted attention from school social workers and others who deal with increasing numbers of immigrant children.

CURRENT ISSUES IN SOCIAL WORK WITH CHILDREN

Historical Overview

A consideration of current social work practice with children has more meaning when it is viewed in a historical perspective. The practice of social work with children has taken many forms—from its beginnings in court-affiliated clinics for juvenile delinquents in 1909, in which social workers studied cases and treated families, to agency and private practice in the 21st century, in which social workers may work with families, with children in groups, or with individual children (using play therapy and other methods appropriate for young clients). Parent counseling has always been an essential component of working with children, even when children reside with extended family members or live in foster homes. Intervention with a child's biological parent(s) remains central to the work with the child, because of social work's enduring belief about the importance of family identity to the child's sense of personal identity and because of the profession's commitment to the concept of family preservation (discussed in Chapter 2).

During the early decades of this century, social workers intervened with families according to their understanding of the problem, which took the form of a "diagnosis" of social factors contributing to the problem situation (Richmond, 1917). During the next phase of more specialized and regulated practice, many social workers worked under the guidance and direction of psychiatrists in child guidance clinics; the psychiatrists "treated" the children while the social workers "guided" the parents, thus introducing the concept of "parent guidance." In situations in which a family failed or was in danger of failing to meet the child's basic needs, the child welfare system assumed the role of parent surrogate, "doing for the deprived, disadvantaged, dependent child what the effective family does for the advantaged child" (Kadushin, 1987, p. 267). During the 1950s and 1960s, child welfare enjoyed special recognition and status as a specialty area within social work. Later this elite status diminished somewhat, as other professionals became involved in child placement decisions, abuse investigations, and adoption procedures (Kadushin, 1987).

After the promulgation of family therapy in the 1970s and later, social workers tended to view a child's problems as symptomatic of a troubled marriage; therefore, intervention tended to focus on the marital dyad or on the family unit, rather than on individual members of the family. As a result, the child's presenting problem might be downplayed or ignored by family therapists, who considered it just the tip of the iceberg. An important goal in family therapy has been to remove the child from the role of the "identified patient" (Satir, 1983). However well intentioned this goal, more recently there is growing recognition that symptomatic children may have internalized problems and therefore require individual help, regardless of whatever assistance is offered to the parents or to the family unit. Social workers increasingly utilize specialized methods such as play therapy (including the use of art, sand play, music, and storytelling) in their work with young children. It is notable that the American Board of Examiners in Clinical Social Work (ABE) has a specialty and a credential in practice with children and their families as a subspecialty of advanced clinical social work. This specialization clearly recognizes the body of specialized knowledge in this field, as well as the necessity for ongoing supervision and continuing education.

Cutting-Edge Issues in Practice with Children

Practice in the second decade of the 21st century must take full account of the social environment, which has a major impact on families and children. In addition, practitioners must continue to pay attention to children's biological and emotional responses to their life circumstances. Methods of intervention must be grounded in a thorough understanding of *all* relevant contributing factors and adapted to both the individual child's developmental needs and to the possible contributing and/or ameliorating factors in the child's surrounding family and social environment.

The following list of cutting-edge issues, though by no means exhaustive, represents matters of concern to my students, my colleagues, and myself in our ongoing efforts to provide the most relevant and helpful service to children and families in the second decade of the 21st century. The chapters that follow in this book address these issues through case examples and literature reviews, as well as through my own experience and knowledge based on more than 30 years as a social work practitioner and educator.

1. *The impact on children of deteriorating social conditions, such as violence, poverty, and all forms of substance abuse/dependence.* Where and how can we intervene to protect children and enhance the quality of their lives? As reflected in the case of Jacob and Damien, many children in urban areas report that outbreaks of violence involving guns and knives have occurred in their schools. Furthermore, the trip from home to school may be marked by episodes of gang warfare in which innocent bystanders are injured or killed. When children's basic safety is in jeopardy, how can they concentrate and learn in school and complete their basic developmental tasks as well? This situation requires attention on a macro level to involve the community and the schools on behalf of the children. These issues are addressed in Chapters 9, 13, and 14. Mass shootings occurring in schools have led many schools to routinely engage students in practice drills involving hiding under desks and locking and/or barricading classroom doors. Although these practices have the goal of preparing for a possible future crisis, they also convey to many young students the fact that safety is not a guarantee in the school, and this can increase the anxiety levels among students with fragile temperaments. Chapter 9 addresses specific school-based interventions intended to help all students, as well as those who are expressing problematic behaviors.

2. *Selecting intervention alternatives at multiple levels*—with the child, the parent(s), the extended family, the school, the community, and government

(political advocacy). How can individual social workers be expected to intervene in *all* areas simultaneously, as might best serve the needs of a particular situation? In view of extensive individual, family, and social needs, should the profession focus on developing subspecialty areas of expertise? For example, should specially trained practitioners carry out lobbying/advocacy efforts, while family practitioners work with family units and child specialists work with individual children? What would be some advantages and disadvantages of this approach? Although we might like to do it *all,* the maxim "jack of all trades, master of none" bears careful thought as demands for more specialized practice increase. This topic is explored in Chapter 2.

3. *Understanding the long-term effects on children who are exposed to different forms of family dysfunction, such as domestic violence, abuse and neglect, substance abuse, and parental absence and/or abandonment.* When parents are unable to carry out their caretaking responsibilities, there will be an inevitable negative effect on the attachment relationship with their children. Furthermore, developing knowledge about the brain indicates that there are serious effects on the child's brain from early neglect and lack of positive interactions with a caretaking adult (Perry, 1997, 1999, 2006). Social workers must utilize a distinct appreciation of the different forms of attachment relationships and how these can influence a child's later relationships with others. Chapter 6 addresses different interventions with the family for the benefit of the child.

4. *Providing culturally sensitive practice.* How can social workers develop sufficient knowledge about numerous ethnic groups to practice effectively? The immigrant population is increasing rapidly, and based on predicted birth and immigration rates, "minorities" will become the majority by the middle of the 21st century (Shinagawa & Jang, 1998). Practitioners who are Caucasians of Anglo-European heritage (Gibelman & Schervish, 1997), must learn how to engage and interact with parents who have diverse beliefs about parent–child roles and about how to obtain help for their children (Nader, 2008). Practitioners need to develop "cultural curiosity" about parent–child behaviors in other cultures and be willing to learn from their clients (Webb, 2001). An understanding of one's own beliefs forms an essential foundation of practice with diverse clients. This topic resonates in each chapter, and Chapter 16 focuses exclusively on the challenges of immigrant and refugee families and children.

5. *Working with severely traumatized children with posttramatic stress disorder (PTSD) and other responses to trauma.* Children are increasingly suffering the effects of exposure to traumatic events, such as community and family violence, terrorism, natural disasters, and war. This exposure can occur through television viewing, in addition to firsthand experience. Some children respond with symptoms of PTSD, and others express their anxiety through other symptoms, such as depression, generalized anxiety, conduct disorders,

and somatization disorders (Jenkins & Bell, 1997; Nader, 2008). The symptoms of PTSD represent dysfunctional, defensive coping responses to environmental assaults on an individual's level of anxiety tolerance. Trauma has a neurological effect on the brain, and social workers must appreciate this and learn how to provide crisis intervention and other treatments for traumatized children, such as trauma-focused cognitive-behavioral therapy (Cohen, Mannarino, & Deblinger, 2012) and play therapy (Gil, 2017). Chapters 9 and 15 discuss the interpersonal violence involved in bullying and suggests some appropriate school responses. Chapter 14 discusses many of the typical responses to family and community violence and reviews some of the recommended treatments to help children with PTSD (Foa, Keane, Friedman, & Cohen, 2009).

6. *Paying attention to the nature of early attachment relationships and to the studies that demonstrate the critical importance of brain development in early childhood* (Siegel, 2012; Osofsky, 1993, 1997). This work helps us understand why treatment attempts in later childhood and adolescence may require numerous repetitions in order to change behavior. This topic is covered in various chapters, and especially in Chapters 2, 10, and 14.

7. *Utilizing evidence-based research to guide choices about intervention methods in work with children and adolescents.* This requires the practitioner to be aware of research studies that demonstrate effective interventions with children so that clinical practice can be improved through consistent use of methods and practice procedures that have been shown to be effective. The limitations of these approaches with children must also be considered. Because the evidence-based focus has both ardent supporters and those who question its universal effectiveness, clinical practitioners should guide their practice according to their best judgment of what will be effective, and they also should keep track of the results of various treatments to better inform their future work. There is a burgeoning literature on the topic of evidence-based practice, and social workers must stay aware of the latest developments (Baggerly, Ray, & Bratton, 2010; Briggs & Rzepnicki, 2004; Kazdin & Weisz, 2003; Weisz & Kazdin, 2010, 2017; Reddy, Files-Hall, & Schaefer, 2005). Various chapters in the book present and discuss evidence-based practices when these are pertinent.

8. *Acknowledging the changing views about gender identity and how this may affect children's beliefs and their own experiences.* A child's discomfort with his or her gender becomes a family, as well as an individual, issue and is discussed in Chapter 6. Social norms vary on this topic, and stigma and discrimination may be added to the stresses of gender dysphoria. It is important for social workers to be aware of these issues and to be prepared to assist families and children who are struggling with them, as well as to work with professionals in schools and community facilities who are dealing with these children.

9. *Utilizing various self-care strategies to avoid vicarious traumatization and burnout.* The topic of self- care is discussed in Chapter 14, but it should be embedded into the practice of all social workers in various locales, especially those who work with young children. We must learn to take care of ourselves, so that we will not suffer burnout and so that we can continue to take pride in our work.

10. *Appreciating the calming and helpful effects from the practice of mindfulness.* These techniques can be adapted to help children learn to focus (as demonstrated in Chapter 7) and can be employed on a regular basis to help the practitioner become centered and focused on the unique specifics of the job at hand.

CONCLUDING COMMENTS

Social work with children is a demanding, all-inclusive field of practice. No longer can a practitioner focus primarily on a child's inner world, nor will it suffice to intervene exclusively with the child's family or social environment. A multilevel approach is essential to understanding, just as it is essential in planning and carrying out helping interventions.

Social workers must learn to scan a child's world and see the broad picture before determining where and how to initiate the helping process. The skills of listening, observing, and empathizing will assist practitioners, who must be able to see through a child's eyes in order to comprehend the child's situation with both head and heart.

DISCUSSION QUESTIONS

1. How can a social worker avoid becoming discouraged when faced with a child who has been victimized by physical and emotional tabuse and neglect in a home in which both parents use multiple substances?
2. What services would be appropriate to offer within a school setting to recent immigrant children and their families for the purpose of assisting with their adjustment and integration into the community? What form of initial contact would make the children and families most comfortable?
3. Review and discuss the selected cutting-edge issues presented in this chapter, indicating how social work education can respond to these needs. Which issues do you think will prove the most difficult to resolve? Why?

CHAPTER 2

Challenges for Practitioners in Helping Children

Understanding the Multifaceted Role of the Social Worker

A social worker attempting to assist a child does not work in a vacuum. Many other professionals often participate in the helping effort, and frequently the social worker serves as self-appointed case coordinator who facilitates sharing of information among different helpers to promote their collaboration for the child's best interests. Each setting has its own group of professional experts who have their own views regarding the child's problem. In addition, each situation dictates its unique protocol for the involvement of different specialists to evaluate and treat a child with problems. For example, when an 8-year-old third grader threatened to throw himself out of a window at school, the social worker at the emergency walk-in psychiatric clinic to which the child was brought consulted with the staff child psychiatrist, the school guidance counselor, and the child protective services (CPS) worker who was investigating allegations of child abuse in this family (Price & Webb, 1999). These contacts, some "in-house" and others collateral, were as essential for understanding the situation in its totality as were interviews with the child and his mother. Because the social worker had a broad view of the problem situation, she understood the importance of contacting other professionals for their input.

A team approach to helping often serves a child and family well, because each specialist's expertise usually contributes to a fuller understanding of the child's situation. When the social worker subscribes to a multifaceted view of etiology, as discussed in Chapter 1, the participation of other professionals with different perspectives about the child's situation is welcomed and valued. Usually the social worker synthesizes all the relevant information obtained from various sources and organizes it into a biopsychosocial summary, which later will be discussed with the parent(s) and with the child (when feasible) as part of the treatment planning and contracting. This assessment process is reviewed in detail in Chapters 4 and 5.

The following case illustrates the different social work roles of clinician, case manager, consultant, and advocate.

THE CASE OF JOSÉ, AGE 6½

Presenting Problem

José, a 6½-year-old Hispanic foster child, was referred for counseling by the committee on special education of his school because of his traumatic and chaotic background. José had both witnessed and been subjected to domestic violence, child neglect, abuse, and abandonment prior to being placed in foster care at age 4½ with his two younger brothers. In addition, he had recently been diagnosed with diabetes, and the school nurse wanted to be certain that the foster mother was capable of carrying out his medical treatment.

Family Information

Both of José's parents were drug addicts, and all three of their sons had been exposed prenatally to drugs and alcohol. The father was incarcerated for stealing and the mother for selling drugs. Before the mother's incarceration, when the boys resided with her, they were often left alone and neglected. Their initial placement in foster care occurred after the police found them wandering alone in the streets at midnight.

Discussion

Even the bare outline of this case permits us to appreciate the complex, multifaceted role of the school social worker who faced the challenge of gathering together the unraveling threads of this child's life. She wanted to create some sense of unified purpose among the various professionals involved with this child, to enable her to coordinate the planning and to clarify future goals.

The following list identifies the array of personnel who were involved with José's life either directly or indirectly and whom the school social worker hoped to involve in this planning:

- Foster care worker
- CPS worker
- José's pediatrician
- Mother's prison caseworker and/or future probation officer

- José's special education teacher
- The foster mother
- The school nurse

An eco-map (see Figure 2.1) was used to diagram these different helpers; it also included the genogram and relevant family members. (See Hartman, 1978, for details about the construction of an eco-map and a discussion of its use.)

Different Roles of the School Social Worker

In her role as *case manager,* the school social worker obtained reports from the professionals involved with José and convened a case conference to which all were invited. Learning more about the nature of José's medical diagnosis and prognosis helped prepare the worker for her ongoing involvement with this child in her role as his *therapist.* After hearing details from the CPS

FIGURE 2.1. Eco-map of José.

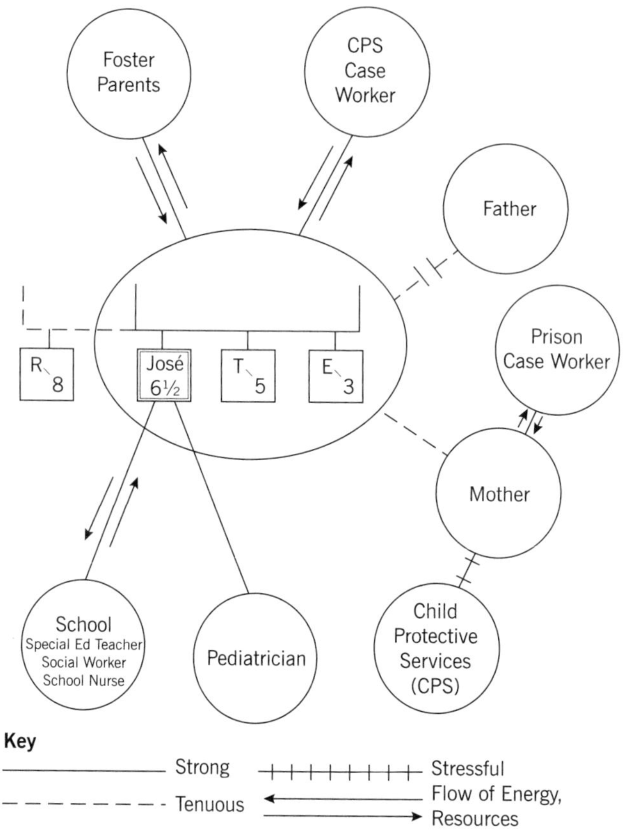

worker about the mother's history of abandonment and abuse of her children, the social worker understood the factors influencing José's untrusting manner of relating to her and others at the school. This information would also be helpful for the school nurse and special education teacher. A child who has suffered chronic neglect and intermittent abuse will often find it difficult to trust other adults, no matter how kind their interaction efforts.

In contrast, the worker served as *consultant* to the pediatrician, who had only minimal information about this child's problematic family background. She served as an *educator* to the foster mother, who needed to learn about diabetes and the necessity for daily care, dietary monitoring, and injections. She also provided information about José's hyperactivity and short attention span, which had become apparent to his teacher.

Because of the worker's concern about José's mother's rehabilitation, she took on an *advocacy* role in recommending that the mother receive counseling and parenting education in prison and drug and alcohol treatment prior to her discharge. The worker also advocated for the children to begin visiting their mother on a regular basis to prepare them for possible future reunification of the family.

Different Settings

In addition to working with many collaborators in a variety of roles and functions, the professional social worker involved with children must also demonstrate versatility in working with clients in a wide range of locations. The tenet of "meeting clients where they are" usually refers to tuning in to their psychological/emotional states. However, it can also refer to meeting the clients on their *physical* terrain. This means that social workers who deal with children's problems work in all locations where children live, learn, and play and where they receive care and counseling when they are injured, neglected, abandoned, or otherwise troubled. Thus social workers help children in hospitals, schools, foster homes, residential treatment centers, family agencies, mental health clinics, and shelters for the homeless. Although each setting has its own focus and specific procedures for helping, certain basic principles and a core of knowledge about child and family behavior and needs must guide the practice of all social workers who help children, regardless of the setting in which they provide services.

COMMITMENT TO A CORE OF VALUES AND CODE OF ETHICS

Professional social work education trains students to become practitioners who demonstrate disciplined "use of self," appropriately applying theoretical knowledge and practice skills. However, knowledge and skills, though necessary, are not sufficient for the task of helping. The situations in which social workers are engaged often require difficult decisions in which no single "right answer" applies. The workers must consider ethical principles and weigh the pros and cons of various possible outcomes in the effort to serve everyone concerned most effectively.

The Code of Ethics

Values serve as guides or criteria for selecting good and desirable behaviors. Most social workers agree about the basic values of client participation, self-determination, and confidentiality (Lowenberg & Dolgoff, 1996; Congress, 1999; Reamer, 2013). However, the complexity of a client's situation can often make decisions very difficult. Ideally, clients participate in decisions affecting their own lives; however, when interests of family members conflict, and/or when abuse and neglect of a minor is a possibility, then the social worker may have to make a recommendation based on his or her judgment regarding the best interests of the child. For example, in the case of José, just discussed, it might be very difficult to determine whether the boy's mother will be able to take care of him and his siblings after her prison discharge.

The National Association of Social Workers (NASW) adopted its first code of ethics in 1960, to provide social workers with principles to help them resolve ethical dilemmas encountered in practice (Reamer, 2006). This code of professional ethics identifies and describes the ethical behavior expected of professional practitioners (Lowenberg & Dolgoff, 1996). Among the principles emphasized are confidentiality, self-determination, and expectations pertaining to standards of professional behavior. The most recent code of ethics (NASW, 2017) continues the general tone of the previous version, therefore requiring sensitive interpretation and case-by-case application in ambiguous conflict situations.

Although the code articulates the value base of the social work profession, it does so with a high level of abstraction that fails to provide specific guidelines for the resolution of ethical dilemmas. Thus, even when students and practitioners subscribe to this code, its implementation may be unclear and subject to differing personal interpretations. The code (NASW, 2017, pp. 2–3) states this plainly:

> The *Code* offers a set of values, principles, and standards to guide decision making and conduct when ethical issues arise. *It does not provide a set of rules that prescribe how social workers should act in all situations.* Specific applications of the *Code* must take into account the context in which it is being considered and the possibility of conflicts among the *Code*'s values, principles, and standards. *Ethical responsibilities flow from all human relationships, from the personal and familial to the social and professional.* . . . Ethical decision making is a process. In situations when conflicting obligations arise, social workers may be faced with complex ethical dilemmas that have no simple answers. (emphasis added)

Issues of Confidentiality/Consent in Work with Children

Questions of ethics often become especially tricky when practitioners try to apply these considerations to children. For one thing, neither society nor the helping professions have taken a stand regarding whether children should have the same rights of privacy and confidentiality as do adults, especially regarding parents' access to information about their children's counseling/therapy. Actually, the federal Family Educational Rights and Privacy Act (Public Law 93-380, 1974) gives parents the right to inspect their children's medical and school records; therefore, social workers cannot legitimately promise confidentiality to children. Moreover, because social work with a child *always* involves work with a parent or guardian, the issue of confidentiality becomes entangled with the question, Who is the client? The parent or guardian has both a need and a right to know in a general way about the course of the child's progress and ongoing problems. In addition, the seasoned practitioner realizes that it is counterproductive and impossible to promise confidentiality to a child. Ironically, this type of promise is the last thing many children would expect anyway, as they know that their parents or guardians "check up" on their work in school and other areas of involvement. Why should counseling/therapy be any different?

My own view about confidentiality as applied to children is that it is a concept more relevant to youngsters over 12 years of age, and even then, it has the same limitations about parents' legal right to access the records of their children under the age of 18. I believe that it is far more useful in most situations to encourage the sharing of information between a child and parent, albeit in a sensitive and general manner that does not divulge details that would be embarrassing to the child. Sometimes the achievement of improved parent–child communication represents a major goal in the helping process. Of course, in situations involving parental physical or sexual abuse of the child, the situation becomes very tricky, and usually a lawyer ultimately decides what information will be revealed and the circumstances for doing so.

Another ethical issue pertinent to working with children is whether a child has the "right" to refuse treatment in the same manner as does an adult who is not a danger to self or others and who is not legally mandated to receive treatment. Can a 5-year-old decide what is in his or her own best interests? At what age *can* a child decide? Anyone who works with children knows that almost *all* children begin as involuntary clients. They may realize that they are unhappy, but in most cases they have no idea that there are people who can help them with their worries and troubles; furthermore, they are wary of adult strangers and uncomfortable about talking with them. When the social worker introduces him- or herself to the child as a "worry person" or a "helper" who knows how to help children with their troubles and worries, the child who has been repeatedly disappointed or betrayed by adults may find the offer to help impossible to believe. Gaining such a child's trust will take time.

For all these reasons, my personal recommendation is that the social worker request that the responsible adults continue to bring the child for appointments, even when the child seems unwilling. This initial "resistance" will almost always be converted into eager participation once the child experiences the reality of a relationship in which he or she is listened to and valued and in which toys and play are a part of the process.

Ethnic/Cultural Sensitivity

When we meet someone for the first time, our initial impressions automatically register such personal characteristics as age, gender, and race, in addition to factors about the individual's personality and mood. When the person resembles ourselves, we may make certain assumptions about him or her, based on our own views regarding the shared characteristics. Of course, all middle-aged white women (for example) are not alike; however, the likelihood of shared empathy increases with similarity of personal characteristics.

What does this mean, then, in view of the fact that "children of color are the most rapidly increasing group in the U.S. population, [that they] are the largest risk group for disabilities and developmental delay related to conditions associated with poverty, and that *most professionals who work with this population are from the dominant culture*" (Rounds, Weil, & Bishop, 1994, p. 12; emphasis added)? Lieberman (1990, p. 101) states that "right from birth, babies become reflections and products of their culture" and notes that child-rearing traditions and values about parent–child roles and attitudes are strongly shaped by cultural beliefs.

Since 1973, the Council on Social Work Education (CSWE) has mandated that social work education include instruction concerning the lifestyles and culture of diverse ethnic groups as an integral part of social work education (Devore & Schlesinger, 1996). Subsequent policy statements have reiterated and expanded on this position (CSWE, 1984, 1992a, 1992b, 2002, 2008, 2015), with the result that courses in the baccalaureate and master's curricula must reflect content regarding cultural diversity for groups distinguished by ethnicity and race, as well as by gender, age, religion, disability, and sexual orientation (Carrillo, Holzhalb, & Thyer, 1993). The implementation of this mandate takes many forms; the work of Lieberman (1990), Rounds et al. (1994), Devore and Schlesinger (1987, 1996), Green (1999), Lum (1996, 1999, 2003), Congress (1997, 1999), Fong (2004), and Webb (2001) contributes helpful guidelines for practice with children of color and their families. These and other writers emphasize the importance of self-awareness regarding one's *own* culture as a foundation for understanding the culture of others. The core technique of the "conscious use of self" requires workers "to be aware of and to take responsibility for their own emotions and attitudes as they affect professional function" (Devore & Schlesinger, 1987, p. 103). This, of course, includes the worker's cultural beliefs. Honest, critical self-examination should occur in conjunction with learning in social work courses and in the field practicum and should continue as the mark of professional behavior as long as a social worker engages in practice.

NASW also has standards on cultural competence, and these involve the requirement of self-awareness, cultural humility, and the commitment to embracing culture as central to effective practice. The latest standards (NASW, 2015) build on the previous foundation and specify a broader conception of culture that moves beyond race and ethnicity to include sexual orientation, gender identity and expression, and religious identity or spirituality.

Tools for Self-Assessment and Improved Understanding of Cultural Differences

Some specific tools and references that can assist students and practitioners in examining their own cultural beliefs include Ho's (1992) "ethnic competence–skill" model, Cournoyer's (1991) overview of a variety of self-assessment measures related to cultural diversity, Chadiha, Miller-Cribbs, and Wilson-Klar's (1997) questionnaire of similarities and differences, and Paniagua's (1998) 10-item Self-Evaluation of Biases and Prejudices Scale. The latter two are reprinted in Webb (2001).

The "culturagram" (Congress, 1994) provides the social worker with a tool for understanding the unique cultural background, beliefs, and circumstances of diverse families. Use of the culturagram encourages appreciation of the impact of the culture on a family, even as it discourages stereotyping of members of a specific cultural group. Because children in culturally diverse families often struggle to reconcile the values and beliefs taught at home with those they observe in the wider community, it is important for social workers to understand the family's backgrounds and the belief systems to which their children have been exposed. The process of constructing and using the culturagram can result in the practitioner's greater empathy for ethnic/cultural differences. Other steps toward improving ethnic/cultural sensitivity, as summarized by Rounds et al. (1994), include acknowledging and valuing diversity, recognizing and understanding the dynamics of difference, and acquiring cultural knowledge.

Attunement to Cultural Differences

The recommendation that practitioners have an in-depth understanding of the cultural background of their clients has been qualified by Lieberman (1990), who reassures us that "it is impossible to be culturally sensitive as a general quality because this would demand an encyclopedic ethnographic and anthropological knowledge well beyond the reach of most of us" (p. 104). She suggests instead that we "think of cultural sensitivity as a form of *interpersonal sensitivity*, an *attunement* to the specific idiosyncrasies of another person"

(Lieberman, 1990, p. 104; first emphasis in original, second added). Insofar as social workers always try to imagine walking in the shoes of their clients, this attunement effort will result in practice that attempts to understand the clients' subjective world as it respects and honors the clients' attempts to carry out the cultural/ethnic traditions that they have inherited and that form the intrinsic core of their identity. As Erikson (1963) has stated, "the ego identity is anchored in the cultural identity" (p. 279). Because of this we must adhere to Fong's (2004) recommendation to include culture habitually and systematically as an integral part of making assessments and planning interventions.

THE ESSENTIAL KNOWLEDGE BASE FOR WORK WITH CHILDREN

We have all been children ourselves, and many social workers also have firsthand experience with children in their role as parents. To assume, however, that personal life experience will prepare one for the type of complicated work described in the case of José is as foolhardy as suggesting that anyone who likes to eat can prepare a gourmet five-course meal! Liking food on the one hand, and memories of childhood on the other, can provide the motivation and even the foundation for success in either venture, but specialized training and study are necessary to move beyond the novice stage of either cooking or working with children.

A solid foundation of basic knowledge is essential for social workers and other practitioners whose work deals with young children and their families. This base of essential knowledge, as mentioned in Chapter 1, includes a grounding in the "normal" course of child development, as well as in deviations from this course (i.e., childhood mental and emotional disorders). The knowledge base also includes information about the ways family dynamics, developmental phases, and events affect children (and vice versa). With this foundation, for example, the practitioner will be able to evaluate the significance of severe nighttime fears when they occur in a 9-year-old child as opposed to a 3-year-old. The knowledgeable practitioner who understands the importance of attachment relationships and appreciates the interplay between the child's temperament and stressful events may discover through skillful questioning that the 9-year-old may have overheard arguments between the parents after she went to bed that led her to the conclusion that a parental divorce was imminent. This "discovery" of the source of the child's fear is not made by accident; it occurs because the social worker is well versed in normal child development milestones, which indicate that nighttime fears are atypical of a 9-year-old child in the absence of traumatic experience or upsetting family events. Nighttime fears, by contrast, are common in 3-year-olds, and the knowledgeable social worker will counsel the parents of the 3-year-old about their typical occurrence at this age, at the same time offering guidance about ways to comfort the child to keep the anxiety within tolerable limits.

Understanding of Child Development

Basic Information

Courses in social work with children usually do not teach the basics of child development, because instructors assume that students have acquired this knowledge in undergraduate psychology courses or the required core graduate courses in human behavior and the social environment. When this content has not been adequately covered or mastered in coursework, practitioners can engage in self-study, using books and conferences to increase their knowledge. An annotated list of references on the topics of children's biological, psychological, and social development appears at the end of this chapter. In addition to these references from the professional literature, there are numerous works written for the public that summarize basic information on child development. Some of these are also included in the list at the end of the chapter.

Attachment and Bonding

The seminal writings of John Bowlby (1969, 1973, 1977, 1979, 1980, 1988) highlight the essential role of attachment and bonding "as a basic component of human nature" (1988, pp. 120–121). "Attachment" refers to an enduring, reciprocal bond of affection that focuses on a specific person or persons. The child's attachment figures are typically the parents or primary caretakers, who play a critical role in the nature and quality of the child's attachment relationships. For example, the child with a "secure" attachment relationship with his or her parents feels confident about leaving the safe proximity of this "secure base" to explore his or her environment, knowing that the parents will respond comfortingly when he or she returns and wants reassurance. However, in situations in which parents are inconsistent and/or unreliable toward the child, the resulting relationship may be characterized as an "anxious/resistant attachment" (Bowlby, 1988) or "ambivalent/resistant attachment" (Davies, 2011). This results in the child's exhibiting intense separation anxiety; when the parent/caretaker returns, the child resists contact and interaction. Bowlby also identifies another form of insecure attachment, "avoidant attachment," characterized by the child's actual *expectation of* rejection from his or her self-involved caretakers or parents, who may use threats of abandonment as a means of controlling him or her. The child defensively adopts a stance of self-reliance, as if the attachment is not important (Davies, 2011). This type of interaction understandably leads the child to become mistrustful of others, because he or she expects or fears abandonment in future relationships with other adults.

Still another form of insecure attachment, identified by Main and Solomon (1990) as "disorganized/disoriented attachment," refers to children who seem confused and conflicted about attaching to the parent. Many of these parents themselves have histories of trauma, abuse, and violence, which may be somehow conveyed to their babies, who appear to be frightened by their anxious and fearful parent.

Many of the children known to social workers show signs of attachment difficulties. Children who have experienced inconsistent care and who demonstrate avoidant, ambivalent, or disorganized attachment to their parents resist engagement with social workers (or other helpers) because of their inability to trust adult strangers (James, 1994). These children, with backgrounds devoid of consistent loving relationships, require extreme patience, sensitivity, and understanding. Remkus (1991, p. 144) quotes the leading attachment theorists in stating, "failure to establish a secure attachment relationship limits the emotional, cognitive, and social development of the child (Sroufe & Waters, 1977; Sroufe, 1979a, 1979b; Ainsworth, 1979; Ainsworth & Bell, 1971; Mahler, Pine, & Bergman, 1975)." Davies emphasizes that the quality of attachment affects future development in a fundamental way.

Parents, usually mothers, bear a major responsibility for the quality of children's attachment (Freud, 1970). However, when parents are overwhelmed with multiple stresses, they may be unable to respond lovingly and consistently to their needy children. Indeed, a parent may not be able to bond to his or her own child because of the parent's *own* attachment-deprived history. Unfortunately, as in the case of José, the parent–child relationship may become angry and abusive when the parent cannot focus on the child's needs.

DSM-5 (American Psychiatric Association, 2013) describes the criteria for the diagnosis of *reactive attachment disorder of infancy or early childhood,* which occurs due to deficient care and leads to marked disturbance in the child's social relatedness. This condition, which begins before age 5 and must have been present for more than 12 months, causes the child to react in two different ways: (1) to rarely or minimally seek comfort and (2) to rarely or minimally respond to comfort when distressed. Students and practitioners who work with children with attachment and trauma disorders will benefit from studying the literature on trauma and its impact on development (Eth & Pynoos, 1985; Herman, 1992; van der Kolk, 1987, 1989; Wilson & Keane, 2004; Nader, 2008; Oppenheim & Goldsmith, 2007).

Mental and Emotional Disorders of Children

Social workers deal with children in a variety of circumstances (foster placement, underachievement in school, and a parent's terminal illness, to name only a few). Referrals may occur because of the circumstances of the situation (e.g., foster placement) or because the child's extreme behavior alerts someone about the child's need for help. Children express their anxieties in various ways, and the social worker or other practitioner to whom a symptomatic child may be referred must be knowledgeable about the different manifestations of childhood symptoms to be able to make an assessment that will result in a helpful treatment plan. The worker's knowledge of normal child development serves as a baseline against which to evaluate the troublesome behaviors presented by the child. It is obvious that the more we understand about normal variations in development, the more we can determine which behaviors and reactions are indicative of problems in children.

In addition to understanding "normal" behavior, however, the practitioner needs to understand the deviations from the normal developmental course. The concept of "psychopathology" affixes a label to a set of behaviors; in the case of children, such labeling may seem pejorative and even ill advised in view of the reality of their rapid development. Nonetheless, practitioners must be familiar with the extremes of human behavior as manifested in children, so that they can recognize severely troubled children who require specialized interventions. An ability to apply the diagnostic categories of DSM-5 does not preclude understanding the multifaceted etiology of a child's problem. However, refusal to recognize that children can exhibit serious behavioral disturbances may lead to neglect based on the ill-founded resistance to applying medical/psychiatric classifications to children. Wachtel (1994) states that "fear of pathologizing children has led to an excessive 'normalizing' of children who could really benefit from . . . psychotherapeutic work" (p. 8). Chapter 4 includes further discussion of the process and tools of child assessment.

Resilience and Coping in Children

Because human behavior is the product of multiple influences, we note with relief that a noxious environment does not *always* bring disastrous results to the children. As discussed in Chapter 1, the concepts of "resilience" and "coping" attest to the ability of some children to thrive and do well despite factors that defeat many of their peers in seemingly similar circumstances. The work of E. James Anthony demonstrates that some children not only survive but actually do well despite all odds to the contrary. Often, the influence of *one* adult makes enough impact to tip the balance of a negative environment in a child's life. Although these "invulnerable children" (Anthony & Cohler, 1987) are exceptional, their life experience argues for the positive impact of professional helpers on the lives of at-risk children who are "vulnerable." Davies's book on child development (2011) presents the concepts of risk and resilience/protective factors in understanding the balancing of multiple influences on development. Diverse applications of a resilience-based model of practice appear in Fraser (1997) and in Norman (2000). For example, Fraser gives examples of risk and protective factors in child maltreatment, in school failure, in the development of delinquency and conduct disorders, and in childhood depression.

Research points to yet another possible factor in resilience, that of biology (Cicchetti, 2008). These findings suggest that genetic elements sometimes can serve as protective factors in some individuals who experience adversity. This means that extreme social experiences such as child abuse or neglect can produce either pathological or adaptive responses.

Understanding of Family–Child Influences

Family Dynamics That Affect Children

The family's critical role in shaping a child is widely accepted by both professionals and the lay public. From the moment of birth, the mood and circumstances of the infant's mother and significant relatives provide the setting in which the child will feel safe and protected or insecure and threatened. The status of the family itself can influence the attitudes of various members about the infant's birth. For example, a first-born planned child will experience a different reception than will a fifth-born unplanned baby. However, birth order is merely one of many factors to be considered in evaluating the family's reactions to the infant. A first-born child of a 14-year-old unmarried mother may be resented because its birth was unwanted, whereas a fifth-born infant in some families may be highly valued for unique reasons having to do with the history of that family and the unique circumstances of the parents and the siblings at the time of birth. Every family is different, and the meanings of relationships cannot be assumed.

The Changing Structure of the 21st-Century Family

Numerous changes have occurred in the format and composition of families in the 21st century. The traditional conception of the "nuclear" family with a mother, father, and children who all live together until the children grow up now includes numerous variations that may include single-parent families, remarried and stepfamilies, gay and lesbian families, and families in which kin members take on the care of children (McGoldrick, Carter, & Garcia-Preto, 2010; Walsh, 2012). The family still plays a critical role in raising children, but the children may face special challenges in adapting to multiple and changing caregivers, as well as in adapting to stepsiblings, stepparents, and diverse relatives (Walsh, 2012). Lidz (1963) describes the impact of the family on the child as follows: "The family forms the first imprint upon the still unformed child and the most pervasive and consistent influence that establishes patterns that later forces can modify but never alter completely" (p. 1).

The Reciprocity of Child and Family Effects

When a family is troubled (e.g., by marital conflict, health problems, or employment concerns), it passes along its tensions to a child, who may, in typical egocentric thinking, conclude that he or she created the difficulty. Sometimes the "problem" in a family *does* originate with the child; this may be true, for example, with a child who has attention-deficit/hyperactivity disorder and who presents management problems at home and at school (this kind of situation is discussed in Chapter 6). When the family is viewed as a system, however, a problem for one member brings problems to all. Therefore, the practitioner needs to think about this reciprocity in trying to understand all the ramifications of the presenting problem. Wachtel (1994, p. 71) comments as follows:

> In assessing the role of family dynamics we try to determine what events may have shifted some stable patterns in the family or what might be going on developmentally in the lives of the children that is affecting family interactions. Understanding the effect of developmental or other changes on the family system involves having a well-articulated sense of the predominant transactional pattern of the family. . . . Understanding how the psychodynamic issues of the child relate to those of other family members is another important aspect of a systemic assessment.

In short, the family has an impact on the child, and the child has an impact on the family. We shall see various examples of both dynamics at work in the cases throughout this book. However, the facts that *all* families experiencing extreme stress do not generate problematic behaviors in *all* the children in their families and, conversely, that families with problematic children do not *always* exhibit disturbed familial functioning speak to the subtleties and vital importance of considering both individual and family strengths and resilience in evaluating the specific impact of events on different individuals and families.

The Effects of Family Crisis

Many children come to the attention of social workers and other practitioners at a time of family crisis, such as the divorce of their parents, the military deployment of one of the parents, or their family becoming homeless. It is essential that practitioners have an understanding of the impact of stress and trauma on children and know the principles of crisis intervention so that they will be able to help in a timely way. Such help may reduce the likelihood of later development of the serious symptoms of PTSD. The use of the "tripartite crisis assessment" (Webb, 1999, 2007; see also Chapter 4, this volume) can assist the social worker in evaluating the resources in the social environment and in formulating appropriate long- and short-term goals.

NECESSARY COMPETENCES IN WORK WITH CHILDREN

Accessing the Network of Children's Services

Practitioners who work with children must know how to make appropriate referrals to meet the special needs of the children in their care. Anyone who has contact with children in a professional role, for example, may become aware that a child in his or her office shows signs of physical abuse; in addition, children sometimes disclose experiences of physical or sexual abuse to their social workers. Chapter 14 discusses the assessment of both physical and sexual abuse. It is mandatory for practitioners to report such evidence or disclosures. All social workers who have contact with children must be familiar with the laws in their states regarding their responsibility and the procedures flowing from a child's disclosure or suspicious evidence of physical or sexual abuse.

In addition, there may be times when referrals to crisis services, to CPS, or to hospital facilities will be necessary to meet the special needs of a child. Because of the unpredictable multiple needs of children, social workers must learn about the referral policies of the relevant agencies in their locale to make their clients' access to services as smooth as possible.

The current political environment in the United States threatens deportation for undocumented immigrants and refugees. This situation creates a climate of intense fear and anxiety among the many thousands of refugees who are without the necessary documentation to avoid being arrested and deported. Chapter 16 discusses this matter in detail, and it is incumbent on all social workers to develop methods for helping these families who are living in a state of uncertainty and crisis.

Blending Generalist and Specialized Practice

It is apparent that some of the tasks described in this chapter fall into the category of "basic skills," familiar to beginning-level social work students, whereas other skills require specialized knowledge, more typical of the training of the "advanced generalist" or "clinical" social worker. Unfortunately, many of those who work with children do not obtain specific levels of training, as is apparent in the child welfare field, in which "it has been found that many Child Welfare workers lack the specialized knowledge and skills necessary to function in complex case situations" (Maluccio, 1985, p. 743; Maluccio, 2006). The requisite ecological perspective and multifaceted role expectations implicit in work with children mean that practitioners must make extra efforts to offer services that balance focus on the family and the child (Walton, Sandau-Beckler, & Mannes, 2001; Webb, 2007).

Ideally, work with children combines simultaneous attention to the impact of the person on the environment and that of the environment on the person, as characteristic of generalist practice (Sheafor & Landon, 1987). In addition, it must be grounded in knowledge of "normal" child and family development and in familiarity with the deviations from the usual developmental course, as described previously. Practitioners must be able to refer children for more specialized services when these are indicated, as well as to convene case conferences including professionals from different disciplines. Clearly, this work is demanding and challenging. The next two sections discuss methods for helping workers meet this multifaceted challenge.

AVOIDING POTENTIAL PITFALLS IN WORK WITH CHILDREN

Children's dependence, honesty, playfulness, and openness have a special appeal for many social workers, who decide to work with children because they genuinely like young people and want to help them. This admirable motivation for helping can sometimes obscure the snares implicit in this work, which must be recognized and avoided by all practitioners whose work focuses primarily on children.

The "Rescue Fantasy"

Probably most social workers who are engaged in work with children have at one time or another experienced a strong desire to "rescue" a child from a situation that appears to be clearly detrimental to the child's healthy development. Perhaps a 10-year-old girl is cast in the role of the "parentified child," taking care of several younger siblings after school and trying to keep the peace when her alcoholic parents begin to argue at dinner. The social worker knows that the child should be more involved with after-school activities, peers, and schoolwork, and she resents the parents' obliviousness to their daughter's age-appropriate needs. The social worker knows that this child would love to be involved in cheerleading and that she has already qualified for the squad. However, this would involve rehearsals every day after school, which would conflict with the child's family responsibilities. The social worker writes the mother a note, stating that she has arranged transportation home for the girl after daily practice and that she hopes the mother will support her child's special interest in this wholesome activity. What is wrong with this scenario? Will it work? What did the social worker overlook in her eagerness to be helpful to the child client?

At least two errors threaten the success of this well-intentioned plan: (1) The worker has moved too fast, and (2) the worker has "taken over," without involving the child's parents in the planning. In cases such as this one, when workers want to help and can see a clear-cut method to do so, it is hard for them to slow down, put on the glasses with wide-angle lenses, and include significant others in "their" treatment plan. Remembering that the child is part of a family system in which he or she carries out a designated role, a worker must consider the impact on the entire system when that role changes. Obviously, in the example given here, the ability of this child to be away from home every day depends on someone else's providing babysitting, and any plan that does not allow for this cannot succeed.

Competing and "Triangulating" with the Parents

Another typical pitfall in work with children demonstrated in this example is the danger of the worker's aligning with the child and either consciously or unconsciously becoming the "good" parent in situations in which the child's own parent appears to be deficient or even "bad." This attitude is always doomed to failure, because the parent will soon begin to resent the worker and will find "reasons" to discontinue the child's counseling/therapy. Unfortunately, the worker is usually not aware of the impact of his or her actions until it is too late. Palombo (1985) states that "children may arouse intense infantile longings in the therapist [and] the therapist comes to be considered by [the child] as [a] substitute parent and induce in the therapist a parenting response rather than a purely therapeutic response" (p. 40). In my opinion, the needier the child, the more likely it is the worker will respond to the impulses to become the "good" parent and rescue the child. In the absence of supervision and/or careful self-monitoring of practice, the countertherapeutic activity will proceed unchecked.

SUPERVISION AND SELF-MONITORING OF PRACTICE

Because the process of helping is interactive and involves the use of self in the helping relationship, and, furthermore, because it is difficult to be objective about one's own actions, supervision provides an opportunity for social workers to review their work and to learn about their own strengths and weaknesses in carrying out the helping process. As mentioned previously, the complexity of work with children makes supervision critically important, both for student social workers and for more seasoned practitioners. The two current registries of clinical social workers require a minimum of 2 years of post-master's-level supervision, and it is not uncommon for workers who wish to enhance their learning to arrange peer supervision groups or to arrange for private supervision if their place of employment does not offer this opportunity

When the worker/counselor/therapist becomes aware of a problem or impasse in the helping process, it is the worker's responsibility to try to understand the reason for the breakdown. In a previous publication (Webb, 1989), I reviewed some techniques that can be helpful in unlocking an impasse. Often such a difficulty stems from a similarity between the worker's own family background and that of the client he or she is trying to help. When these similarities are not recognized, the worker may unknowingly respond to the client (or to a member of the client's family) as if this person were a sibling or parent from the worker's own past. It must be emphasized that considerations of this type do not mean that supervision becomes therapy. "The *educational goal* of supervision argues against this occurrence and insists that the focus begin and end on the *work*" (Webb, 1983, p. 44; emphasis in original). Palombo (1985) challenges us to cast aside the past in our clients' best interests:

> We grow in our acceptance of our patients and we increasingly understand and accept ourselves. We grow also as with time and experience, our knowledge is transformed into therapeutic wisdom, but over and above that, we grow as we accept the challenge to question the old, the tried and the true when it no longer works. (p. 47)

CONCLUDING COMMENTS

Social work practice with children presents many problems. The young client usually cannot determine what is best for him or her, and often it is the social worker who must weigh all alternatives and consider multiple possibilities. Fortunately the social worker does not have to carry out his or her duties alone, as many helping professionals often play a role in providing the best possible outcome for the young child. The social worker must learn to operate as a member of a team in order to ensure that the child's needs are being met. Ideally the parents will be part of that team, as the child's family and its values and goals should be considered in any treatment plan. Thus the social worker must consider many factors and intervene with multiple systems in effectively providing services to young children.

DISCUSSION QUESTIONS AND ROLE-PLAY EXERCISES

1. How can the social worker best guide a parent whose child says that he or she does not want to go for "help"? How can the social worker try to engage this child, once the parent brings the child to the office? Role-play both of these situations at least three different times, with different players illustrating different types of resistance and engagement methods.
2. If you have been assigned a new case involving a family from a culture about which you know nothing, what can you do in preparation for your first meeting with the clients? What can you do in the initial session with the clients to enhance your relationship with them? How can you know what the experience was like for the client?
3. Suppose that, in the case conference about José, it becomes apparent that the foster care worker is vehemently opposed to the possibility of future family reunification following the mother's discharge from prison. The school social worker, knowing how much José misses his mother, favors a plan to reunite the family. How can the school social worker continue to collaborate with the foster care worker in the face of this disagreement about goals? Role-play a case conference with the school social worker and the foster care worker in which they each express their objections and in which a compromise is finally reached.
4. How can a social worker best utilize supervision for his or her own learning? Please respond in terms of the "ideal" situation.

RECOMMENDED TEXTS ON CHILD BIOLOGICAL, PSYCHOLOGICAL, AND SOCIAL DEVELOPMENT

Brazelton, T. B. (1992). *Touchpoints: Your child's emotional and behavioral development.* Reading, MA: Addison-Wesley.—This book summarizes Brazelton's several previous works for parents. Written by a pediatrician who has both medical and psychoanalytic training, it includes information about child development from physical, cognitive, emotional, and behavioral points of view.

Brazelton, T. B. (2001). *Touchpoints: Three–six. Your child's emotional and behavioral development.* Reading, MA: Addison-Wesley.—A more intensive review of the preschool stage of development.

Davies, D. (2011). *Child development: A practitioner's guide* (3rd ed.). New York: Guilford Press.—This book applies developmental knowledge to the assessment and treatment of children and families; illustrated with numerous case vignettes, it emphasizes a transactional approach in discussing risk and protective factors in infancy, early childhood, and middle childhood.

Erikson, E. H. (1993). *Childhood and society* (rev. ed.). New York: Norton.—Erikson's book, which has become a classic, outlines the eight stages of human development from birth to adulthood, emphasizing the developmental tasks at each stage. Erikson's conceptualization expands on Sigmund Freud's by viewing the individual in interaction with the social environment.

Faber, A., & Mazlih, E. (2012). *How to talk so kids will listen and listen so kids will talk.* New York: Scribner.—Considered the ultimate "parenting bible" by the *Boston Globe*, this book offers suggestions to parents about effective communication with their children.

Fraiberg, S. (1959). *The magic years.* New York: Scribner's.—This classic work, written by a social worker/child analyst, gracefully conveys solid knowledge about the preschool years in a readable style that belies its wealth of information.

Freud, A. (1963). The concept of developmental lines. *Psychoanalytic Study of the Child, 18,* 245–265.—Anna Freud's view of child development emphasizes the push for growth that is intrinsic to human nature.

Freud, S. (1963). *The sexual enlightenment of children* (P. Rieff, Ed.). New York: Macmillan. (Original work published 1907)—Although many practitioners today consider Sigmund Freud's work culture-bound and sexist, he must be recognized as a pioneer who first gave attention to the concept that children can have sexual feelings and who formulated a theory of childhood psychosexual development based on his retrospective work with adult patients.

Greene, R. W. (2001). *The explosive child: A new approach to understanding and parenting easily frustrated, chronically inflexible children* (2nd ed.). New York: HarperCollins.—Strategies for dealing with rebellious, oppositional and defiant behavior.

Greenspan, S. T., & Greenspan, N. T. (1991). *The clinical interview of the child* (2nd ed.). Washington, DC: American Psychiatric Press.—A useful guide for new practitioners and a helpful review for more experienced clinicians.

Ilg, F. L., Ames, L. B., & Baker, S. M. (1981). *Child behavior* (rev. ed.). New York: Harper & Row.—This book is a classic guide and manual for parents, written by the cofounders of the Gesell Institute at Yale University.

Kagan, J. (1984). *The nature of the child.* New York: Basic Books.—An overview of child development by a child development specialist.

Piaget, J., & Inhelder, B. (1969). *The psychology of the child.* New York: Basic Books.—This work establishes the framework of cognitive development of the child, pointing out basic differences in the thinking of children that affect their understanding of the world and their communications with adults. It is *essential* that practitioners working with young children understand and apply this conception of children's cognitive development in their work with children.

Siegel, D. J. (2012). *The developing mind: How relationships and the brain interact to shape who we are* (2nd ed.). New York: Guilford Press.—Explores the infant–parent early relationship and the biological context of attachment research.

Siegel, D. J., & Bryson, J. P. (2012). *The whole-brain child: 12 revolutionary strategies to nurture your child's developing mind.* New York: Bantam Books.—The authors present strategies for child rearing that encourage children's healthy brain development and positive emotional and behavioral development.

Thomas, A., Chess, S., & Birch, H. G. (1968). *Temperament and behavior disorders in children.* New York: New York University Press.—This landmark work documents the intrinsic childhood temperamental qualities that endure throughout life and resist modification by parents and other caretakers.

Vernon, A., & Al-Mabuk, R. (1995). *What growing up is all about.* Champaign, IL: Research Press.—A guide to child and adolescent development.

PART II

THE PROCESS OF HELPING CHILDREN

A Running Case Illustration of a Child in a Single-Parent Homeless Family

CHAPTER 3

Building Relationships with All Relevant Systems

Social workers often must reach out to needy children and families even when their attempts to help are ignored or refused. Families that are overwhelmed and burdened with survival concerns may prioritize their needs differently than do professional "helpers," who want to jump in and "rescue" dependent young children whose lives appear to be at risk because of adverse familial and/or environmental influences. The parents in such families may not agree with the professionals' views about their families' needs, thereby causing the helpers to struggle between a parent's right to self-determination and "the best interests of the child." Unfortunately, these are not always synonymous, and the practitioner may feel torn between conflicting responsibilities to two sets of clients—that is, the children and the parents.

These dynamics ebbed and flowed in the case of Barbie Smith, who grew to the age of 10 in a family with a mother who was in prison for extended periods and a father who was physically abusive to her and her mother and with no positive role model who could instill hope for a better future. Barbie's life had always been unstable, with homelessness and irregular schooling her prevailing realities. The girl's situation demonstrates the challenge of helping children when their everyday environment victimizes rather than nurtures them. These are the unfortunate circumstances for many children for whom social workers attempt to provide services. I use Barbie's case to illustrate the gap between the ideal and the possible, as I describe, over the next three chapters, the process of helping children. This process begins with the challenge of establishing initial relationships with reluctant or resistant family members; it continues with formulation of the biopsychosocial assessment of the child and then focuses on planning services to help in a manner that respects the family members' right to make choices in their own behalf.

THE CASE OF BARBIE, AGE 10

The ache for *home* lives in all of us, the safe place where we can go as we are and not be questioned. It impels mighty ambitions and dangerous capers. . . . [We hope] that . . . home will find us acceptable or, failing that, *that we will forget our awful yearning for it.* (Angelou, 1986/1991, p. 64; emphasis added)

Even a child who has had only *brief* periods of time in a secure "home" environment can experience this feeling of longing. Barbie stated at the beginning of the videotape/DVD *No Place Like Home* (Hunt, 1992): "I'm afraid that we're never going to get a home again of our own. It scares me." Barbie's life as depicted in this tape consisted of a series of moves from one motel or shelter to another, with no stability. Barbie's older brother, David, age 16, said, "It's not that bad. Instead of renting a house, we rent our own motels." Barbie, however, complained that she was getting tired of packing. A photo of her hugging a doll as she buried her bowed head in the doll's clothing (Figure 3.1) conveys the sadness and resignation that permeated her life. It also depicts how an attachment object, such as a doll, can provide some comfort in the life of a homeless child.

FIGURE 3.1. Barbie Smith, as she and her family were packing for yet another move. Photograph by James E. Nicoloro. Reprinted by permission of the photographer and the Smith family.

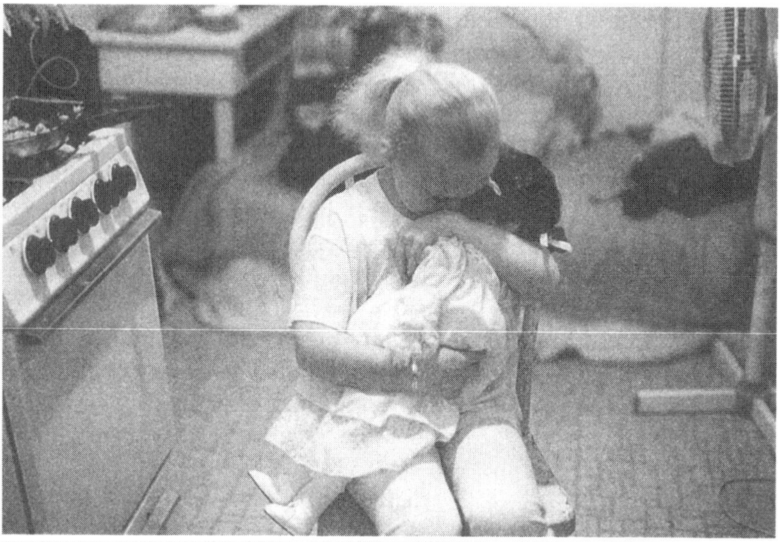

Background on the Case

At the beginning of the videotape, Barbie's mother confirmed that the family had moved seven times over a 6-month period, resulting in Barbie's attending *five different schools* during this time! The reason for the numerous moves was not at all clear, except for some reference to drug-infested neighborhoods. Barbie was eventually enrolled in a school for homeless children, where she came to the attention of a filmmaker, Kathryn Hunt, who obtained the mother's permission to tape the family and their various future moves over a period of time. I saw the resulting video at a professional meeting as part of a presentation about the special school, First Place School in Seattle, Washington. I immediately recognized that Barbie's experience as a homeless child was like that of many other disadvantaged children, and I believed that the tape would be useful for teaching purposes. Furthermore, I decided to establish contact with Barbie's family to obtain their permission to write about them in this book. Many months later, having finally obtained the signed releases and some of Barbie's school records, I struggled with the task of presenting this family's situation in all its complexity, while also trying to depict their lives with sensitivity and compassion. Their separate and *prior* decision to be videotaped had already resulted in full disclosure of their identity and life circumstances. Nonetheless, I will use only their first names and a fictitious last name, "Smith," in this discussion.

Family Information [obtained from school records and from the videotape]

Relatives in the Home

Child client	Barbie, age 10, third grade; reading and writing below grade level. Physically abused in foster care at age 6.
Mother	Lori, age 34, unemployed; former bartender and drug abuser. Prison record for possession of drugs and firearms.
Brother	David, age 16, Lori's son by a previous partner (father's whereabouts unknown). School dropout; working on general equivalency diploma (GED).

Relatives Outside the Home

Sister	Donna, age 18, Lori's daughter by another previous partner (father died of kidney disease). School dropout. At time of referral, living away from family because mother disapproved of her boyfriend; later returned to live with family. Had kidney and heart problems.

Father Jim, age unknown, occupation unknown. Lived out of state; physically abused Lori and Barbie, according to Lori's and Barbie's statements on video. At time of referral, parents had been separated for 3 years and divorced for 1 year. Barbie had not seen her father since the divorce, although he maintained occasional telephone contact with her.

There were no known extended family members. The family was Caucasian; religious affiliation was unknown. Financial support came from Aid to Families with Dependent Children and food stamps.

Referral

The social worker at the shelter where the Smith family was then residing spoke to Mrs. Smith about a special school program for children like Barbie, who do not have permanent homes. Because this program provided transportation, Mrs. Smith agreed to take the bus with Barbie the next day to complete the necessary registration forms to enroll Barbie in the school. This school program was created to educate children who are "in transition" and to assist their families with counseling and other services. The application process, conducted by a social worker, included a detailed history of the child and the family. Mrs. Smith cooperated fully with this process and openly shared information about her past incarceration and drug abuse, stating with pride that she had been "clean" since her release from prison 3 years earlier. She also revealed that Barbie and her siblings had each been physically abused in the separate foster homes in which they were placed while she was incarcerated.

IDENTIFICATION OF THE NEED FOR SERVICES

We can assume that homeless families have multiple problems and needs, including not only housing but also concerns related to their overall welfare, schools for the children, employment for the adults, and so forth (Phillips, DeChillo, Kronenfeld, & Middleton-Jeter, 1988; Choi & Snyder, 1999; Jackson, 2000; Vostanis & Cumella, 1999). In the case of Mrs. Smith, her reason for contacting the special school program for homeless children was to arrange for her daughter's education, which had been highly erratic during the previous 6 months. Every time the family had relocated, Mrs. Smith had enrolled Barbie in the nearest school. Mrs. Smith was not aware that the First Place program was different from the others in that an array of services would now be available to her and her family.

Mrs. Smith as an "Unintentional" Client

Although philosophy of support to *families* seems appropriate and necessary to meet the educational needs of homeless children, Mrs. Smith came to First Place to arrange for her youngest child's education rather than to obtain any other kind of help for herself and her other children. Her willingness to give family information to the intake worker reflected her belief that this was an expected part of the application procedure rather than that she was applying for counseling or other forms of help. Indeed, the filmmaker (who later gained Mrs. Smith's trust over a period of time) clarified that, because of the children's previous experiences of abuse in the foster care system when Mrs. Smith was in prison, she was wary and mistrustful of "the whole helping system." Thus it is understandable that she never attended any of the parent support group meetings that were held at First Place, even when transportation and babysitting were available. Another reason for her noninvolvement may have been her history as a former felon—a status that could have stigmatized and set her apart in the group and prevented her feeling comfortable in sharing parenting and other life concerns with other single mothers. Perhaps these obstacles could have been anticipated and resolved if the social worker had met individually with Mrs. Smith prior to the group's first meeting.

A Necessary Focus on Clients' Perceived Needs

Mrs. Smith's failure to avail herself of counseling services at the school highlights how important it is for social workers to understand the *client's* point of view regarding their own needs for service. We cannot assume that *our* views about the client's needs match the individual's own assessments of the kinds of services they need or want. In addition to schooling for Barbie, Mrs. Smith's top priority was to find permanent housing for her family. She succeeded in this goal approximately 2 months after Barbie began at First Place, resulting in Barbie's subsequent transfer to a neighborhood public school. Yet another school for Barbie!

In addition to housing, Mrs. Smith was concerned about obtaining medical care for Donna, who had kidney and heart ailments and who lived with the family sporadically. Also, Mrs. Smith was obligated to meet regularly with her parole officer and to have contact with the local department of social services to receive financial assistance. Dore (1993) notes that in work with poor families, "assistance in obtaining concrete resources is central, not adjunctive, to the helping process" (p. 552). Mrs. Smith proved able and willing to seek out the help she wanted for her family without assistance from professional helpers. She did not, furthermore, identify a need for counseling for herself or for her children, even though she knew that they had been abused.

Figure 3.2 is an eco-map illustrating the various agencies with which Mrs. Smith had regular contact during the 2-month period in which Barbie was enrolled at First Place School. None of these agencies, except the school, appeared to offer services related to helping with the emotional or

FIGURE 3.2. Eco-map of the Smith family.

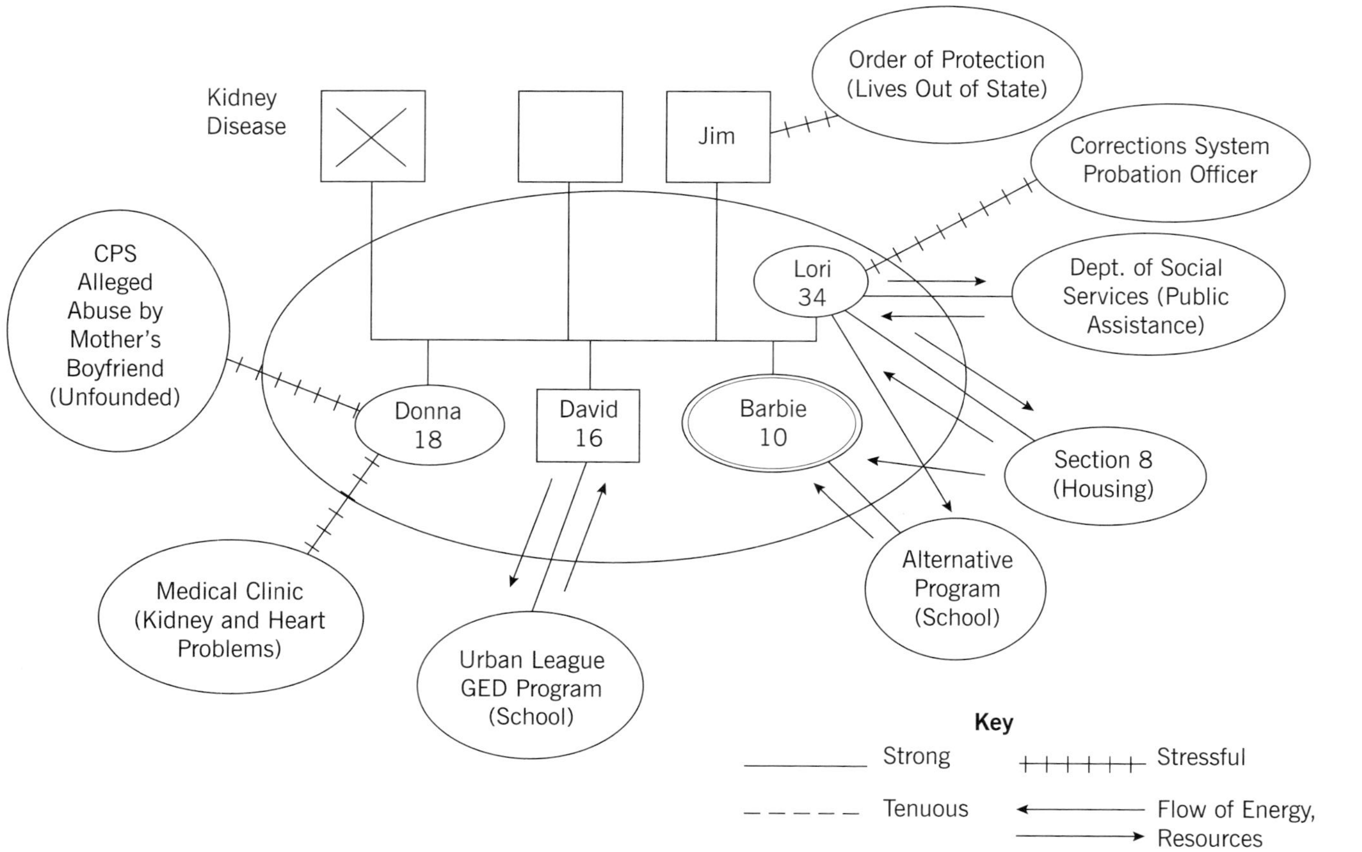

interpersonal issues of individuals or the family unit. Because this family had experienced numerous problems—spousal and father–child physical abuse; divorce and subsequent absence of the father; lengthy and stressful periods of maternal separation and child placement; conflict between the mother and a daughter (Donna); two children who dropped out of school (David and Donna); and the mother's drug abuse, imprisonment, and felony record—it seems obvious that some type of counseling in the form of family intervention and/or parent support would have been appropriate in attempting to interrupt the intergenerational transmission of dysfunctional interaction patterns that lead to violence, unhappiness, and dependence. Although provision of concrete services was essential, it brought only short-term relief and did not address the prevention of future repetition of the same difficulties. The lack of *long-term* planning, goal setting, and counseling with the members of this family deprived them of the opportunity to extricate themselves from the cycle of homelessness and poverty that characterized their lives when they initially became known to First Place School.

In retrospect, how and by whom might counseling services have been offered and implemented in this situation? Certainly there was no lack of professional helpers involved in this case, as shown in the eco-map. Unfortunately, however, there was *no collaboration in goal setting* among the helpers, with the result that Mrs. Smith probably felt scattered and unfocused in her efforts to help her family. The discussion that follows presents the "ideal" management of this case, in the hope that this retrospective analysis will lead to more effective interventions with others like the Smiths, who have multiple problems, multiple needs, and few resources with which to cope with the difficulties of their lives.

INTERAGENCY COLLABORATION ON BEHALF OF CHILDREN AND FAMILIES

The move away from the philosophy of "child rescue" to viewing intervention as "family-supportive and family-strengthening" argues for delivery of services in a family's home or natural community environment (Whittaker, 1991; Tracy, 2001). Ideally, a model of intervention that avoids fragmentation of services while facilitating greater participation of parents in the care of their children would be desirable for homeless families (Lourie & Katz-Leavy, 1991; Choi & Snyder, 1999). How might services have been better coordinated in this case? To put that question in context, we need first to consider Mrs. Smith's degree of openness to receiving help.

Work with the Unintentional Client

Mrs. Smith appears to have been uninterested in *counseling* for herself and her family, although she did everything in her power to obtain financial, medical, and educational services on her family's behalf. Both of her daughters had received some form of counseling following their abuse in foster care 3 years earlier, and Mrs. Smith had participated in drug rehabilitation while she was in prison. She may have felt that these matters had been "taken care of." Although Mrs. Smith may have felt burdened in carrying the full weight and responsibility of meeting her family's needs, she did not seem to perceive the need for counseling for herself. She may have associated counseling with being "weak" or "mentally ill" or "addicted." It was also possible that she was overwhelmed and even depressed; we know that depression is more prevalent among persons at the lowest socioeconomic level (Dore, 1993; Kirby, n.d.). Moreover, Mrs. Smith's own childhood history of sexual assault (which she mentioned on the videotape) and her repeated experiences of victimization in her marriage could have resulted in "learned helplessness" (Hooker, 1976), feelings of hopelessness (Beck, Rush, Shaw, & Emery, 1979), and the inability to conceive of any possible improvement in her life (Browne, 1993). It certainly was sadly revealing and somewhat shocking when Mrs. Smith stated on the tape that she could not project what she wanted for Barbie's future, and Barbie, in turn, stated that she wanted to be just like her mom!

It was not clear whether Mrs. Smith's probation officer knew about her struggle to obtain housing or whether anyone had ever made any efforts to help her obtain employment. She indicated on the school intake form that her difficulty in obtaining permanent housing was related to her "record." If this was indeed true, this could have led to feelings of discouragement and anger. This situation merited exploration with the probation department and the housing authority, and one of the helpers involved in this case should have offered to make a phone call to clarify this matter.

Efforts to engage Mrs. Smith in counseling for herself would probably have failed unless they were tied directly to issues related to something of concern to *her*, such as Barbie's schooling. In presenting strategies for working with an involuntary client, Rooney (1988) suggests a "let's make a deal" proposal, in which something the client wants is paired with an issue considered essential by the worker. This permits the client to exercise some choice, thereby enhancing his or her autonomy and reducing possible resistance. An example of how this might have been presented to Mrs. Smith follows:

WORKER AT BARBIE'S SCHOOL: Mrs. Smith, we're concerned about Barbie's delayed skills in reading and writing. In addition, she does not have a very good sense of self-esteem, because her skills are not on the same level as other children her age. We're prepared to help her with the academics, but it will only work if you help her with her feelings about herself.

MRS. SMITH: How can I do that? I'll help in any way I can, but I don't really know what you mean.

WORKER: Maybe I can make a suggestion. I know how Barbie admires you; when we talk in school about what the children want to do when they get older, Barbie says that she wants to be just like you. That is a great compliment, since I know that your life has not been easy!

I wonder if we could help Barbie in a kind of roundabout way, by arranging some job training for *you*. A lot of the mothers of our students never had a chance to develop job-related skills, so we're going to have some special classes to help mothers just like you to figure out what kind of job training they want and then help them get it.

MRS. SMITH: I really don't like to go out at night and leave the kids alone in that place. It's full of pimps and addicts. Besides, I don't really see how doing this would help Barbie.

WORKER: Barbie needs to have more faith that girls can be successful in their lives. We don't want her to "give up" and think that she is "stupid" when she is only 10 years old and never had a chance to stay at one school long enough to learn.

We're going to have the job meetings in the morning. You can ride the bus with Barbie, and tell her that you're trying to figure out what you want to do with the rest of your life because you want a better life. You'll not only be helping yourself, but you'll be helping Barbie.

MRS. SMITH: OK. Just tell me when the first meeting is and I'll be there.

WORKER: It's day after tomorrow. We're going to start Barbie's special tutoring the same day. It's really important for you to tell Barbie that you and she are both going to try your best to improve your lives. If she knows that *you* are enthusiastic, it will help her feel optimistic. And I'm going to keep track of how you like your class. So, I'll meet you after your class finishes day after tomorrow.

School-Based and Shelter-Based Service Models

As the preceding dialogue suggests, the issue of job training for single mothers is critical for homeless women if they are to overcome poverty and move beyond the extremely limited financial assistance provided by welfare. It seems logical for such employment counseling and training to take place in a school setting, as statistics indicate that two-thirds of homeless parents never graduated from high school (Nuñez, 1994). Another option for intergenerational education is the model of shelter-based education programs as implemented by the Homes for the Homeless project and study (Nuñez, 1994), which have demonstrated that both children and parents become more enthusiastic about school and education after as short a period as 8 weeks in family-based educational programs. The project's philosophy is that "it is education, rather than housing, that holds the greatest potential for ameliorating the deplorable crisis [of homelessness]" (Nuñez, 1994, p. 29). Other authors (Dupper & Halter, 1994) have pointed out the lack of parents' involvement in their children's schooling as a key factor in the poor school attendance of many homeless children. Therefore, stimulating mothers' interest in furthering their *own* education can bring positive benefits to their children.

The facts that Mrs. Smith's two older children had both dropped out of school and that Barbie was absent for 15 out of 31 school days during the 2-month period in which she was enrolled at First Place suggested that Barbie was at risk of following in her siblings' footsteps. We do not have any information about Mrs. Smith's own schooling history. However, it seems clear that *all* the Smiths would have benefited from educational counseling and training for future employment. Shelter-based services, as recommended by Nuñez, unfortunately do not reach homeless families like the Smiths, who often reside in motels rather than shelters and who move frequently.

A school-based model of help, with the school social worker assuming an outreach role with homeless families in transitional housing, holds promise. However, it needs to be backed with transportation, career counseling, liaisons to welfare and probation counselors or officers, health services, and all social service providers with which homeless families have contact. It also requires that the social worker have a small enough caseload, as in the Homebuilders program (Kinney, Haapala, & Booth, 1991), to allow time to work intensively with each family for the period necessary to initiate some positive changes. Other intensive family-centered crisis models recommend that workers serve no more than six families at a time for an average of 8–10 hours per week (Tracy, 2001).

Commitment to Case Management and Collaboration

Homeless families headed by single women tend to have fewer and less stable support networks than do families headed by poor women with housing (Bassuk, 1993; Choi & Snyder, 1999). Because they may have exhausted the willingness or ability of their extended family members and friends to help them, these single mothers must rely on social agencies to meet their basic needs. Unfortunately, many agencies fulfill the minimal requirements of client service without considering a holistic approach to their clients' situations. Thus, in Mrs. Smith's case, her probation officer tended to focus primarily on whether she was drug-free without attending to her additional need for housing or employment or to her children's needs. Many practitioners would consider the coexistence of two unemployed teenagers in a shelter accommodation in a one-bedroom motel as a disaster waiting to happen! However, when agencies shortsightedly address only the narrow concerns mandated by their specific purpose, more extensive preventive goals fall by the wayside.

The need for a case coordinator or case manager in this situation is evident, just as it was in the case of José (Chapter 2). Without this coordination, in fact, the helping efforts the Smiths did receive lacked the combined positive impact the family members would have experienced from a group of social service professionals organized to mount a united effort on their behalf (Schlosberg & Kagan, 1988; Choi & Snyder, 1999).

There is no doubt that coordinating the various helpers in the Smiths' case would have taken time and effort. A single meeting, however, attended by the various personnel involved with this family, *together with the mother,* would have provided the opportunity to set realistic goals for each family member. The anticipated long-term benefits to the family of such collaboration would have made the effort worthwhile and ultimately cost-effective. The lack of such planning and oversight deprived this family of the opportunity to benefit substantially from the separate helping efforts offered by the separate agencies involved with the family at the time of Barbie's referral to First Place School. (Updates regarding the circumstances of the family 2 years and 6 years later and about Barbie at age 28 appear at the end of Chapter 5. They compellingly portray the chronic hold of homelessness and its relentless intergenerational transmission in the absence of counseling and long-term educational/employment intervention for all family members.)

ESTABLISHING PROFESSIONAL RELATIONSHIPS

The Smiths' case, like most, would have required that the social worker relate to many different individuals—both clients and other professionals—in the process of carrying out the social work role.

Relationships with Clients

Several decades ago, Perlman (1979) identified the main features of professionals' relationships with clients as stemming from their purpose, their time-limited and client-centered nature, and the implicit expectation that the professional will exercise responsibility and self-control in carrying out his or her role. This means that the worker–client relationship is quite different from social relationships because it is essentially unbalanced, with the primary focus on the client and on the purpose of the contact. The power of the professional relationship flows from the client's experience of personal validation through being the full center of another person's attention.

Carl Rogers's client-centered approach to therapy (see Rogers, 1951) emphasizes the special qualities of warmth, acceptance, empathy, caring/concern, and genuineness as essential attributes of relationships. In a helping relationship, when the worker listens carefully to the client's concerns and communicates both verbally and nonverbally an attitude of acceptance, the client feels validated and "safe," thereby setting the foundation of the worker–client alliance. Fox (2001) sums this up by stating that "the relationship is the keystone of the helping process" (p. 53). Landreth's model of "child-centered play therapy" (2002a, 2012) subscribes to many of these same values in child therapy, using play as the method of interacting and communicating with the child. Whether the client is a child or an adult, the engagement process must rest on a relationship of respect and trust as the foundation for work on setting appropriate goals.

Initiating Relationships by Telephone

Face-to-face contact offers the best opportunity for two people to meet and begin the process of getting to know one another, because people communicate nonverbally through body language such as eye contact, posture, gestures, and dress, in addition to words. In telephone conversations, these visual cues are absent, and the speakers must rely primarily on words and tone of voice.

When I decided to contact Mrs. Smith to obtain her permission to write about her family, I obtained her phone number from the filmmaker, Kathryn Hunt, with whom the family had a very positive relationship. Because my call occurred on the evening before the family was being evicted from the apartment they had lived in for almost a year, they were in the midst of packing and preparing to move (the same situation Ms. Hunt depicted in the video). I had to make several calls before I reached Mrs. Smith, and in the process I spoke briefly with David and with Barbie. Ms. Hunt had told Mrs. Smith that I would be calling and about the purpose of my call. Mrs. Smith had told Ms. Hunt that she would agree to my request, but I wanted to speak with her personally and ask her to sign release forms.

Because I had already seen all members of the Smith family in the videotape (Hunt, 1992), I had their physical appearances in my mind as I was speaking to them. My initial comments to Barbie, to David, and to Mrs. Smith when I spoke to each of them referred to the video and to my (telephone) relationship with Kathryn Hunt. My mention of Ms. Hunt's name was critical in the family's acceptance of me. I also identified myself as a professor of social work in New York, despite the risk that they might have negative feelings about social workers. This did not register as important in any way I could determine, because they (especially Barbie) were excited that I was calling from *New York*, and my association with Kathryn Hunt ensured their willingness to speak with me.

My contact with Mrs. Smith surprised me in its intensity. When I said something to her about how impressed I was by her struggle to keep her family together, she began crying and spoke almost nonstop for at least 10 minutes. It was hard to understand everything she said because of her sobbing and her clipped, rapid speech; nonetheless, I sensed her strong need to reveal some of her own sad history and to vindicate herself. I shared with her my feelings of regret that I was so far away and therefore unable to offer any firsthand assistance to the family. This did not seem to trouble Mrs. Smith, as her opening up to me seemed to serve the purpose of ventilation rather than to indicate any expectation that I would help. I experienced Mrs. Smith as being very accessible to forming a helping relationship and would not consider her as "reluctant" or "uninvolved" when she engaged with someone who listened to her with empathy.

Initiating Relationships with Child Clients

In beginning work with a child client, the practitioner needs to set the tone for a type of adult–child relationship that is different from others the child has experienced. The child usually expects the worker to relate to him or her as a teacher or parent usually does, with corresponding expectations about how the child should "behave." Because the nature of the helping relationship is so very different and unfamiliar to most children, it is the worker's responsibility to say something to the child, in language that the child can understand, about the nature of the helping process. A statement about who the worker is ("I'm a [lady, man, doctor] who helps children and parents with their troubles and worries") and about how the worker will help ("Sometimes we talk, and sometimes we play") gives the child the framework for this unique relationship, even though he or she probably does not comprehend it fully. It is also important to have some preliminary discussion with the child regarding the reason for the child's contact with the worker, as this has usually been a source of conflict and anxiety for the child and the family. Children, like adults, deserve to be treated with honesty and respect as the basis for an effective helping relationship.

Using Toys to Engage and Work with Children

As will be apparent in many examples of intervention with children in this book, the preferred method for engaging and working with children involves the use of toys and play. Most children have limited verbal abilities, but they communicate their worries and anxieties very graphically through their play. Therefore, it is essential for social workers to have familiarity with and a degree of comfort in using toys with children so that they can interact effectively with their young clients (Webb, 2007, 2011, 2015). I have conducted workshops across the United States and abroad focused on helping social workers and other practitioners learn the rudiments of communicating with children through the symbolic language of play. Although mastery of the complexities of play therapy requires specialized knowledge and training, I believe that every social worker can and should have some minimal knowledge about working with children using play techniques. Given the likelihood of having to work with young children in family sessions or in schools, foster care, residential settings, hospitals, mental health agencies, and family service agencies, social workers must be prepared to use both verbal and nonverbal communication in their interactions with child clients.

Figure 3.3 lists the basic play materials that should be available in every office to facilitate appropriate interactions with children, and the Appendices list some suppliers of these materials. Students who are beginning their careers and expect to work with children should acquire play materials that they can carry with them in a tote bag, so that they will not be dependent on the presence of supplies in the various offices in which they are doing their internships. In previous publications (Webb, 1999, 2007, 2015), I have reviewed various play materials and their use in work with young clients. In this book, examples of the use of drawings can be found in Chapters 4, 6–8, and 11–14. An example of puppet play is given in Chapter 7, and examples of the use of

FIGURE 3.3. Equipping the "average" office for work with children.

Drawing materials

File folders with variety of colored papers.
(Papers include special colored paper to depict different skin colors.)
Colored markers (washable; two sets, one "thin," one "fat").
(The fat markers are available in diverse colors so children can realistically portray their ethnic identity.)

Cutting and pasting

Scissors, two sets with blunt ends. Glue.
Stapler for making "books." Scotch tape.

Dolls and puppets

Bendable family dolls (available in Hispanic, black, white, and Asian).
Most sets include mother, father, boy, girl, baby.
Optional varieties of hard plastic and wooden dolls include a variety of workers, the elderly, and the physically different.
Hand puppets available as family puppet figures.
Animal puppets (in selecting animals, choose two or three "aggressive" and two or three "neutral").

Miniature doll furniture

Kitchen (small table, chairs, refrigerator, stove, sink).
Bedrooms (double bed and single beds). (Other rooms available.)

Games

Card game: Feelings playing cards.
Board game: Talking, Feeling, and Doing Game.

Optional items

Play-Doh (four colors). Doctor kit. Tape recorder.
Toy telephones (2). Blocks, beginner set.

family dolls are provided in Chapters 7 and 12. A videotape/DVD demonstrating play techniques is also available (Webb, 1994b).

Trying to engage young children in a helping relationship without the use of toys and play materials would be as unthinkable as trying to communicate with a deaf person without the use of sign language! A young child may have a rudimentary understanding of verbal communication, and a hearing-impaired person may be able to communicate in writing or may have some knowledge of lip reading, but neither situation respects the basic principle of "starting where the client is." Children (and the physically challenged) have too often been overlooked and treated like inferior beings. The concept of "adultcentrism" (Petyr, 1992; Tyson, 1995) calls attention to the fact that many practitioners expect children to respond as if they were adults. It argues that children should be accorded the rights that are due them, beginning with the use of communication methods (i.e., play) that are "user-friendly" to child clients.

Relationships with Other Professionals

Any social worker who provides services to children will, of necessity, have reason to interact with other professionals. Depending on the circumstances of the case, it may be necessary and appropriate to collaborate with the following range of persons who may have contact with the child:

- The child's teacher
- The school psychologist
- The child's special education teacher
- The child's physician
- The child's caseworker/guardian *ad litem* (i.e., a lawyer or other individual assigned to protect the child's legal interests)

Necessary procedures must be followed prior to any discussion with other professionals. A social worker must have signed releases from a child's parent(s) prior to engaging in any contact with others involved in the case. In addition to obtaining these releases, it is a good idea to discuss with the parent(s) just how much information about the family they are comfortable having the worker disclose (Wachtel, 1994). For example, parents may understand the importance of the worker's learning about test results (either medical or educational) to clarify the agreed-upon purpose of helping their child with self-esteem issues. However, they may not see the utility of the worker's sharing information about his or her psychosocial assessment and intervention with school personnel. Wachtel (1994) points out how helpful it can be for the teacher to be able to reinforce certain goals with the child in the classroom, so that the teacher, parents, and worker are all emphasizing the same objectives. When this approach is presented to parents as in their child's best interests, the parents usually will permit the worker to use his or her professional judgment regarding what to share with others. When working with families of diverse cultural backgrounds, the worker should be aware that the family may feel shamed because of the child's problematic behavior, and/or they may be very uncomfortable about revealing details about the family members, especially when different children may have different fathers and/or when the family resides with grandparents or other relatives. As mentioned in Chapter 1, social workers should be sensitive about cultural differences and try to learn about the values and expectations regarding parent–child behavior in the specific family with which they are working.

As a rule, a worker should exercise restraint about sharing family information that is not directly related to helping the child. Other professionals do not necessarily subscribe to the same code of confidentiality as that of the social work profession, and once personal matters move into the "public" domain, the clients' right to privacy can no longer be guaranteed. A continuing focus on the *purpose* of sharing information will help determine what and how much to share; the best interests of the clients should be the guiding ethical principle in each instance.

CONCLUDING COMMENTS

The quality of relationships between clients and a social worker and among the various helpers in a specific case often determines the success or failure of the helping contact. Positive relationships can inspire motivation and hope for change, whereas negative relationships can reinforce feelings of futility and even hostility. Because of the *purposive* focus of the helping relationship, a client can begin to believe that something different can happen and that he or she will receive assistance in planning and creating a life change. Listening carefully to the client's vision of what he or she wants is the key to the worker's understanding and empathy. Weick and Pope (1988) point out that the client's views may be different from what the worker envisions and that true client self-determination flows from the worker's appreciation and respect for the inner meaning of the client's reality.

This principle of respect for the client applies to work with children in the necessity for adults to communicate with children in *their* language of play rather than expecting children to use words exclusively. A relationship between a social worker and a child client therefore makes special demands on the worker, who must join with the child on his or her developmental level, while simultaneously attempting to comprehend the meaning of the child's play so that the worker can respond helpfully within the play metaphor.

Similarly, the need to convey respect applies when working collaboratively with other professionals. There may be differences in language and viewpoints between a social worker and other professionals, such as teachers or physicians. The very attempt on the worker's part to understand how another professional views the client's situation conveys an attitude of appreciation for the contribution of the other individual. If terminology or language differences interfere with understanding, it is appropriate for the worker to ask for clarification.

Workers who use family and small-group modalities are familiar with the need to maintain a neutral stance and to listen and observe each member without forming alliances with any one person. The same principle applies in work with the various individuals involved in many helping situations. The goal of objectivity does not imply coldness but rather the ability to relate to different people according to their own specific needs and to keep the purpose of all relationships clearly in mind.

DISCUSSION QUESTIONS AND ROLE-PLAY EXERCISES

1. Imagine that you are the school social worker assigned to work with the Smith family. Consider where, how, and with which family member(s) you would structure the *first* meeting. Give reasons for your decision.
2. Role-play several alternative scenarios of the initial meeting with the Smith family, such as the following:
   - With Mrs. Smith and the worker, at the school.
   - With Mrs. Smith, Barbie, and the worker, at the school.
   - With Barbie and the worker, at the school.
   - With the entire family, at the shelter. After the completion of these alternatives, discuss the different types of information obtained in each format and the relative degree of pressure on the worker in each interview situation.
3. Again, imagine that you are the school social worker. What other professionals would you want to contact in connection with your work with Barbie and Mrs. Smith? How would you approach Mrs. Smith to gain her approval of these contacts? Role-play this exchange.

CHAPTER 4

The Biopsychosocial Assessment of the Child

Most social workers rely on assessments and treatment plans to guide them in their work. The process of helping a child depends on understanding as fully as possible *all* the factors that have contributed to and that maintain a problematic situation; this understanding helps a practitioner formulate, propose, and implement an appropriate remedy. Because "the problem" as presented by the parents, by the school, or by others often represents only the tip of the iceberg, leaving a great number more contributing factors beneath the surface, the social worker must look up, down, and all around while trying to analyze the totality of the problem situation. For example, parents may refer a child because of his or her troublesome behavior, but the "real" problem may be their disturbed marriage, to which the child is reacting. In Barbie's situation (Chapter 3), Mrs. Smith identified Barbie's educational needs, but not the family's lack of stability and multiple problems.

Before recommending a course of action for a child and family, a social worker must have a clear sense of the strengths and weaknesses of the vessel in which all parties are traveling, as well as of the possible detours and obstacles that may be encountered in trying to reach the destination. It is also essential to know about the possible rescue resources available in the event of an emergency. The biopsychosocial assessment functions like a compass and a nautical chart that assists the worker in helping the child and family navigate toward their goals.

WHAT IS AN ASSESSMENT?

The assessment has been described as "the thinking process that seeks out the meaning of case situations, puts the particulars of the case in some order, and leads to appropriate interventions" (Meyer, 1993, p. 3). Another definition refers to assessment as "the worker's professional opinion about the facts and their meaning" (Northen, 1987, p. 179). Although the assessment process is time-consuming and often difficult because of its complexity, it may reveal exciting discoveries. The worker, like an explorer or a detective, uncovers as much as possible about the presenting problem to determine its history, magnitude, and ramifications. This *appraisal* component of assessment requires that the worker analyze the interrelationship among biological, psychological, and sociocultural factors as these pertain to a client's life situation. Traditionally, social workers have emphasized the *psychosocial* components of the presenting problem (psychological factors and environmental/cultural influences). In recent years there has been more recognition of the potential importance of biological factors, such as temperament and prenatal influences, and the effects of abuse and neglect on children's brains and their future development and ability to relate.

The reason for conducting an assessment is to try to understand why a problem exists so that a remedy can be recommended. Sometimes an assessment leads a social worker to identify the need for specialized medical, psychological, or educational evaluations and to make appropriate referrals. For example, in assessing the factors contributing to Barbie Smith's poor school performance (Chapter 3), the school social worker might have considered the possibility that her academic delays were perhaps related to fetal alcohol/addiction syndrome, based on the assumption that her mother had used substances during her pregnancy with Barbie. The fact that Barbie changed schools so frequently may have been only partially responsible for her academic difficulties. Had timely testing been completed and specific disabilities revealed, Barbie's educational planning could have targeted remediation of her specific learning deficits.

Important Points about Assessment

1. Collecting data during the initial phase of work does not mean that the client's pressing needs for immediate help are put on hold while the worker systematically and single-mindedly goes about formulating the biopsychosocial assessment. *Assessment and intervention typically occur simultaneously.*

2. The assessment process is not over when the biopsychosocial summary is written. *Assessment is an ongoing process* and therefore subject to elaboration and revision throughout the contact with the clients.

3. Assessment of children is always tentative, because children's development is in flux. *Child evaluations, therefore, should be repeated periodically to allow for normal developmental changes.*

THE ASSESSMENT PROCESS

The purpose of conducting an assessment is to understand the multiplicity of factors that are contributing to the presenting problem, so that an agreement can be made about how to alleviate it. According to Mash and Hunsley (2007, p. 4) "there is a general consensus regarding the need for assessment strategies not as an endpoint, but as a prerequisite for planning, implementing, and evaluating effective and efficient services for children." The following basic questions must be considered in planning the steps of the assessment:

1. Who/what is to be assessed? (Child? Parents? Entire family or subsets of the family? Peers? Neighborhood?)
2. In what order should the assessment be conducted? Should parents, child, or the whole family be seen first? And what general guidelines should be followed in contacts with each party?
3. What collateral information should be obtained? (School, medical, psychological, legal reports?)
4. What assessment tools should be employed? (A few of the options for selection are developmental history and family background; tripartite assessment forms; traumatic exposure screening, genograms, eco-maps; DSM-5; psychological and educational testing).
5. How should the relevant data be summarized?
6. How should the assessment be reviewed with parents and others?

The remainder of this chapter focuses on these questions.

DETERMINING WHO/WHAT IS TO BE ASSESSED

Determining the "unit of attention" is a basic task in beginning work in any case situation. Most individuals live in families, and these families, in turn, are subject to both the favorable and the harmful influences of their surrounding environment. A systems viewpoint recognizes that every part is influenced by the whole to which it belongs, just as the whole, in turn, is affected by its individual members. Chapter 1 discussed and diagrammed an ecological perspective on etiology, upon which this chapter expands. In several previous books (Webb, 1991, 1999, 1993, 2002a, 2007, 2015), I have presented different versions of a tripartite concept of assessment, taking account of three groups of factors that interact in any assessment:

- Factors related to the individual.
- Factors related to the problem situation.
- Factors related to the support system.

When a child comes to the attention of a social worker, it is imperative that the worker keep these three general categories of factors in mind as he or she tries to understand the complex dimensions of the problem situation. Like a juggler tossing balls into the air sequentially and keeping them aloft, the worker must possess the ability to divide his or her attention among the numerous people and events related to the particular case. Figure 4.1 diagrams the interactive components of a tripartite assessment.

I have developed three different forms to guide the worker in obtaining, organizing, and recording information preparatory to formulating a biopsychosocial assessment. These are presented and discussed in the section on assessment tools later in this chapter. The amount of information to be collected can seem overwhelming, especially to the beginning social worker, who may not immediately comprehend its relevance. It is important to stress that the purpose of data collection is to guide the worker in setting goals and planning intervention strategies. Therefore, although my assessment model is comprehensive so that it can apply to a wide range of problem situations, each separate assessment need not include information on *all* the items listed

FIGURE 4.1. Interactive components of a tripartite assessment.

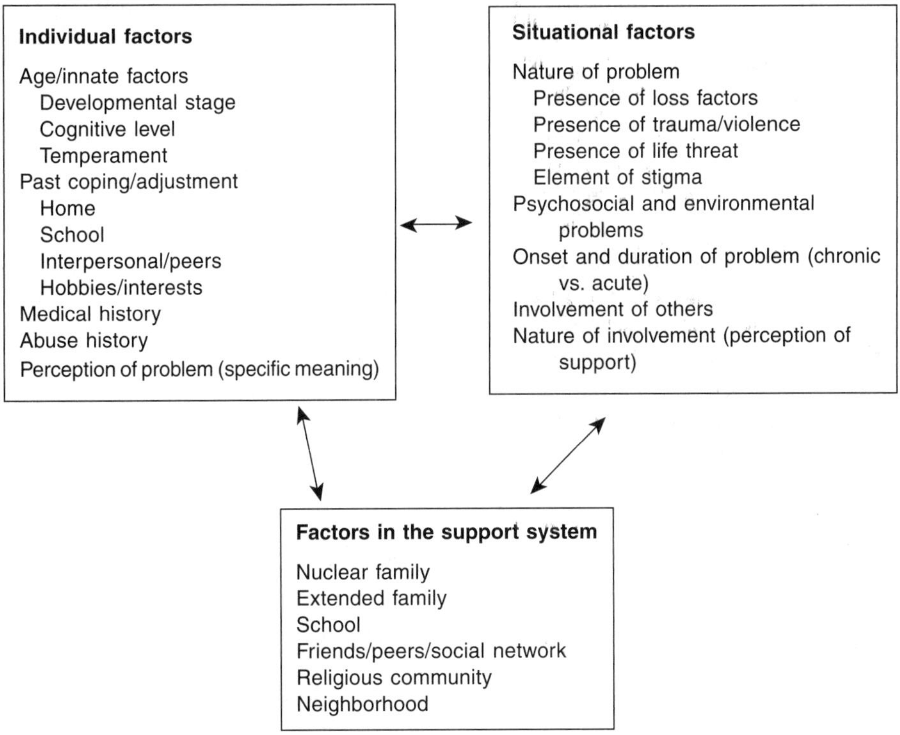

on the forms. *The worker's judgment about the relevant factors in each case situation guides the assessment process accordingly.*

OBTAINING COLLATERAL INFORMATION

Information about a child and family usually comes from numerous sources, in addition to the personal observations and interviews of the social worker. These other sources of data include reports of the clients' past contacts with other agencies, as well as summaries of past and current school, medical, and legal contacts. *Releases must be signed by the client (or the client's parents) before the worker can request collateral information.* Sometimes a client arranges to have reports sent directly to a worker, after signing necessary releases for the reporting agency. However, more typically, in the first meeting with a client or parent the intake worker determines the collateral information that is relevant, discusses this with the client or parent, and obtains his or her signature prior to requesting the information.

In cases involving children, some agencies routinely ask parent(s) to sign releases to obtain the child's school and medical records. Occasionally a parent objects to having the school know that a child is receiving counseling, and if the problem is not school-related, there is no necessity to obtain school records. For example, a child with a sibling/family conflict may be doing well in the academic sphere, and thus school and medical records would be superfluous. However, in cases in which the worker believes that school records are essential for completing the assessment, he or she may need to discuss this necessity with the parents and encourage them to reconsider. Often it is helpful for the worker to reassure the family that only information relevant to the child's problem will be shared with the school.

Sometimes a worker wants to speak with a child's teacher and make a school visit. Sometimes a home visit is appropriate to observe a child's interaction with a babysitter or to assess the atmosphere in the home. Often a telephone conference with the child's pediatrician is helpful, especially if the child has somatic complaints or a coexisting medical problem. When the child's troublesome behavior is the focus of concern, the worker may ask the parents and the teacher to fill out a behavior checklist (see "Assessment Tools" later in the chapter). Again, the decision about what information to obtain depends on the circumstances in each case and the worker's judgment about what information will lead to improved understanding.

ORDER AND GENERAL GUIDELINES FOR ASSESSMENT

The Usual Order of Assessment for a Child Client

It is a truism that first impressions may be lasting. Therefore, a social worker must consider carefully the impact of seeing one family member before another.

The worker's observations and impressions weigh heavily in the assessment process, and when the worker interviews one family member prior to another, that individual enjoys the possible advantage of having his or her point of view heard *first*. Sometimes the worker inadvertently forms an alliance with the family member seen first, thereby putting members who are seen later at a disadvantage. Ideally, the worker remains neutral and objective, regardless of the order in which clients are seen.

The usual order of assessment, when the presenting client is a child, is as follows:

1. The worker meets with the parent(s). In situations of separation or divorce, contact with the noncustodial parent may involve a separate interview or a telephone conference.
2. The worker conducts two or three play evaluation sessions with the child.
3. The worker sees the entire family when the problem situation seems to have reverberations for other family members. (This step may be postponed until later or, in some cases, may never occur.)
4. (Optional) The worker contacts the child's teacher by telephone and, depending on circumstances, makes a school visit and/or requests school records. (See the previous section, "Obtaining Collateral Information.")
5. The worker refers the child for psychological or educational testing, if appropriate.
6. The worker obtains a report from the child's pediatrician. (See the previous section, "Obtaining Collateral Information.")

General Guidelines for Contacts with the Parent(s)

There are several important reasons to see the parent(s) first when the child is under 10 years of age:

- To form an alliance with the parents (essential for ongoing work with the child).
- To obtain a developmental history of the child, including matters the parent(s) may not wish to discuss in the child's presence.
- To prepare the parent(s) to prepare the child for the assessment sessions.
- To obtain signed releases for all collateral contacts.

General guidelines for pursuing the first three of these goals follow.

Forming an Alliance with the Parent(s)

Working with children requires that the worker include parents as essential partners in helping their children. When parents are not included, the worker walks the dangerous ground of ignoring the very roots of children's identity and being. Insofar as a child's identity consists of his or her dual inheritance from a male and a female parent, the child instinctively attributes the basis of his or her identity to those two people. Even when a parent is unknown, the child has fantasies about that parent, which may reflect the child's expectations about his or her own future life.

Most parents are imperfect, insofar as they are human, and some are so disabled by their own upbringings that they do not know how to parent effectively. Work with children is complicated by the fact that the counselor must deal not only with appealing youngsters who may be "victimized" but also with parents who, out of ignorance or desperation, may have substantially contributed to their children's problems. Blaming a parent, however, is *never* productive and may ultimately result in a worker's inability to help a child. Even in the most compellingly incriminating situations of parent neglect, abuse, criminality, and/or abandonment, we must not minimize parents' ongoing influence on their children. A child who was unwanted, resented, and abused by a parent must constantly cope with the meaning of this rejection. Eventually the child must come to some understanding about the abuse related to the parent's own deficiencies, but this realization usually does not occur until adulthood. Parents are major influences in their children's lives, both in reality and as symbols. Workers, therefore, must put all judgments aside and find ways to include parents in the process of assessing and helping.

Obtaining the Child's Developmental History

The assessment of a child is difficult because of the many factors that may contribute to the child's presenting problem. Obtaining the developmental history serves two purposes: (1) It provides a template against which to measure the course of the child's emotional and physical growth, and (2) it gives a sense of the family environment into which the child was born and in which he or she has developed. The developmental history form presented later in this chapter is one of several assessment tools. The history should be obtained either from a parent or from someone else who has been intimately involved in the child's upbringing.

In addition to the specifics of the child's development, the worker learns a great deal from the *manner* in which the parent or other caretaker conveys the information. Does he or she seem to take pride in the child's development, or is the child pictured as "difficult" and annoying? Sometimes a parent can remember very little about the child's early life, which suggests that the parent was or is not very tuned in to the child. Possibly a mother's difficulty recalling details results from her past postpartum depression or drug/alcohol abuse, and the worker may appropriately inquire about these factors.

For example, in the process of obtaining information from Mrs. Smith about Barbie's language and social development, a sensitive school social worker would have empathized with Mrs. Smith's life circumstances during

Barbie's early childhood. The worker's caring attitude might have encouraged this mother of three children and victim of spousal abuse to openly acknowledge her use of drugs and alcohol as a means of dealing with her depression and stress. Had Barbie been present during the intake, Mrs. Smith might not have felt comfortable disclosing her own addictive behavior. Barbie was 10 years old at the time of the referral to the special school program for homeless children, and Mrs. Smith brought her daughter with her when she visited the school to enroll her. Under these circumstances, it is usually possible for the school social worker to arrange a private meeting with the mother to obtain the history and release forms while the child visits the classroom.

Preparing the Parent(s) to Prepare the Child for the Assessment

Although this was not what happened in Barbie's case, a parent often applies for services for a child and meets with an intake worker without the child's being present. An example is the case of Tammy, age 4 (see Chapter 7), whose serious separation problem in nursery school prompted her teacher to suggest that the mother obtain some counseling to alleviate the child's unhappy, withdrawn behavior.

In situations such as this, when a parent meets with the worker first, the worker then can help the parent think about how to prepare the child for subsequent meetings with the worker. Parents often want to avoid telling their child anything ahead of time, possibly because they themselves feel uncomfortable about "the problem" and because they do not know what to say to the child. I have found that parents are very relieved when I give them explicit suggestions. First, I propose that they tell their child that, because they have been concerned about the fact that they can't seem to help him or her, they have found and spoken with somebody who "helps children and families with their troubles and worries." I further suggest that the parents tell the child that they will be bringing the child to see this person, who has toys and who helps children "sometimes by talking and sometimes by playing with them." I assure parents that, if necessary, they may remain with their child during part or all of the session, depending on the child's level of comfort. I also convey my experience that most children greatly *enjoy* the assessment sessions, so that the parents will approach their child with an optimistic spirit.

General Guidelines for Assessment Sessions with the Child

It is usually advisable to see children for two or three play evaluation sessions. The child's behavior with a stranger during the first session may not be typical, and, in any case, the worker will need to see repeated examples of the child's behavior before coming to any conclusions.

The First Session

The most important task of the worker in the first session is to establish a relationship with the child in which the child feels understood, listened to, and respected as a person. Initially the child will expect the worker to be like other adults, such as parents or teachers, so the worker must make a point during the first session of clarifying the helping role. The worker may ask the child something like this: "Did your mother explain to you who I am, and why she brought you here?" (Most children do not answer this question clearly.) As suggested in Chapter 3, the worker can then say something like the following: "I am a [doctor, lady, man] who helps children and their parents with their troubles and their worries. Do you know what 'worries' are? [Pause for child's response.] Sometimes we'll be talking, and sometimes we'll play."

PREPARING THE OFFICE FOR CHILD EVALUATION SESSIONS

Evaluation sessions differ from the less structured play therapy or helping sessions that may follow the assessment. Just as the social worker beginning with an adult client usually follows an interview guide in obtaining specific information during the intake, the play therapist or social worker who is meeting a child client for the first time needs to prepare in advance and have planned activities and appropriate materials on hand. The worker selects these to serve the dual purpose of (1) making the child client feel comfortable (by offering age-appropriate play material) and (2) providing the worker with information that will assist in understanding the nature and scope of the child's difficulties. Therefore, the office setup for an evaluation session with a 9-year-old differs from that for a 4-year-old because of the types of play materials that the worker makes available to each child.

In evaluation/assessment sessions I have a limited number of toys in view to avoid overstimulating the child and causing scattered play. Table 4.1 outlines suggested play materials for assessment sessions with children of different ages. This table is only a general guide and should not be used rigidly. Work with children requires spontaneity, flexibility, and a tolerance for surprise; the overriding obligation is to respond to the uniqueness of each child.

SUGGESTED ACTIVITIES FOR THE FIRST SESSION

I provide drawing materials to children of all ages and routinely ask them in the first session to make two specific drawings: (1) the Draw-A-Person and (2) the Draw-A-Family. When a child spends a long time on the first drawing and appears to have expended a great deal of effort on this task, I do not ask him or her to complete another drawing during that session. On the other hand, some children can readily complete both a Draw-A-Person and a Draw-A-Family quickly, with energy and enthusiasm. I then invite these children to do a third drawing that can be anything they wish (optional drawing). My videotape/DVD *Techniques of Play Therapy* (Webb, 1994b) illustrates different responses of three children in initial sessions to my request that each child make some drawings. The youngest child, Trey, age 3½, refused to draw anything; 5-year-old Willie spent more than 10 minutes completing his Draw-A-Person (Figure 4.2); and the third child, Natalie, age 4½, completed a Draw-A-Person, a Draw-A-Family, and an optional drawing within a 5-minute interval (Figures 4.3–4.5).

The worker must be attuned to the child's ability, level of energy, and degree of anxiety. Requests for specific drawings should be tailored to the child's responsiveness. Future sessions will provide additional opportunities to obtain further drawings from the child. *The worker should keep in mind that establishing a relationship with the child is the primary goal in the first session and that the toys and activities are means to that important end.*

After a child has completed one or more drawings, I usually suggest a change of activity. If the child is age 7 or younger, I introduce a set of small family dolls and doll furniture and suggest that the child might like to make up a story about this family. Children over age 7, especially boys, may not want to play with dolls, so I offer puppets or superheroes or army men or "therapeutic" (i.e., special/structured) board or card games to boys and/or older children.

TABLE 4.1. Suggested Play Materials for Assessment Sessions with Children of Different Ages

Materials	Ages 3–5	Ages 6–7	Ages 8–10
Colored paper	×	×	×
Colored markers	×	×	×
Scissors	×	×	×
Glue, Scotch tape	×	×	×
Play-Doh	×	×	
Clay		×	×
Small, bendable family dolls	×	×	
Dollhouse furniture (especially kitchen and bedroom)	×	×	
Blocks	×	×	
Animal puppets	×	×	×
Feelings playing cards (see Figure 3.3)		×	×
Talking, Feeling, and Doing Game (see Figure 3.3)		×	×

FIGURE 4.2. Willie's Draw-A-Person. From Webb (1994b). Copyright © 1994 The Guilford Press. Reprinted by permission.

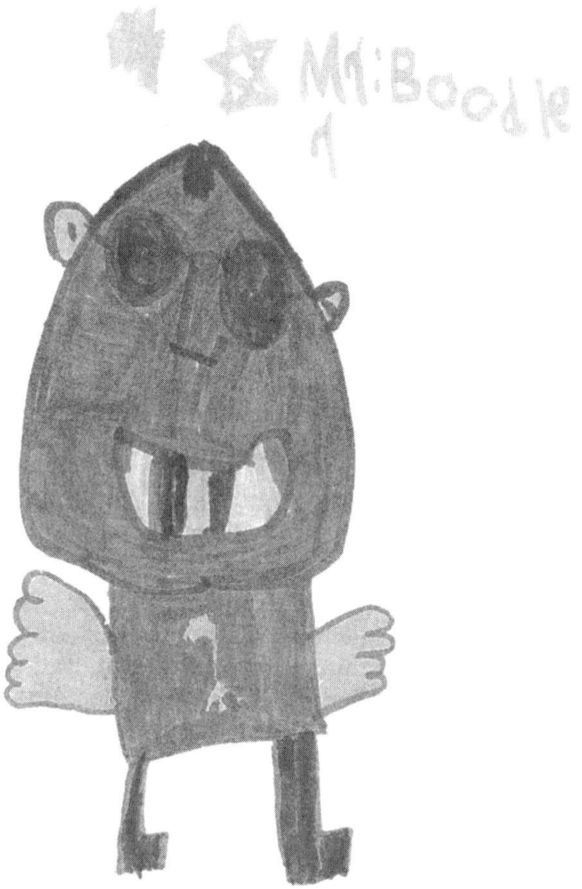

Subsequent Sessions

During the second and third play assessment sessions, I follow a pattern similar to that of the first session. That is, I usually begin by asking the child whether he or she would like to draw and then introduce other toys and activities. Of course, the child remembers the first session and often comes to subsequent meetings eager to resume a play activity he or she enjoyed in the first session. The worker should take special note of such requests, as they may have special significance for understanding the child's circumstances.

FIGURE 4.3. Natalie's Draw-A-Person. From Webb (1994b). Copyright © 1994 The Guilford Press. Reprinted by permission.

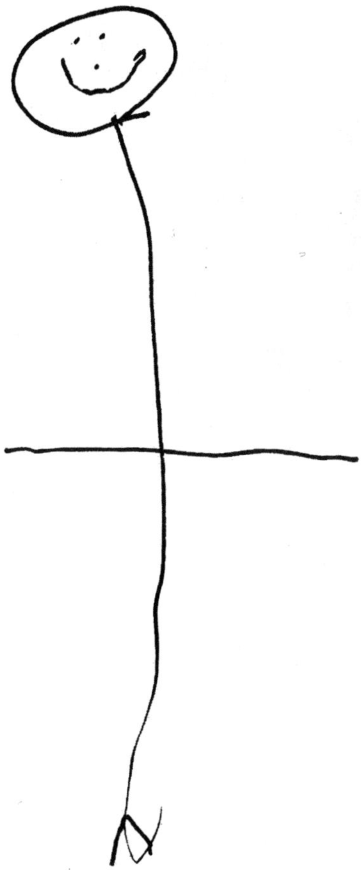

What to Observe in the Child Evaluation Sessions

During the evaluation, the social worker is trying to learn as much as possible about the child by watching the child's play and how he or she relates. After each play session, the worker should take some notes about the following aspects of the child's behavior:

1. *Developmental factors: Age-appropriateness of child's play.* What developmental tasks/issues and concerns are typical of the "average" child of the age under consideration? The worker should evaluate the child's play (including drawings) in terms of evidence of age-appropriate or inappropriate content.

FIGURE 4.4. Natalie's Draw-A-Family. From Webb (1994b). Copyright © 1994 The Guilford Press. Reprinted by permission.

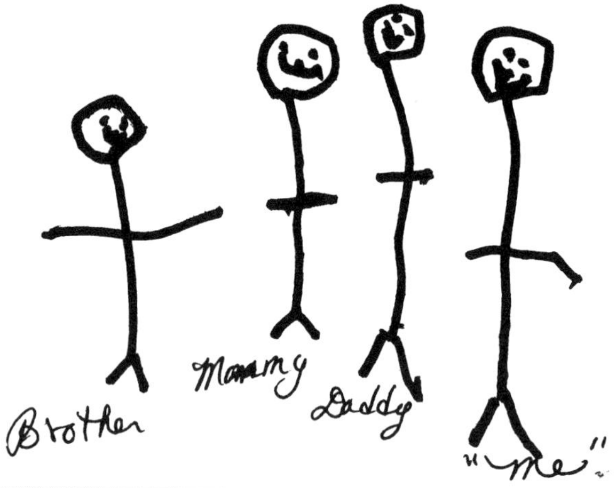

FIGURE 4.5. Natalie's optional drawing. From Webb (1994b). Copyright © 1994 The Guilford Press. Reprinted by permission.

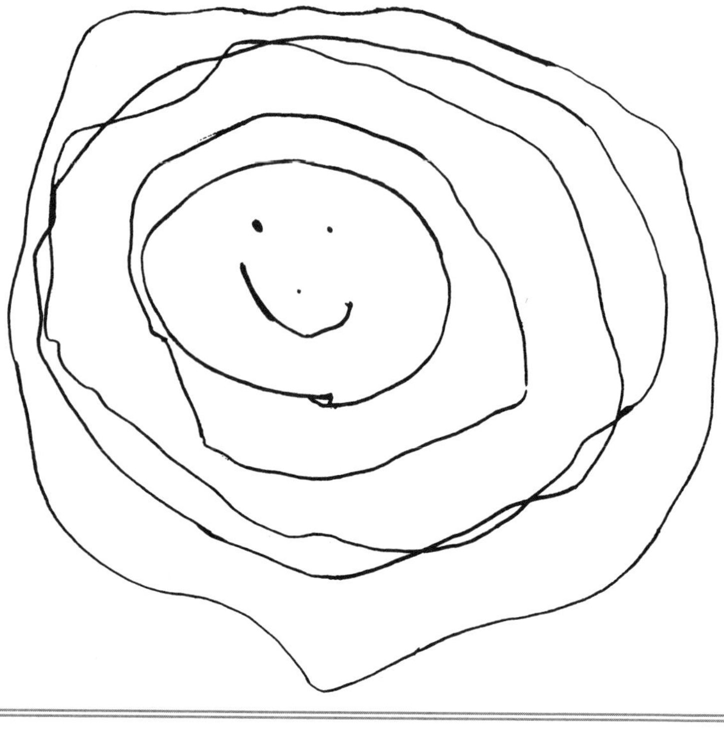

2. *Mood/quality of child's play.* How can this child's play be characterized on the dimension of creativity–constrictiveness? Happy or sad? Aggressive or passive? Did the mood varied over the course of the session(s)? In instances in which constriction is noted in the child's play, does this appear to be evidence of anxiety or of the child's temperament? Has the child's overall mood vary from session to session?

3. *Themes in child's play and possible areas of conflict.* What significant themes can be noted in the child's play? How often do those themes occur? And what factors in the child's life might they stem from? (This last question is merely speculative; however, *numerous* occurrences of aggressive or abandonment play themes, for example, should be noted for further exploration, as should other themes, such as nurturance.) Are there similarities or differences between the types of conflicts or problem situations presented by the child in play and those noted in the parent's or caretaker's earlier reports?

4. *Separation anxiety/ability to relate to worker.* What indications of separation anxiety are noted in the child's actual separation from parent or caretaker in the first session? Do themes in the child's play or interruptions in the play reflect separation concerns? How does the child relate to the social worker? Consider behavior at different points in time, especially variations in the child's responses within each session and among successive sessions.

5. *Ability to concentrate in session.* How distractible is the child? Can he or she focus on a task until completion? Does the child seem to be attending to noises outside the room?

Figure 4.6 provides a form for reviewing and recording these elements in the child's play.

When the worker has completed the evaluation sessions with the child and obtained all other necessary reports (see the section "Obtaining Collateral Information"), he or she meets again with the parents to give them a verbal summary of the assessment and recommendations and to involve the parents in setting goals and formulating a treatment plan.

ASSESSMENT TOOLS

Many different tools are available to assist the worker in forming an assessment of a child and family. Few workers (if any) will use *all* the tools described here in any one case. The nature of the agency often dictates the use of specific assessment methods, such as the DSM in a mental health clinic or a genogram in a child welfare or family services agency. Although we may all agree that

FIGURE 4.6. Assessment of the child's behavior in play sessions.

Date ______________ Which session ________________________

Child's age __________ (years) _______ (months)

1. Age-appropriateness of child's play (check one)

   Regressed _____ Average _____ Advanced _____

   Notes:

2. Mood/quality of child's play (check all that apply)

   Happy _____ Sad _____ Anxious _____ Scattered _____ Creative _______

   Aggressive _____ Passive _____ Other (describe) ______________

   Notes:

3. Themes in child's play (check all that apply)

   Abandonment _____ Nurturance _____ Anger _____ Fear _____

   Loneliness _____ Danger _____ Other (describe) ________________

   Notes:

4. Ability to separate from parent/caretaker

   Appropriate for age _____ Inappropriate _____

   Notes:

5. Ability to relate to worker:

   At beginning of session _____ In middle _____ At end _____

   In second session _____ In third session _____

   Notes:

6. Ability to concentrate in session

   Good _____ Moderate _____ Distractible _____

   Notes:

From *Social Work Practice with Children, Fourth Edition*, by Nancy Boyd Webb. Copyright © 2019 The Guilford Press. Permission to photocopy this figure is granted to purchasers of this book for personal use or use with clients (see copyright page for details). Purchasers can download enlarged versions of this material (see the box at the end of the table of contents).

"the more information we have, the better" about an individual child, time constraints often prevent the completion of a comprehensive assessment. Reality dictates that the worker choose the assessment tools that promise to produce the most useful information in formulating a specific evaluation within a reasonable time frame.

Among the possible choices of assessment tools are the following:

- Developmental history form (Webb; described below)
- Tripartite assessment forms (Webb; see Figures 4.8, 4.9, and 4.10)
- Assessment of risk and protective factors (Davies, 2011)
- Child PTSD Symptom Scale (CPSS; Foa, Johnson, Feeny, & Treadwell, 2001)
- Genogram (McGoldrick & Gerson, 1985; McGoldrick, Gerson, & Petry, 2008)
- Eco-map (Hartman, 1978)
- Culturagram (Congress, 1994, 2008)
- Educational and psychological testing
- Specific drawing exercises (Malchiodi, 1998, 2006; Di Leo, 1973)
- Projective questions
- The latest version of the DSM (DSM-5; American Psychiatric Association, 2013).

Developmental History Form

The developmental history form I have created for my practice and teaching (Figure 4.7) includes a sweeping view of the child's life from birth to the present, concluding with an appraisal of the child's ego strengths and weaknesses. The developmental history constitutes the core of the assessment, pointing to areas of developmental delay, difficulties in separation/individuation, the child's school history, and affective social development. Appraisal of the child's development depends on the worker's solid knowledge of typical developmental norms. As discussed in Chapter 2, this knowledge base is essential in work with children.

The experience of relating information about the child's life sometimes makes a parent very contemplative. The review can, in itself, help a parent comprehend significant pieces of the child's life in a manner that is meaningful to him or her. This occurred, for example, in the intake with Tammy's mother (see Chapter 7), who began to realize as I questioned her about Tammy's friends and babysitters that she had never permitted Tammy to be cared for by anyone other than herself or her own mother. The fact that Tammy's mother was currently having difficulty getting pregnant a second time seemed to cause the mother to cling to her little girl, even as the child was reciprocating by clinging to the mother. Children can sense their parent's anxiety, and this, of course, makes them feel uncomfortable.

FIGURE 4.7. Developmental history outline.

I. *Identification and description of child and family* (outline). Give ages, birthdates, genders, and occupations of all family members. These may be separated into (1) relatives in the home, (2) relatives outside the home, and (3) nonrelated persons living in the home.

II. *Presenting problem* (one or two sentences, in the parents' own words). State the problem that brings the child to the agency, the referring source, and the source's statement of the problem.

III. *History of problem.* Include how problem got started (onset, duration, intensity) and circumstances under which the problem manifests itself.

IV. *Family background* (including three-generation genogram). Indicate ethnicity, religion, socioeconomic status, educational and occupational data, and some conceptualization of patterns of interaction within the family, especially with regard to the child.

V. *Specific developmental history*
   A. Family atmosphere into which the child was born
      1. Marital situation
      2. Financial situation
      3. Was pregnancy planned or unplanned?
      4. Parental attitudes toward children; maturity for parenting
      5. Physical living situation—space?
      6. What kind of community environment?
   B. Delivery
      1. Abnormalities, difficulties, unusual procedures
      2. Gender of child (parental/sibling reactions)
      3. Birth weight
   C. Infancy
      1. Physical development (feeding, toileting, activity level, motor development)
      2. Emotional responsiveness and sensitivity
      3. Quality of mothering (maternal availability for positive, fulfilling relationship); who was the primary caretaker?
      4. Parental perception of child's temperament (easy–difficult)
   D. Early childhood
      1. Language development
      2. Separation–individuation (18–36 months)
         - Physical separation (any delays in development?)
         - Maternal reactions to toddler's greater independence
         - Outside factors affecting mother and child (medical, psychological, social)
      3. Other factors affecting child's early emotional development
         - Sibling births
         - Separations from parents
         - Medical problems/health-related difficulties
         - Unavailable or severely deprived parents
      4. Reactions to nursery school or other separation
      5. Discovery of anatomical sexual differences (reactions)
      6. Exposure to sexual activity or materials
      7. Exposure to traumatic events

(continued)

FIGURE 4.7. *(continued)*

8. Affective/social development
9. Fantasy life and play

VI. *School history*
1. Separation reactions
2. Ability to learn, concentration, cognitive development
3. Superego formation (clear sense of right and wrong)
4. Any noted difficulties in behavior or learning
5. External factors (teachers, moving, etc.)

VII. *Ego strengths and weaknesses*
1. Friends
2. Hobbies/special interests
3. Frustration tolerance, ability to delay gratification
4. Previous symptoms or difficulties

VIII. *Current functioning* (one or two sentences describing child's present adaptation).

In contrast to Tammy's insightful mother, who was able to make meaningful connections between her child's behavior and her own anxieties, other parents may have difficulty remaining focused on their child during the intake. This appeared to be the case in my lengthy telephone call with Mrs. Smith, when I asked her to tell me about Barbie's life before she started school. Mrs. Smith began crying and talking about *herself,* and specifically about how unsupportive her family was and how she eventually had decided to "pay back to others what they had done" to her, even though she knew now that it was wrong. I am still not sure about the meaning of this statement other than as a possible explanation for her drug-dealing activities, which had led to her imprisonment. I sensed during that phone conversation how very needy Mrs. Smith was. Had I been attempting to obtain a developmental history of Barbie, it might have been necessary to focus first on Mrs. Smith because of her own numerous problems. Once such a parent feels validated and respected, he or she may be more able to focus on the related experiences of his or her child.

Tripartite Assessment Forms

During and following the collection of data for the developmental history, the worker begins to weigh the significance of the numerous events and experiences in the child's life. I have developed three forms to help the worker in completing a tripartite assessment (Figures 4.8–4.10). These forms organize the data into distinctive categories that further assist in identifying pivotal influences on the child's life.

(text resumes on page 79)

FIGURE 4.8. Individual factors in the assessment of the child. This form is one part of a three-part assessment of the child, which also includes an assessment of situational factors (Figure 4.9) and an assessment of the child's support system (Figure 4.10).

1. Age _____ years _____ months _____ Date of birth ____________

   Date of assessment ____________

   a. Developmental stage:
      Freud __________
      Erikson __________

   b. Cognitive level:
      Piaget __________

   c. Temperament:
      Thomas and Chess __________

2. Past coping/adjustment
   a. Home (as reported by parents): Good ___ Fair ___ Poor ___
   b. School (as reported by teachers and parents): Good ___ Fair ___ Poor ___
   c. Interpersonal/peers (as reported by parents and self): Good ___ Fair ___ Poor ___
   d. Hobbies/interests (list) ____________

3. Medical history (as reported by parents and pediatrician)—describe serious illnesses, operations, and injuries since birth, with dates and outcome ____________

   ____

4. Abuse history
   a. Physical: No _____ Yes _____ Reported (Y or N) _____ Child's age ________
      Single episode _____ Repeated _____ Perpetrator ____________
      Outcome (give details) ____________

      ____
   b. Sexual: No _____ Yes _____ Reported (Y or N) _____ Child's age ________
      Single episode _____ Repeated _____ Perpetrator ____________
      Outcome (give details) ____________

      ____

5. Exposure to traumatic events (give details with dates and outcome) ________

   ____

   ____

   ____

6. DSM-5 diagnosis, if available ____________

   ____

   ____

   ____

7. Child's personal perception of problem: What is the specific *meaning* of the problem situation to the child at this time? ____________

   ____

   ____

   ____

Note. This form is one part of a three-part assessment of the child, which also includes an assessment of situational factors (Figure 4.9) and an assessment of the child's support system (Figure 4.10). From *Social Work Practice with Children* (4th ed.). by Nancy Boyd Webb. Copyright 2018 by The Guilford Press. Permission to photocopy this figure is granted to purchasers of this book for personal use only (see copyright page for details).

FIGURE 4.9. Situational factors in the assessment of the child. This form is one part of a three-part assessment of the child, which also includes an assessment of individual factors (Figure 4.8) and an assessment of the child's support system (Figure 4.10).

1. Nature of problem
   a. Presence of loss factors
      Separation from family members (list relationship and length of separation) ______________
      ____
      Death of family members (list relationship and cause of death) ______________
      ____
      Loss of familiar environment (describe) ______________
      ____
      Loss of familiar role/status (describe; temporary or permanent?) ______________
      ____
      Loss of body part or function (describe, with prognosis) ______________
      ____
   b. Presence of trauma/violence
      Witnessed: Verbal ______ Physical ______
      Experienced: Verbal ______ Physical ______
   c. Presence of life threat
      Personal (describe) ______________
      To family members (describe, identifying relationship) ______________
      ____
      To others (describe) ______________
      ____
   d. Presence of physical injury or pain (describe) ______________
      ____
   e. Element of stigma/shame associated with problem (describe) ______________
      ____
2. Psychosocial and environmental problems (list problems) ______________
   ____
   ____
3. Onset and duration of problem
   a. Chronic (give details, including child's age at onset and frequency of occurrence) ________
      ____
      ____
   b. Acute (give child's age and duration of problem) ______________
      ____
      ____
4. Involvement of others
   a. Nature of involvement (describe) ______________
      ____
   b. Perception of support: Sufficient ______ Insufficient ______

From *Social Work Practice with Children, Fourth Edition,* by Nancy Boyd Webb. Copyright © 2019 The Guilford Press. Permission to photocopy this figure is granted to purchasers of this book for personal use or use with clients (see copyright page for details). Purchasers can download enlarged versions of this material (see the box at the end of the table of contents).

FIGURE 4.10. Assessment of the child's support system. This form is one part of a three-part assessment of the child, which also includes an assessment of individual factors (Figure 4.8) and an assessment of situational factors (Figure 4.9).

1. Nuclear family members
   a. How responsive are they to the child's needs? Not at all ____ Somewhat ____ Very ______
   b. To what extent is the child included in discussions about "the problem situation"?
   Frequently ____ Never ____ Sometimes ____
   c. Do parents tend to show a judgmental attitude toward the child's behavior?
   Yes ____ No ____

2. Extended family members
   a. How frequently are they in contact with the child?
   Rarely ____ Monthly ____ Weekly ____ Daily ____
   b. Describe nature of the relationships, indicating who is the most supportive relative to the child
   c. To what extent do the views of the extended family differ from or agree with those of the nuclear family on matters pertaining to the child? (give details)
   ____

3. School/peers/social network
   a. Child's grade in school ________
   b. Child's friendship network: How many friends does child have?
   Many ____ "A few" ____ None ____
   c. Would child like to have more friends than he or she has? Yes ____ No ____
   d. How many days after school, on the average, does the child play with another child?
   Most days ____ Once or twice ____ Never ____

4. Religious affiliation
   a. Does the child/family participate in religious services?
   Yes ____ (If yes, give name of religious group:) ______________________
   No ____
   b. If yes, indicate how frequently the child/family participates:
   Weekly ____ Major holiday observances ____ Rarely ____

5. Neighborhood/school activities
   a. Is the family involved with neighborhood/school activities? No ____ Yes ____
   b. If yes, describe ______________________________________
   ____

From *Social Work Practice with Children, Fourth Edition,* by Nancy Boyd Webb. Copyright © 2019 The Guilford Press. Permission to photocopy this figure is granted to purchasers of this book for personal use or use with clients (see copyright page for details). Purchasers can download enlarged versions of this material (see the box at the end of the table of contents).

Applying Developmental History/Tripartite Assessment Principles in the Case of Barbie

Before I continue with the description of various assessment tools, it may be instructive to consider how the tasks of obtaining a developmental history and conducting a tripartite assessment might have been carried out in the case of Barbie Smith. First, I want to emphasize that, in the case of a child as disadvantaged as Barbie, the most useful way of beginning an assessment may be to consider the child's strengths. On the *No Place Like Home* videotape (Hunt, 1992), Barbie presented as an appealing youngster who had not yet been destroyed by the difficult circumstances of her life. She was open about her feelings, conveying resignation about her homeless circumstances and past beatings. Yet she demonstrated the ability to be playful and to enjoy herself when she went roller skating and when the filmmaker allowed her to experiment with a camcorder. Barbie had not only "survived" her difficult childhood; she had matured into a preadolescent with an appeal that caught the interest of a filmmaker and myself. She had learned to take basic care of herself; in the videotape she is shown washing her own hair, cooking a simple meal, and even serving it to her mother. In many respects, she seemed old for her years, especially when she applied eye makeup prior to going skating, as if she were preparing for a "date"—behavior that probably imitated her mother and sister. Barbie is, in fact, an example of how negative experiences do not always result in a negative outcome; she showed great resilience and ability to carry on with her life.

Although Barbie had experienced the separation from both her mother and her father during her preschool years, these losses had not caused her to mistrust other adults. Any social workers or other professional helpers entering Barbie's life needed to acknowledge the girl's strengths while also questioning whether and how this youngster could have a more fulfilling life than that of her mother and how to ensure that this child would not be swept along in the relentless current of poverty, dependence, and constricted beliefs about her future options as a woman.

Information Obtained about Barbie at Time of Referral

The intake interview at the time of Barbie's entry to the special school program for homeless children required (or involved) numerous forms and releases. In addition to information about the family's current living situation, details were obtained about Barbie's health and educational history. The forms did not include information about the child's developmental history, but the social worker nonetheless obtained some information about Barbie's experience in foster care while her mother was in prison for possession of firearms and possession and manufacture of methamphetamines.

According to the information given by Mrs. Smith at intake, she began using drugs when Barbie was about 3 years old, and she was imprisoned for 20 months when Barbie was between 5 and 7 years old. During that period all three children were placed in foster homes in which, according to Mrs. Smith, the girls were molested and beaten. These charges were investigated and later dropped by the district attorney. The girls received counseling for about 2 years, and Mrs. Smith stated that she herself had also been in treatment several times. She claimed during the intake that she had been drug-free since she was released from prison, when Barbie was about age 7; she was employed as a bartender for a while following her release.

The intake also revealed information about Barbie's father. Barbie's parents were married when she was 4 years old, having lived together for 2 years prior to her birth. They separated a year later and were divorced when Barbie was 9. According to Mrs. Smith, her former husband had physically abused her and the children, and she had taken out many court orders of protection against him. He later moved out of state, and Barbie had not seen him since she was 9, although he maintained occasional telephone contact with his daughter.

Reconstruction of Significant Factors in Barbie's Developmental History

In this case, as in many presented to social workers, comprehensive information was (and still is) lacking, and a social worker would have had to make professional judgments despite many missing pieces. Because homeless children require prompt emergency services, it is understandable that the school did not get *detailed* facts about the child's history beyond the preceding 2 years. Actually, the information obtained by the intake worker exceeded the minimum required on the form.

I devised a time line, listing pivotal events of each year of the child's life from her birth to the time of the Hunt videotape for the purpose of reconstructing the important events in Barbie's development. There was virtually *no* information about the period from Barbie's infancy until she was 3 years old, when her mother stated that she began using drugs. We can speculate that this period may have been characterized by Mrs. Smith's alternating states of feeling overwhelmed by the care of three young children and trying to medicate herself with drugs or alcohol. If Mrs. Smith used amphetamines, these would have had a stimulating effect on her mood, and, typically, according to Straussner (1993, p. 311), alcohol serves a sedating function for users of amphetamines. We do not have any information about Mrs. Smith's *alcohol* use, but a colleague of mine—a professor who teaches courses on alcohol and other substances—commented about the similarity between Barbie's facial features (as depicted in the publicity photo for *No Place Like Home*) and those of children with fetal alcohol syndrome (U.S. Department of Health and Human Services, 1993, p. 203). This observation is pure speculation.

Whether or not Barbie's mother was using alcohol prior to her admitted substance abuse when Barbie was 3 years old, we can reasonably question the quality and consistency of Barbie's early parenting experiences. The marriage of Barbie's mother and father was tumultuous and lasted only a year, and Mrs. Smith's incarceration soon after their separation, when Barbie was 5, suggests that the family circumstances were chaotic and not conducive to a child's need for emotional calm and stability. The nature of the attachment relationship between Mrs. Smith and Barbie is not known, but the absence of a mother for 2 years and her father's departure from the home would inevitably affect a 5-year-old child, who was placed in several foster homes where she was abused during this time.

Pivotal elements in the assessment of individual factors in Barbie's development (see Figure 4.8) included the following:

1. *Abuse history* (item 4 in Figure 4.8). Details are lacking, but Mrs. Smith referred to *multiple* instances in which Barbie's father physically abused both her and the children. On the videotape, Barbie asked pointedly, "Just because he hit us, that doesn't mean he doesn't love us, does it?" This question is typical of abused children with ambivalent/anxious attachment who are not certain from one moment to the next whether their parent will hug them or hit them. In addition to physical abuse by her father, Mrs. Smith stated that Barbie was physically and emotionally abused in foster care. Details about this are unknown. Often children who are abused by multiple adults come to mistrust *all* adults, and some begin to believe that abusive behavior is the norm.

2. *Exposure to traumatic events* (item 5 in Figure 4.8). Barbie's early life was characterized by the "loss" of both parents, as well as the loss of her familiar intact family. We do not know what Barbie was told at age 5 when she "lost" her mother to the prison system. She also "lost" her sister, brother (separate foster homes), and father at the same time, and her father never returned to live with the family after her mother was released. Screening for a possible diagnosis of PTSD (Foa et al., 2001) could have revealed the presence of intrusive or avoidance symptoms or negative alterations in thoughts and feelings, or increased reactivity following these multiple experiences of abuse. Clearly, Barbie would qualify for a diagnosis of "complex trauma" (Courtois & Ford, 2009) based on her history of repeated traumatic stressors of neglect and abandonment by caregivers during her early childhood, with the resulting potential of serious impact on her future development.

The assessment of the child's support system (see Figure 4.10) was also revealing. There appeared to be very few supports available to the Smith family in the usual form of extended family members or religious or community affiliations. Mrs. Smith spoke on the tape about her poor relationships with her own family, and she conveyed an attitude of anger and resentment toward them. She had a friendly manner, however, and she appeared to have some male friends, who were shown on the tape helping the family move. In view of the frequency of the family's moves (seven times during a 6-month period), it was remarkable that this mother had the stamina to persevere in her determination to keep her family together. She verbalized this goal frequently, and this may have reassured Barbie about her own personal worth and value. Barbie admired her mother and wanted to be like her. The child seemed unaware of her mother's deficiencies and failures, choosing instead to identify with her strengths. The mother's strong love for Barbie had helped the child endure repeated experiences of abuse and loss. Given the severity of Barbie's early life experiences, it was truly remarkable that she related as well as she did to adults. No information was available about her relationships with peers, however, which certainly would have been compromised by the family's frequent moves. Homeless children typically demonstrate lowered self-esteem and difficulty in making friends (Timberlake & Sabatino, 1994).

Risk and Protective Factors

Davies (1999, p. 45) points out that the identification of risk and protective factors is a critical part of any assessment. Although the presence of protective factors may balance and offset risks, if more than three risk factors exist, "the child and parents are more likely to become overwhelmed, resulting in a developmental or psychiatric disorder in the child" (Davies, 1999, p. 49).

Risk Factors

This term refers to influences in the individual and the surrounding social environment that increase the probability of negative future outcomes for children (Kirby & Fraser, 1997). Davies (2011, p. 65) identifies the following three types of risk factors:

- Vulnerabilities in the child, such as mental retardation or chronic illness.
- Impaired parenting.
- Socioeconomic and institutional factors, such as lack of access to medical care or chronic exposure of the family to poverty and social disadvantage.

We note that in Barbie's case two of the three risk factors were present, namely impaired parenting and chronic poverty.

Protective Factors

The quality of parenting is probably the most important mediator of risk for children, but positive relationships with other adults also can serve a protective function. Barbie appeared to have a secure attachment relationship with her mother, despite her mother's shortcomings, and, in addition, she seemed to benefit from the ongoing attention of the filmmaker. Other protective factors for this girl included her general good health, good looks, and an easy temperament.

Resilience

Davies (2011) wisely emphasizes that risk factors do not determine a child's fate. Studies have shown that only about one-third of any population of at-risk children actually experiences a negative outcome (Wolin & Wolin, 1995) and that the remainder seem to survive without major developmental disruptions (Kirby & Fraser, 1997). These "survivors" were referred to as "invulnerable children" by Anthony and Cohler (1987); authors now use the label "resilient" (Garmezy, 1985; Rutter, 1987; Gitterman, 2001; Norman, 2000). As mentioned in Chapter 1, there is research suggesting a biological difference in the genes of 'resilient' children that may serve to protect them from adverse influences that would put other children at risk (Cicchetti & Blender, 2004). This fascinating possibility is still under study.

Although risk and protective factors appear to be oppositional, Fox (2001) maintains that resiliency actually develops from the interaction between the two sets of factors. He states, "The key in the development of resiliency is not in avoiding risk, but rather in accommodating to it successfully" (p. 140). Table 4.2 specifies common risk and protective factors.

TABLE 4.2. Common Risk and Protective Factors for Serious Childhood Social Problems: An Ecological and Multisystems Perspective

System level	Risk factors	Protective factors
Broad environmental conditions	Few opportunities for education and employment Racial discrimination and injustice Poverty/low socioeconomic status	Many opportunities for education, employment, growth, and achievement
Family, school, and neighborhood conditions	Child maltreatment Interparental conflict	Social support Presence of caring/supportive adult
	Parental psychopathology Poor parenting	Positive parent–child relationship Effective parenting
Individual psychosocial and biological characteristics	Gender Biomedical problems	"Easy" temperament as an infant Self-esteem and self-efficacy Competence in normative roles High intelligence

Note. Adapted from Kirby and Fraser (1997, p. 20). Copyright © 1997 National Association of Social Workers, Inc. Adapted by permission.

Although Barbie's mother had made negative choices for herself and her family in the past, when she was involved in producing and taking drugs, at the time of the video she appeared to be making repeated efforts to survive and to keep her family together. She was demonstrating good coping and resilience in the face of severe adversity. During the period of the video, Barbie admitted to being discouraged by the many moves, yet she continued to function and to be open to new relationships.

Genogram

The genogram, probably one of the most useful of assessment tools, enables the worker to diagram on one page all the members of both the nuclear and the extended family, together with identifying information about them (e.g., ages, occupations, marital status, dates and manner of deaths, and the quality of relationships among various family members). Readers wanting instruction in the construction of genograms can consult McGoldrick and Gerson (1985) and McGoldrick, Gerson, and Petry (2008).

"Reading" a genogram can reveal the following helpful information about a child and family:

- The similarity or difference between the position of the child in his or her nuclear family and the corresponding position of a parent in his or her family of origin.
- Relative(s) for whom the child was named.
- Repetition of problems across the generations (e.g., learning disabilities and alcohol dependence).
- Patterns of "cutoffs" when family conflict is not resolved.
- Patterns of closeness, dependence, and lack of separation linking family members, regardless of age or marital status.

The worker usually constructs the genogram together with the parent(s). If the child is present, this process can provide important information regarding how much the child knows about extended family members. If the child is *not* present, it may be helpful to involve the child in constructing a separate genogram later; however, the worker should keep in mind that developmental considerations probably prevent a child under 6 years of age from being able to conceptualize family relationships on paper. Gil has developed a *play genogram* (McGoldrick et al., 2008) that involves inviting children to choose a miniature figure to represent each of the family members illustrated on the paper-and-pencil genogram.

The school for homeless children in which Barbie Smith was enrolled did not routinely construct genograms with the families of students. My attempt to produce a genogram of the Smith family is based on the scant information presented on the videotape and the intake forms. Because no information was available about members of Mrs. Smith's family of origin, the genogram consists of only two generations. Some of the data may be inaccurate; these would have had to be confirmed or corrected by Mrs. Smith during the process of working with her.

Because the genogram of the Smith family is so sketchy, I have combined it with an eco-map to illustrate the various helping agencies with which the family was involved (see Chapter 3, Figure 3.2). In many homeless urban families like the Smiths, the helping system serves as an essential substitute for the extended family, whose members may be unable or unwilling to offer financial or other support.

Eco-Map

Together with the genogram, the eco-map (Hartman, 1978) offers a visual representation of the persons and potential resources and depicts the family's connections with their environment. As shown in Figure 3.2 for the Smith family, the genogram diagrams family relationships, whereas the eco-map illustrates contacts with social agencies and other community resources. The eco-map also usually contains an abbreviated genogram in its center, showing the members of the household in which the clients reside.

Culturagram

As a family assessment tool, the culturagram (Congress, 1994, 2008) offers social workers an important method for recognizing and individualizing the impact of ethnicity on culturally diverse families. The families with which social workers interact usually come from many different cultural backgrounds, and a tool such as the culturagram can assist in understanding each family's unique heritage and belief system. Chapters in this book that deal with children from minority, immigrant, or mixed cultures include the cases of Jacob and Damien (Chapter 1), José (Chapter 2), Pedro (Chapter 9), Maria (Chapter 10), Vanessa and Vernon (Chapter 13), and Alexa (Chapter 16). Each of these children lived in a home in which language, beliefs, values, and connections with the community were influenced to varying degrees by the cultural history of his or her family. Sometimes the children of immigrants serve as interpreters for their parents, thus reversing usual parent–child roles. At other times, the parents' expectations about acceptable child behavior differ from the prevailing norms; this puts undue pressure on the children, who are caught between two worlds (see Webb, 2001, and Chapter 16, this volume, for a further discussion of cultural factors in parent–child relationships).

The culturagram provides a structured method for recording a family's cultural history and beliefs, and as such it is an essential resource in assessment and intervention with culturally diverse families.

In the case of the Smith family, information about the ethnicity of the family was incomplete. The school program Barbie attended obtained data about languages spoken in the home and about the ethnicity of various family members. Barbie's school record identified her as a native-born English speaker, with only English spoken in her home. With respect to ethnicity, the Lapp, Lettish (Latvia), and Jamaican categories were checked in the record as applying to "spouse partner," but we do not know whether these applied to Barbie's father or to other men in the home. No categories were checked as applying to Mrs. Smith's ethnicity. Barbie's light blonde hair, blue eyes, and pale skin resembled her mother's and sister's coloring and seem characteristic of persons with northern European origins. We have no information about the family's religious or cultural practices.

DSM-5 Diagnosis

DSM-5, the latest edition of an assessment tool produced by the American Psychiatric Association (2013), is a system of classifying observable symptoms and behaviors into discrete diagnostic categories. Many practitioners (Johnson, 1993a; Rapoport & Ismond, 1990) are concerned about affixing diagnostic labels to children, whose development is in flux and whose "disorders" may be reactive to family and environmental stress rather than indicative of intrinsic pathology. Furthermore, scientific validation is lacking for many of the DSM categories used in practice with children, and some concepts applicable to adults have been extended to children without adequate recognition of the essential biological and psychosocial differences between children and adults (Johnson, 1994; Garmezy, 1985).

These reservations notwithstanding, DSM classifications are widely used in clinical practice and probably will become even more so in the current environment of managed care, in which DSM diagnoses are required for reimbursement. Johnson (1993a) points out that "neither social work nor any other discipline, so far, has produced [an alternative to the DSM] that has gained wide acceptance" (p. 144). Therefore, we must use it "by default" until a more satisfactory system emerges.

My own view is that the DSM is a useful assessment tool for identifying and understanding certain psychological disorders and other conditions. I would never employ *only* the DSM, however, in formulating an assessment, because the developmental history, the genogram and eco-map provide essential information that is not included in the DSM. The use of the DSM may be limited in schools, because they are educational, rather than mental health settings. However, school social workers need to be familiar with the various diagnoses, especially those related to learning problems, because children who are having adjustment difficulties in school may require an evaluation for possible learning disorders.

DSM-5 has eliminated the five "axes" (American Psychiatric Association, 2013) that had been included since the DSM-III of 1980 to cover different domains of information to assist the practitioner in specifying the nature and scope of the difficulty under examination. The third edition of this book included a speculative multiaxial diagnosis of Barbie Smith, and this is repeated here because it demonstrates the various factors that can be considered in formulating an appropriate treatment plan:

- *Axis I. Clinical Disorders; Other Conditions That May Be a Focus of Clinical Attention:* 315.00—Reading Disorder (pending formal tests); 315.2—Disorder of Written Expression (pending formal tests).
- *Axis II. Personality Disorders; Mental Retardation:* V71.09—No diagnosis.
- *Axis III. General Medical Conditions:* Deferred, pending medical exam.
- *Axis IV. Psychosocial and Environmental Problems:* Problems with primary support group (parental divorce, past physical abuse by father, erratic contact with father); problem related to the social environment (inadequate social support); educational problems (academic problems); occupational problems (mother's unemployment; housing problems (homelessness, unsafe neighborhoods); economic problems (poverty, inadequate welfare support); problems related to interaction with the legal system/crime (mother on probation).
- *Axis V. Global Assessment of Functioning (GAF):* GAF = 50 (current and past year).

It is my belief that pulling together the information obtained at intake with a DSM framework would have alerted the school staff as to specific problem areas that might have been contributing to Barbie's learning difficulties. Although the main function of school is to educate, a special program targeted to homeless children must, of necessity, attend to the basic needs of the students and their families before the children's education can proceed. Barbie's special needs would have been listed explicitly on DSM Axes I and IV. Axis V would have indicated that Barbie's general level of functioning was fairly low, both currently and during the past year (estimated at 50, with the range from 0 to 100). Because the child's problem situation had not changed during the preceding year, the important question about the chronicity of her difficulties would have been highlighted. Barbie's mother stated at intake that Barbie had received special education services within the preceding 3 years, so these records would have had to be obtained to compare Barbie's present academic functioning with her former level and to maintain some continuity in making future educational plans.

Educational and Psychological Testing

The following types of tests commonly used with children (Barker, 1995) may be recommended either by the intake worker or by the child study team to obtain more detailed information about the child:

- Tests of academic attainment
- Intelligence tests
- Personality tests
- Behavior checklists
- Tests assessing specific psychological conditions, such as anxiety, depression, self-esteem, and sustained attention

The social worker does not test the child but must understand when to make a referral and how to explain the need for specialized testing to the child and the parent(s). We do not know which, if any, of these types of tests were completed with Barbie at the time of referral.

Tests of academic achievement are usually part of children's regular school records, as they are often performed on an annual basis to determine the children's appropriate class placement. Intelligence tests are not performed routinely in most schools, and they have been criticized in the past decade as being culturally biased. Nonetheless, they give a rough estimate of a child's native ability, and they are especially useful in suggesting the need for additional specialized testing for possible learning disabilities when a sizable discrepancy exists between the verbal and performance subsections.

Personality tests such as the Children's Apperception Test (CAT) attempt to elicit responses that reflect the child's inner world and mental state. This is a projective test, adapted from the adult Thematic Apperception Test (TAT). Both present the client with a series of ambiguous pictures onto which the client "projects" his or her personal meaning.

Another assessment measure sometimes employed as part of the assessment process is the Child Behavior Checklist (CBCL) (Achenbach & Edelbrock, 1983; Achenbach, 1991), on which a parent or teacher responds to questions about his or her perceptions of a child's behavior. This measure results in several different opinions, which may be useful in pinpointing a specific setting or person with which or whom the child's behavior is considered most troublesome. The Achenbach and Edelbrock (1983) CBCL is widely used in the child welfare field to track outcomes of services. A 2-day roundtable attended by 30 researchers was held in 1997 to share experiences in using this tool and to summarize and publish this knowledge for the benefit of others in the field (LeProhn, Wetherbee, Lamont, Achenbach, & Pecora, 2002).

Another behavior checklist with separate forms for parents and teachers has been developed by Conners (1969, 1970).

An intake worker who is concerned about a child's depressed mood may ask the child to fill out a questionnaire about the level of his or her depressed feelings (the Children's Depression Inventory; Kovacs, 1978). Of course, this presumes that the child can read or that the child is willing to respond to questions read by the worker. Pfeffer (1986) lists a series of questions to ask in evaluating a child's risk of suicide. In situations in which I have serious questions about a child's depression and possible suicide risk, I communicate this to the parent and strongly suggest an immediate psychiatric consultation. Another self-report checklist, the State–Trait Anxiety Inventory for Children (Spielberger, 1973), assesses children's anxiety, and other scales exist for assessing the preschool child's home environment (Caldwell & Bradley, 1979).

In my own practice, I rarely use these various checklists. I prefer to base my assessment on my observations of the interactions among the child, the parent(s), and myself, as well as on the actual statements of the child and the family and on the various reports from collateral sources. When social workers begin their work with a child and a family, the workers must focus on getting to know them as people; requests to fill out forms can feel rather impersonal and cold. However, because these checklists and tests may be used by school psychologists, it is important for workers to know about their contents and purpose. A manual of typical tests used in child assessment (e.g., Goldman, Stein, & Guerry, 1983) can serve as a useful resource.

Children's Drawings

As previously discussed, I routinely invite children to complete several drawings during their assessment sessions. Because I am a social worker and not a psychologist, I do not "score" these drawings, as would a psychologist analyzing a Draw-A-Person test or a Kinetic Family Drawing. Whereas the psychologist examines the child's drawings and evaluates them with respect to the child's personality and developmental level, I follow the guidelines used by art therapists in using drawings in assessment and therapy (Di Leo, 1973; Oster & Gould, 1987, pp. 21–28, 41–43, 47–48; Malchiodi, 1998, 2006). Some of the elements to be noted in the child's drawings include the size and position of the figures, the absence or exaggeration of body parts, the use of color and shading, the nature of facial expressions, and the general mood of the drawing. In addition, the child's attitude in producing it (e.g., labored, rushed, perfectionistic, or self-critical) should be noted.

Family drawings can reveal a child's feelings about different family members. We can note who is drawn largest and which family members are closest to one another. Sometimes a child will tell a story about the drawing that can reveal significant family dynamics. It is important, however, *never* to make any assumptions about the family from only one drawing. The child's pictures are only a part of the overall assessment, and other corroborating information will always be necessary before making any conclusions.

Projective Questions

Commonly used by social workers and others in initial sessions with children, projective questions seek to elicit a child's feelings about his or her family and life. Examples of typical projective questions are as follows:

1. "If you had three wishes, what would you wish for?" (When a savvy child responds that he or she would want a thousand more wishes, the worker needs to specify that this will not be possible, and that the child must specify what he or she wants.)
2. "If a baby bird fell out of the nest, what might happen?" (The child is expected to complete the story.)
3. "If you were going on a rocket trip to the moon, and you could take only one person with you, who would you want to go?" (The child's response is expected to reveal the most important person in his or her life, but it may also reflect the child's judgment about who would be most helpful in this special situation.)

The child's responses to these and other projective questions should be explored by the worker in an unhurried, interested way. The child should be given the explicit message that there is no one "right" answer and that the worker is asking the questions to get to know the child better.

SUMMARIZING THE RELEVANT DATA

During the process of gathering information about a child and family, the worker continually weighs the significance of his or her findings and immediately starts to generate hypotheses about what is wrong and how to help. This analysis, synthesis, and speculation constitute an ongoing process that continues *throughout the life of the case*. However, during the early evaluation of a case, most agencies expect the worker to formulate a biopsychosocial assessment summary in writing. According to Kadushin (1995), "Gathering data does not in itself yield an assessment. Data must be organized, interpreted, integrated with theory, and made meaningful to derive an assessment" (p. 63). The three tripartite assessment forms (Figures 4.8, 4.9, and 4.10) will help the worker organize the data preparatory to formulating a summary statement regarding the significant features of the case.

Hepworth, Rooney, and Larsen (2002, pp. 198–216) recommend a multidimensional assessment to deal with the client's identified problems and concerns. I have prepared a retrospective assessment summary for Barbie Smith during the period of her enrollment in the First Place School program, with special attention to factors relevant to a *child* assessment. The categories of the assessment are as follows:

- The nature of the client's problems.
- The coping capacities of the client and significant others; assessing strengths and obstacles, risks and protective factors.
- The other persons or systems involved in the client's problems.
- The available or needed resources.
- The client's motivation to work on the problems.

A SAMPLE BIOPSYCHOSOCIAL ASSESSMENT SUMMARY: BARBIE SMITH

Date of birth: 6-6-82

Date of evaluation: 2-10-93 (hypothetical)

Age at time of evaluation: 10 years, 8 months

Reason for Referral

The family was referred to the First Place School, a special education program for children in transition, by the shelter in which they were currently residing. The mother was seeking schooling for Barbie, then in third grade. The family had moved seven times in 6 months and had been befriended and videotaped by a filmmaker, Kathryn Hunt, during this period. Ms. Hunt had also recommended this school program to Mrs. Smith.

Family Description

This female-headed household consists of a mother and three children, all born of different fathers. The mother has a history of imprisonment for the possession of firearms and methamphetamines, but she claims to have been "clean" since her release 3 years ago. She is estranged from her family of origin and has no contact with the children's fathers, one of whom is deceased and another of whom lives out of state (Barbie's father). The family receives public assistance and has been living in various shelters and welfare motels. They move because of inability to pay the rent and dissatisfaction with the neighborhood, which the mother describes as populated by addicts and pimps.

Family Composition

Lori (mother), age 34, unemployed (former bartender)

Donna (daughter), age 18, school dropout, in and out of home (living with boyfriend when away)

David (son), age 16, school dropout

Barbie (daughter), age 10, third grade

The Nature of the Client's and Family's Problems

This homeless family seems beset by one crisis after another. The mother, a former addict, appears to be highly motivated to help her younger daughter obtain schooling, but her ability to organize her life in a way that will achieve this goal is questionable. Although the mother is not seeking help for herself, she clearly plays a pivotal role in this child's ability to pursue a normal developmental course. Therefore, it is essential to engage and help the mother with her numerous problems. The mother's energies are totally absorbed in searching out places for the family to reside.

Mrs. Smith alludes (on the Hunt videotape) to serious problems with her family of origin. She herself has been abused, and although we know no details about this, she appears to have suffered emotional damage that merits attention. This mother is trying to the best of her ability to hold her family together, but she seems to be under great stress and may be at risk for depression and/or resumption of drug abuse.

Mrs. Smith, while professing "distrust of the system," nonetheless maintains an open attitude toward persons on the periphery, such as the filmmaker and myself (by telephone). This suggests that despite her feelings of anger and hurt, she has not closed herself off completely and may be still reachable.

Barbie's problems seem to be secondary to the situation of her family. Her delay in academic performance is understandable in view of her extremely erratic school attendance. If Barbie spends a consistent period of time in one school, we can better evaluate her true ability. With regard to the housing situation, Barbie's mother states that the girl sleeps with her lights on because of roaches and that she is beginning to have nightmares.

Coping Capacities of Client and Family: Assessing Strengths and Obstacles and Risks and Protective Factors

Both Barbie and her mother demonstrate an unusual ability to deal with the uncertainties of their lives. We lack in-depth information about how they deal with stress, but the video portrayal suggests both resignation and determination on Mrs. Smith's part. At one point, she questions whether she may have brought her difficulties upon herself—a statement that demonstrates some capacity for self-reflection.

Neither Barbie nor her mother likes the uncertain quality of their life. Persons who live in a continual state of crisis are sometimes described as "borderline," but we have insufficient information on which to base this or any other diagnosis. However, the possibility of a mental disorder, in addition to a diagnosis of drug addiction, will need to be considered in evaluating Mrs. Smith's coping methods. She has a lot of strength, but she also seems to be under great stress.

Barbie's coping capacities are more difficult to determine. She is about 2 years behind her expected grade level, which probably has a negative impact on her self-esteem. After Barbie's first 2 months at First Place, her teacher wrote as follows:

> Barbie seems very defensive about her low skill level. She often seems angry and wants to control others. She may need counseling. *She really is a sweet little girl. She needs a lot of nurturing and patience.* (emphasis added)

Everything in the teacher's comments is understandable, in view of this child's life experience. Her lack of academic skills makes her anxious and defensive, and she responds with anger and an attempt to control others. So much of her own life has been beyond her control that she tries to exert whatever influence she can on others.

Despite Barbie's harsh past and present life, she still elicits positive feelings in adults, indicating a probability that she will be able to respond to a helping relationship.

Other Persons or Systems Involved in Client's and Family's Situation

Several agencies are involved with this family, but there is no evidence that they are in contact with one another to coordinate the case planning. The housing authority was instrumental in making Barbie's referral to the school. Mrs. Smith has ongoing contact with the public assistance agency and also with the corrections department, as she is on probation. Both of Barbie's siblings also have had special school affiliations, and her sister reports monthly to a medical clinic for chronic kidney and heart problems.

Barbie's school records have not yet been obtained. She has changed schools so often that the records have not kept up with her. This situation presents serious problems in terms of academic planning targeted to Barbie's specific needs.

Available or Needed Resources

1. The family's most pressing need at this time is for decent housing in a safe neighborhood. The housing should afford a quiet place for Barbie to do her homework and read.

2. Case management/coordination is essential to bring the various helping agencies into contact with one another. The school could appropriately assume this role, as Barbie's academic success will depend on various family circumstances, including her mother's ability to remain drug-free and supportive to her children.

3. Academic tutoring is needed for Barbie. This should follow a review of previous tests and completion of current tests to target Barbie's special needs.

4. Counseling is also indicated for Barbie. Ideally, this should occur on both an individual and a group basis. Barbie would benefit from individual counseling to deal with her feelings about her past traumatic experiences, such as being in foster care, the abuse she suffered from her father and while in foster care, and her father's apparent abandonment of her. Group therapy with other homeless children will serve the function of mutual support and self-esteem building. The group members can identify themselves as "survivors" and reinforce one another's positive coping strategies.

5. Job counseling and training are needed for Mrs. Smith. [*Note:* Suggestions about approaching Mrs. Smith on this matter were discussed in Chapter 3.]

6. Individual counseling is also indicated for Mrs. Smith. (The success of this will depend on the worker's establishing a positive relationship pertaining to a concrete service, such as putting Mrs. Smith in contact with a resource for housing or job training.) Mrs. Smith has many issues to work out, including her conflicted relationship with her family of origin, her problematic relationships with men, and her history of addiction and homelessness. It is important to highlight how hard Mrs. Smith is trying to keep her family together, as this is her strength and the key to motivating her. Basic trust in the helping relationship will build slowly.

7. Mrs. Smith should be encouraged to attend Narcotics Anonymous or other group counseling focused on addiction. In order to maintain her sobriety, Mrs. Smith needs to establish new friends and activities that are not drug-related.

8. Educational and/or occupational counseling may well be needed for Barbie's older siblings. We do not know enough about either one to suggest specifics, but as they appear on the Hunt videotape, neither seems to be headed toward a productive work career.

Client's and Family's Motivation to Work on Their Problems

Motivation is unknown at present. The problems as listed here are not recognized as such by Mrs. Smith or Barbie. The key to progress with the members of this family will be to engage them in a trusting relationship, based on Mrs. Smith's interest in providing schooling for Barbie and on keeping her family together. Barbie, as a 10-year-old girl, requires education and social opportunities with her peers. Acknowledgement of Barbie's needs and of how these are connected to the family's problems must occur within the context of a trusting helping relationship. Then contracting about how to work on the recognized needs can occur naturally. This is discussed in the next chapter.

Note. This assessment is based on observations from the videotape (Hunt, 1992) and on reports of various individuals who had contact with the Smith family. It is *not* based on any play sessions with Barbie nor on firsthand contact with her or her family.

FEEDBACK/REVIEW WITH PARENTS AND OTHER PROFESSIONALS

Engaging the Parent(s) in the Feedback/Review Process

It is the responsibility of the person formulating the assessment to share it with a child's parent(s) and with other professionals involved in the case. In the case of Barbie Smith, I am assuming that the school social worker might have taken the initiative in engaging Mrs. Smith and in convening a case conference to involve all the concerned professionals in establishing mutually agreed-upon goals and a plan for collaboration.

Maintaining contact with Mrs. Smith would have been essential to engaging her, both for Barbie's education and for the potential overall benefits for the Smith family. The worker would have had to stress that "the educational *team*" planned to pay special attention to Barbie's situation because she was a new student and that the team would convene a meeting to make specific recommendations for Barbie. The worker would also have had to emphasize that the *parent's* input into this meeting would be very important and that he or she would thus need Mrs. Smith's help to prepare for the meeting.

Often parents are intimidated by child study meetings in which "professionals" use unfamiliar terminology in talking about *their* children. The worker would have had to emphasize that he or she would need to meet with Mrs. Smith several times to prepare for this meeting and might have suggested that Mrs. Smith ride the school bus to come to these special individual planning meetings. The purposes of the individual meetings with Barbie's mother would have been to establish a relationship with her, to learn more about Barbie's history, and to give Mrs. Smith a private review of the recommendations about her daughter prior to the case review meeting. The worker could have offered to record and summarize the various recommendations for Mrs. Smith after the meeting.

Releases for sharing of information among the numerous agencies involved with a family are routinely signed when a child enrolls in a special school program such as First Place. During the one or two individual meetings with a child's parent(s) prior to the case conference, the social worker emphasizes how important it is for all these separate people to cooperate on behalf of both the child and the family.

When a parent does not keep the agreed-upon appointment with a social worker, a note should be sent home with the child stating the worker's concern and repeating the necessity of the parent's input with respect to the upcoming meeting. The note should offer the prospect of a home visit if the parent is unable to come to the next scheduled meeting. Actually, a home visit is often very helpful because of the opportunity it affords the worker to see the environment in which the child is living.

The Case Conference

The case conference provides the opportunity for professionals involved in separate aspects of a case to meet in person to discuss the multidimensional elements of a given family's situation. In the case of the Smith family, had such a conference taken place, the probation officer and the housing authority worker might have put their heads together to resolve the prejudice Mrs. Smith faced in obtaining housing because of her history as a felon. Furthermore, the probation officer and the school social worker might have explored Mrs. Smith's employment prospects, with the possibility of recommending testing for her to ascertain her interests and abilities.

Once such a meeting has taken place, it is much easier to coordinate the case through ongoing telephone contact. The impact on Mrs. Smith if such a meeting had taken place can only be guessed, but it would, of necessity, have been self-affirming because of the time and care these numerous professional helpers would have devoted to helping her and her family.

CONCLUDING COMMENTS

Assessment is a complex and systematic process, requiring discipline, patience, the ability to apply a body of professional knowledge, and sensitivity to clients' strengths and their unique individual and cultural profiles. Depending on each situation, varying attention must be given to biological, psychological, and social factors that interact and merge into a specific situation of human need. The case of Barbie Smith emphasizes the social factors of homelessness and poverty, as these contributed to the psychological distress associated with family dysfunction, abuse, addiction, imprisonment, and school failure.

The purpose of assessment is to point to needs that require intervention. The next chapter deals with establishing goals that flow from the needs identified in the assessment. One aspect of Barbie's case about which more information was needed was the possibility that a learning disability (biological factor) was interfering with her educational progress. Special testing could have provided details about this. I have noted that Barbie seemed to possess a resilient temperament, which had helped her cope with a non-nurturing environment. This strength, similar to her mother's, would have provided a basis for optimism about the prospects of moving beyond the assessment to a series of helping interventions that would have a positive impact on this family's future.

DISCUSSION QUESTIONS AND ROLE-PLAY EXERCISE

1. How can the worker deal with his or her negative feelings about parents who are overwhelmed with multiple problems and who seem oblivious to their children's needs?
2. Discuss the advantages and the disadvantages of using the DSM in assessing children. Consider the impact on Barbie Smith's family of employing this classification. How would you proceed in prioritizing the problem situations noted in Barbie's DSM diagnosis?
3. Examine the four drawings in this chapter (Figures 4.2–4.5). What elements in the children's drawings do you find of interest in terms of possibly conveying information about the children? After obtaining these drawings, what other play materials would you introduce?
4. Role-play a session with Mrs. Smith in which a worker attempts to engage her and prepare her for the case conference about Barbie.

CHAPTER 5

Contracting, Planning Interventions, and Tracking Progress

Every case situation is different, yet human needs are very similar despite these individual differences. Maslow's hierarchy of needs remains as pertinent today as it was over 40 years ago, when he first maintained that we all have certain basic needs that must be met for us to reach our full potential as humans (Maslow, 1970). The first level of needs includes the fundamental necessities of life, such as food, water, and shelter, which ensure our physical survival. The second level of needs consists of safety considerations; the third is to feel loved and to belong; the fourth is the need for self-esteem. The culminating achievement of "self-actualization" occurs after the lower-level needs have been met and the individual realizes the fulfillment of his or her potential as a person.

CONTRACTING: ENGAGING CLIENTS AND IDENTIFYING THEIR NEEDS

According to Maslow's schema, Barbie Smith's life (see Chapters 3 and 4) was characterized by unmet needs on every level. Any helper involved with the Smith family would have had to consider carefully where to start and how to involve Mrs. Smith in the decision-making process. It certainly would have been contraindicated for other people, no matter how good their intentions, to "take over" and disempower Mrs. Smith's decisions about her own family. In fact, any school social worker must understand that a pupil's parent is not a *client* but the parent of a student who may or may not welcome assistance with various family difficulties. For this reason I used the term "unintentional client" in Chapter 3 to refer to Mrs. Smith's uncertain status. The engagement process of a parent like Mrs. Smith involves making an offer to help with matters other than the presenting problem of her or his child's education. *A person becomes a client only after an offer to help has been made and accepted.*

Chapter 3 emphasized the importance of focusing on the client's perception of his or her needs, in preparation for suggesting some strategies that could be useful to engage Mrs. Smith in job-related counseling for herself. The rationale for this relates to the mother's important role as an identification model for her daughter, Barbie. A commitment from the worker to help the family locate decent housing would have been equally important for the well-being of the entire family, and this ideally would have coincided with the effort to upgrade Mrs. Smith's employment prospects. Like the job training offer, the housing issue would have had to be couched in terms of *Barbie's* needs to capture Mrs. Smith's attention successfully. This mother's willingness to discuss her family problems and needs would have depended on repeated emphasis on the interconnection between the family circumstances and Barbie's learning situation. For example, if the school social worker had mentioned to Mrs. Smith the importance of Barbie's having a quiet place to do her homework, this topic would inevitably have brought up the issue of the family's poor housing and lack of privacy. Discussing the family's housing needs in the context of *Barbie's* academic requirements might have been more acceptable to Mrs. Smith than a direct offer of assistance, which she might have perceived as the worker's prejudgment that she was incompetent to take care of this matter herself.

It is not unusual for parents who live in ghetto or substandard environments, such as that in which the Smith family resided, to feel misunderstood by and alienated from middle-class helpers whose life experience differs drastically from theirs. Combrinck-Graham (1989, p. 235; 2006) points out that

> poverty is more than just a low income. Rather, it is an encompassing lifestyle of opportunism and survival . . . and a dangerous life. Poor families, when they ask for help, need acceptance of their situation, recognition of their efforts to make life livable, and assistance in identifying and connecting with any additional resources the sociopolitical system may have to offer them.

When the gap between worker and client appears too great, the client reacts to the perceived lack of empathy by missing appointments, which the worker may subsequently label "client resistance."

Engaging poor families in treatment makes special demands on the worker to understand the problem *from the clients' point of view.* This task

> requires that the clinician understand the *context* in which the problem is embedded . . . [and pay] attention to the concrete needs of the family, lest the reality of their world be invalidated and the therapist lose all credibility. Immediate intervention in this area is possibly the most powerful and most connecting engagement skill, regardless of the discipline of the clinician. (Parnell & Vanderkloot, 1989, p. 447; emphasis added)

It seems probable that Mrs. Smith would have responded positively to an offer to help Barbie through assisting her family to find better housing if the worker making such an offer had indicated respect for her and an understanding of how repeatedly frustrated she had been in her own efforts to accomplish this. Her criminal history as a felon made it difficult for this mother to obtain housing in the absence of a sponsor who would vouch for her dependability in paying the rent regularly. The help of Mrs. Smith's public assistance worker and probation officer (with Mrs. Smith's permission) could have been very valuable in working out some form of guaranteed direct-deposit rental system.

In this multiproblem family, as in others, environmental interventions such as seeking new housing are generally implemented in concert with other interventions. Hepworth et al. (2002, p. 219) point out that "problems, strengths, and resources encountered in direct social work practice result from interaction of intrapersonal, interpersonal, and environmental systems. Difficulties are rarely confined to one of these systems, for functional imbalance in one system typically contributes to imbalance in others."

Mrs. Smith's psychological status was not assessed, despite the many stresses to which she alluded on the video. We do not know whether individual counseling was recommended to her. As reported in Chapter 3, Mrs. Smith chose not to become involved in the various opportunities at the school, which might have addressed some of her own parenting challenges in a group format with other, similarly challenged parents (such as in a parenting support group).

Even more troubling was the fact that Mrs. Smith did not make it possible for Barbie to attend school on a consistent basis. Despite the availability of transportation, Barbie missed 15 out of the 31 school days (almost half) during the 2 months she was enrolled in the First Place program. One wonders how she occupied her time during these days at home in a motel with her mother. Later, the family obtained Section 8 housing, and Barbie transferred to a neighborhood school briefly before leaving for an extended stay with her father out of state. Just imagine the frustration of a 10-year-old girl in trying to make friends, to understand the academic expectations of different teachers, and to adapt to these successive new neighborhoods and living situations!

Choi and Snyder (1999) mention that homelessness can exacerbate existing disorders and contribute to depression and anxiety, thereby making it more difficult for individuals to carry out normal daily functions. A consultant with many years of experience in the addictions field expressed great skepticism that Mrs. Smith would have remained drug-free during the entire time shown on the video, which was the period during which Barbie missed so many days of school. Many former addicts find it formidable to get up in the morning and organize their lives. The consultant also commented that Mrs. Smith actually may have *needed* Barbie and her brother to help her with various daily living tasks. The tape showed Barbie and David preparing and serving their mother a simple meal and also assisting with the laundry. Of course, many children perform routine chores to help their parents, and we do not know for certain whether or not Mrs. Smith had returned to using drugs or alcohol at this time. However, it is unfortunate that she did not insist on Barbie's school attendance and that she was not sufficiently engaged by the school to avail herself of any of its potentially useful services for homeless families or to obtain a referral for counseling services outside the school.

I would like to consider, in retrospect, how the school personnel might have successfully engaged Mrs. Smith at the time of Barbie's first contact with them. I do not intend this to be critical of what was done or not done but rather to use hindsight as a way to learn from experience, in order to highlight engagement methods that may be effective with other homeless and disenfranchised populations.

Mrs. Smith's request when she contacted the school initially was for schooling for Barbie. A wide-angle, ecological view of the child's situation would have challenged the helpers to broaden the mother's view of her daughter's needs to include the notion that helping Barbie would require that she simultaneously help *herself* and the rest of her family.

Successful contracting with Mrs. Smith, therefore, would have involved (1) starting with the mother's request for schooling (i.e., starting where the client was) and then (2) expanding this request to include housing, job training, and supportive counseling to help *all* family members cope with their past and current stresses. All of this would have had to be presented in a manner that recognized and validated Mrs. Smith's strong wish to be a good mother and to keep her family together. Thus *successful contracting helps clients to want what they need.* It culminates in an oral agreement, which then becomes operationalized through putting specific goals in writing.

PLANNING INTERVENTIONS

The Unit of Attention

What would have been the appropriate focus of the Smith case? The people or their environment? The child (Barbie) or her family? A "person-in-environment" ecosystems perspective (Germain, 1973; Gitterman & Germain, 2008; Meyer, 1983; Davies, 1999, 2011; Hepworth et al., 2002) encourages the worker to consider *all* relevant dimensions of the case, including the degree of fit (or lack of fit) between the people and their environments.

Whenever a child is the reason for referral, involvement with the family is mandatory. However, the unique circumstances of each case determine the degree to which either the child or the family becomes the primary "unit of attention." In some situations, such as helping a child process and accept his or her placement or traumatic experience (see Chapters 10 and 14), work with the child is primary, and family counseling is secondary to helping the child. In other situations, work with the family is pivotal to understanding and helping the child. This is true, for example, in families in which divorce (Chapter 11) or a substance use disorder (Chapter 13) is a major factor. Still another method of work involves conjoint sessions with the child and family members. Many variations may also be appropriate, including alternating among individual child sessions, parent–child sessions, and full family sessions. The circumstances of each case determine who is seen and in which combinations, and these circumstances may vary over the lifespan of the case. The preferred model, presented frequently in this book, is one that integrates child and family therapy.

The worker must keep a wide-angle focus on both environmental considerations *and* the persons involved. In Chapter 1, a multisystems diagram of problem situations (Figure 1.1) depicts the interplay of reciprocal influences between the child and his or her physical and social environment. Specific factors, such as the child's temperament and coping style, can mediate and counteract detrimental conditions in an unsafe, nonsupportive environment; conversely, a fragile child with a very reactive temperament may respond poorly even in supportive environmental conditions. Therefore, we must always consider interactive factors—those pertaining to the "fit" between persons and their environment—in assessing problem situations and planning interventions.

Setting Goals and a Time Frame

The establishment of goals follows directly from the client's recognition that help is needed and from his or her agreement to focus with the worker on tackling the specific difficulties together. The goals may be outlined for individual family members and/or for the family as a unit, depending on the situation. Establishing a time frame for completion of certain goals or tasks increases motivation. Goals may be listed as "long term," requiring a protracted period of time (possibly 9–12 months) for their completion, or as "short term," with a designated target date for completion (possibly in 1 month). *It is essential* for the client to participate in the setting of the goals and the time frame, and it is usually advisable to put these in writing.

Keeping Goals Manageable: A Sample Dialogue

A cardinal rule in setting goals is to draft them in a manner that promises achievable results. The worker wants the client to have an experience of success, no matter how small this may be. Furthermore, it is important not to overwhelm the client; therefore, it is essential to begin with a limited number of manageable goals, with the understanding that once success has been achieved with the initial list, others may be added.

The sample biopsychosocial assessment summary for Barbie, given in Chapter 4, lists eight "needed resources" for helping the Smith family. This comprehensive list could have been converted into specific goals during a planning session with Mrs. Smith and Barbie. It would have been important to begin with goals for Barbie that centered on her educational needs and to specify family or personal goals for Mrs. Smith that would also have an impact on Barbie. A dialogue for this hypothetical meeting follows.

WORKER: I know that you are both very eager to have Barbie get a good start and do as well as possible in her new school. We want to do whatever we can also, so the purpose of this meeting is to decide *together* how to help Barbie achieve up to her fullest potential.

MRS. SMITH: Unfortunately, Barbie is behind where she should be for her age. We've moved so much, and she's been in so many different schools. It's not her fault.

WORKER: Of course it isn't her fault. (*to Barbie*) There are other children in this school like you who don't have permanent homes and who have changed schools a lot. In fact, this school was designed exactly for kids like you, and we have some special ways to try to help.

BARBIE: Like what?

WORKER: Several different programs and activities that you will find out about as you go along. The first way is to try to find out just what you do know, so we can help you catch up, wherever you may need to. So, I'm going to start a list of what the school will do, and what each of you can do. (*Divides a sheet of paper into three columns and heads the first column "The School," the second section "Barbie," and the third section "Mrs. Smith."*) Under "The School," I'm going to write "1. Academic tests" and "2. Special tutoring." Barbie will be given a special teacher, who will work individually with her to help her in whatever areas the tests show she needs help. How does that sound? [See Figure 5.1.]

BARBIE: Will I have a lot of homework?

WORKER: We don't expect you to get caught up the first week, or the first month! Yes, you will have homework, but it probably won't be more than an hour or, at most, two a day. (*to Mrs. Smith*) Would you be able to help Barbie figure out a quiet place and a time to do her homework?

MRS. SMITH: That's not so easy. We're in a one-bedroom motel, and the only table is where we all eat.

WORKER: Lots of kids do their homework on the kitchen table. The trick is to cut down on the distracting noise level, like from a TV. Do you think you could set aside a regular time each afternoon that would be "quiet time" for Barbie, and for you also, when there would be no TV and no distractions?

MRS. SMITH: That would be a miracle. But I'll try. Sometimes Barbie doesn't want to go to school when she doesn't do her homework or if she doesn't get it right.

FIGURE 5.1. Goals contract.

Goal: To improve Barbie's school/academic performance

The School	Barbie	Mrs. Smith
1. Academic tests	1. Do homework at least 1 hour every day	1. Arrange 1 hour of quiet time every school afternoon
2. Special tutoring	2. Come to school every day	2. Be sure Barbie attends school every day
Signature: [Worker]	Signature: [Barbie]	Signature: [Mrs. Smith]
Date:	Date:	Date:

WORKER: In this school you don't always have to get it right, but you do have to try. So, Mrs. Smith, I'm writing this in your section: "1. Make a family rule for 1 hour of quiet time every afternoon, when there will be no TV and no noisy talk." The other thing is that you must be sure Barbie comes to school every day. She can't learn or catch up if she isn't here. So, I'll write "2. Be sure Barbie comes to school every day."

Now we have to think about what to put in Barbie's section of this agreement. What do you think, Barbie?

BARBIE: I have to do my homework.

WORKER: Yes. You have to try. And your special teacher will help you. So, I'll write this for you: "1. Do homework at least 1 hour each day." I also think you have to promise to come to school every day unless you are sick. I'm going to write that down as number 2. Actually, I think you'll like it here and *want* to come. We have some special groups for kids to get to know each other, and I'll see you tomorrow and tell you about those.

Sometimes the three of us will meet together, like today, and other times I'll meet alone with each of you. Let's make an appointment when we can all meet together again, so we can see how things are going with everybody's goals. I'd also like to set a separate appointment for Mrs. Smith to give me some background about Barbie.

Obviously, this would have been only the beginning of the contracting process. The next conjoint meeting (which ideally would have been scheduled within a week) would have provided an opportunity for reports of success in implementing the two goals of Barbie's regular school attendance and the homework routine. Later, separate individual meetings with Barbie and Mrs.

Smith could have been used to introduce the offer of individual counseling, as well as support groups for each. Possible future long-range goals and short-term tasks for achieving these are outlined for Barbie and Mrs. Smith.

Barbie's Long-Range Goals

1. To improve school performance
   - Short-term tasks:
     - Attend school regularly
     - Complete 1 hour of homework daily
     - Participate in academic tutoring
2. To deal with her feelings about her family and their homelessness
   - Short-term tasks:
     - Participate in group therapy with other homeless children
     - Participate in weekly individual therapy to deal with past losses and abuse

Mrs. Smith's Long-Range Goals

1. To maintain sobriety
   - Short-term tasks:
     - Attend Narcotics Anonymous
     - Establish new friendships and activities that are not drug-related
2. To obtain job counseling and training
   - Short-term tasks:
     - Participate in vocational testing/counseling
     - Select two or three possible career choices
     - Examine newspapers regularly to check job availability
3. To deal with her feelings about her past history of abuse Short-term tasks
   - Short-term tasks:
     - To make a commitment to individual counseling
     - To participate in group therapy with women who also have abuse histories

These goals are merely suggested and would need the agreement of the individuals involved to enhance their motivation to work on them. Both the process of participation in formulating goals and the experience of achieving success are very ego-enhancing and increase self-esteem. Success in achieving goals, in turn, enhances clients' motivation to work on additional, more challenging tasks.

Various Intervention Options

Let us consider the range of intervention options that might have been pursued with the Smith family, both within and outside the First Place (school) program. Within the school setting, support groups exist both for children and for parents. In addition, individual counseling is available for children, and case management for families. The latter includes networking and coordination with shelter providers, as well as referrals and follow-up to other services (housing, mental health, etc.). A flyer describing the range of services is given to each parent upon the child's admission, so this could have served as a nonthreatening way to review the available services with Mrs. Smith in a follow-up meeting. During this and subsequent sessions, the matter of the family's housing needs and Mrs. Smith's employment counseling or training could have been discussed, as could possible referrals for school or employment counseling for Barbie's siblings.

Individual counseling (therapy) for parents is *not* available through the school's professional staff, and therefore this very important referral for Mrs. Smith would have had to be made to an outside agency. Because this family was already involved with so many other outside agencies, it would have been understandable if Mrs. Smith were reluctant about engaging with yet another person and place. Nonetheless, because help for Mrs. Smith would translate into potential help for her entire family, the matter of finding a counseling program for her that she could accept would have had to be pursued with utmost care and determination. It probably would have been best to make this referral after the relationship with Mrs. Smith was firmly established through provision of other needed services.

Individual counseling for children is available through the school and would have been a vital resource for Barbie. Her issues of past abuse and loss were probably continuing to create anxiety for her, and her family's ongoing lack of stability may well have made her vulnerable to loneliness, depression, and low self-esteem (Bassuk & Rubin, 1986; Choi & Snyder, 1999).

In addition to a relationship with a counselor or therapist, Barbie might have benefited from a mentoring relationship. The literature reports the important role of such relationships in contributing to resilience in high-risk youth (Rhodes, 1994). Barbie's life was lacking in role models other than her mother. She had no known female relatives (other than her sister) and had never been involved in the type of extracurricular activities, such as Girl Scouts or team sports, that would provide her with other models of adult females she might choose to emulate. Studies in Great Britain (Rutter, 1979, 1987) and Hawaii (Werner & Smith, 1982) found that children living in developmentally hazardous settings who sought support from nonparental adults had a lower risk of psychiatric disorders and were more resilient than children living in similar settings who did not seek such support. Anthony's work on "the invulnerable child" also confirms the significance of one positive relationship in the lives of children growing up in very hostile home and/or community environments (Anthony & Cohler, 1987).

Finally, because of her family's frequent moves, Barbie had never had the opportunity to establish friendships with peers. She may have lacked socialization skills and would probably have benefited from being in a group with other children in similar circumstances. Issues discussed in these school-based groups include friendships, conflicts with classmates, loss of former friends and schools, and domestic violence. It is very supportive for children to learn through being in such a group that they are not the only ones who have difficulties such as these.

Teamwork within and between Agencies

Professional collaboration would have been the key to success in the Smith case, as the clients' motivation and ability to work on their own behalf might have been limited. This would probably have been a "labor-intensive" case, requiring a major input from staff members to maintain the clients' motivation. Within the school, it would have been essential for the special education teacher working with Barbie to be aware of the physical limitations of the child's home environment and to know about the agreed-upon contract for protected homework time. In addition, the regular classroom teacher would have needed to know about Barbie's history of extensive school changes, which may have interfered with the girl's ability to make friends and participate in social exchanges appropriate for a 10-year-old.

Regular pupil review conferences could also have alerted all staff members to significant developments in the family that might affect Barbie's ability to concentrate and learn. Examples of such developments might include Mrs. Smith's becoming involved with a new man or Mrs. Smith's arguing with Barbie's sister, Donna, over Donna's choice of boyfriend.

Parnell and Vanderkloot (1989) state that they cannot work with poor, multiproblem families without a team of professionals:

> For members of the team, the involvement of the other members spells relief from the recurrent crises, the chronic problems, and the many occasions when it is necessary to devote whole days to individual clients. Furthermore, the team members function as a support group to one another, and as the nucleus of a resource network. (p. 452)

This kind of collaboration is also necessary among staff members in different agencies who are working with a multiproblem family. Certainly, it would have been within the purview of Mrs. Smith's probation worker to help arrange adequate housing. It would *not* seem appropriate for someone with a history of addiction and possession of drugs to be living in an environment populated by substance users. Similarly, it would seem inappropriate for someone like Mrs. Smith to obtain employment in a bar, where she would probably be thrown into contact with many alcohol-addicted individuals. We do not know how much (if anything) Mrs. Smith's probation officer knew about her life or her background, but a case conference, coordinated by the school, would have provided the opportunity for *all* the professionals involved to meet with Mrs. Smith to share information and to coordinate planning on her behalf.

TRACKING PROGRESS AND TERMINATING

Tracking Progress

Once relationships have been established among the various professionals involved in a case, the process of keeping abreast of developments becomes easier. Ideally, the case conference establishes clear areas of responsibility, so that each member of the "team" knows his or her focus of duty, and no one person feels overburdened by attempting to work alone with *all* the various facets of the case. In the case of the Smiths, the school social worker might have become the case manager, with the understanding that new developments and the concerns of other agencies could be funneled through him or her. This might appear to be a major responsibility in and of itself, but if others shared the tasks of helping Mrs. Smith find permanent housing, job training, addiction counseling, and mental health counseling, then the school social worker would have been freed from becoming involved personally in each of these tasks. The school, after all, was the primary contact point for the child, and the other agencies (probation, social services, housing, mental health, etc.) could share the responsibility of trying to rehabilitate the Smiths and help point them toward a more productive life.

Of course, the danger of having so many different people involved with the Smiths would have been that the family could have become scattered and frustrated because of having too many people to relate to. They also might confuse the appropriate functions of each unless they were given direct guidance. Each professional would need to be clear in communicating his or her specific helping role to the family.

Case review conferences should be held periodically to track the progress of each case. The timing of such reviews should be determined during the original conference. Because of the rapidly changing elements in the Smith case, a plan for a review in 6 months might have been impractical, although in other case situations this is a reasonable period of time. Probably a once-a-month review would have been appropriate for this family.

The Smith family found Section 8 housing after Barbie had been at First Place School only 2 months. They moved, her records were transferred to a regular public school, and the case management role of the special school ceased to exist. In retrospect, a plan to confer with the social worker in the new school and a fallback plan to prevent the family's becoming "lost" would have helped keep both the helpers and this family on track.

Termination

The concept of termination is not applicable in dealing with young children whose development is in flux or with families that have serious and ongoing problems. What happens is that some families drop out of sight for a while and later come to the attention of other agencies, which may be unaware of previous efforts to help the family. The word "termination" assumes that the difficulties presented at intake have been resolved and that there will be no further contacts. It certainly cannot guarantee that similar or different problems will not resurface later. It is quite likely that a child who shows sufficient difficulties to come to the attention of a school social worker in third grade will again present problems in middle school, when physiological development creates stresses that make many youth less able to cope. The fact that a child has a confidential record related to the earlier difficulties may assist the counselor or social worker who meets this child for the first time at age 12. In my opinion, the availability of records offers great aid to professionals who enter a case after much work has already been done but about which the parent(s) may give an incomplete report.

UPDATE ON THE SMITH FAMILY: 1995; BARBIE, AGE 13

The following summary of what happened to the Smiths after the end of the *No Place Like Home* videotape (Hunt, 1992) is based on information from the filmmaker, Kathryn Hunt; on my telephone conversation with Mrs. Smith; and on various conversations with the First Place School personnel, who had signed releases from Mrs. Smith to share this information.

The end of the video announced that Barbie had been sent a one-way ticket and that she had gone out of state to visit her father. Her mother told me that Barbie remained with her father for an extended time (almost a full school year), although the original plan had been for a summer visit only. When Barbie eventually returned to her mother, she told the filmmaker that she had not gone to school during the previous year! However, the school records do indicate an out-of-state registration. The facts about this remain unclear.

During the summer following Barbie's stay with her father, I attempted to contact the family to obtain releases for the first edition of this book. The filmmaker had prepared Mrs. Smith for my call, and Mrs. Smith had indicated her willingness to give me her permission. I spoke to Barbie and David before finally reaching Mrs. Smith. My conversation with her took place the night before they were to be evicted from the apartment in which they had lived for more than a year following Barbie's transfer out of the special school program. Mrs. Smith gave me permission over the phone and indicated her willingness to sign releases, which I said I would send to Kathryn Hunt.

Following their eviction, it took 4 months for the personnel at the school and Ms. Hunt to locate the family. During this time, Mrs. Smith evidently had some trouble with the law and was imprisoned again briefly (I do not know any details). Because I continued to press the school to locate the family, they eventually did so, through the department of social services. I had assumed that if the Smiths were still in the same state, they would be receiving public assistance. The fact that Barbie was *not* enrolled in school (which had been verified) constituted grounds to report Mrs. Smith for neglect, and this information was conveyed to her through a note to her public assistance worker.

Mrs. Smith soon after reappeared at the special school program to enroll Barbie. This time Barbie remained there for a full 6-month period, during which time Mrs. Smith accepted a referral and involved herself in counseling provided by the mental health system. Barbie made considerable academic gains during this period, was tested, and was found *not* to have a learning disability. In other words, her serious academic delays were attributable to her irregular school attendance, rather than to any personal learning disability. At this time Barbie was eligible to continue at that school program for 1 more year, after which she would be too old. However, the availability of the special school program for Barbie was contingent upon her family's continuing homeless status. Were she to transfer to a "regular" public middle school, it would be unlikely that there would be any special services to accommodate her special needs.

Barbie's sister, Donna, was once again living apart from Mrs. Smith and Barbie. She had had a baby and was living alone with her child, because the baby's father was in prison. Barbie's brother had also moved out, and his whereabouts were unknown. At the time of the 1995 update, Barbie had her own room in the motel where she resided with her mother.

UPDATE ON BARBIE: 2002, AGE 18½

In connection with preparing the second edition of this book, I again contacted Kathryn Hunt to see if she had remained in touch with the Smith family during the past 6 years. She said that she had and that these contacts were reciprocal: Sometimes they would contact her, and other times she would telephone them. She gave me a brief overview and offered to call Mrs. Smith to see if she and Barbie would agree to talk with me. After Ms. Hunt notified me that the family would welcome my call, I telephoned and learned that Barbie had recently moved out of state with her boyfriend. Her mother expected to hear from her, and she said that she would pass along my message and ask Barbie if she could give me her telephone number.

At the time the second edition was published, I had spoken with Barbie twice, once soon after her move, when she was living temporarily with her boyfriend's cousins, and several months later, after the couple had moved to live with the boyfriend's parents. During this time the couple had married and were looking forward to the birth of a baby in a few months. The summary below was reviewed and approved by Barbie and her husband, whom I call Mike. Barbie told me that Mike was not comfortable with giving details about his baby for this book, and therefore I mainly focused on summarizing Barbie's life during the years of her adolescence.

After the previous update, when Barbie had returned to live with her mother and was attending First Place School again, the pattern of family instability and frequent changes of residence continued because of her mother's ongoing drug involvement and other periods of imprisonment. Barbie lived for a while with her sister in California, then for another period with her father in the Southwest. Some of this time was relatively stable for Barbie; she attended school and reconciled with her father. He had remarried, had a baby, and was not involved with drugs for about 6 years. In telling me about her father and this period, Barbie said, "Dad gave me rules about what I could and couldn't do. I realized that he loved me. I got to know him and I forgave him. He was kind to me and even let me call my mom from his house." Unfortunately, his ability to remain drug-free did not last, and he returned to prison.

Barbie admitted that she also had been involved with drugs for about 9 years but stated that she had been clean for the last 2½ years. I thought that this could not be an accurate memory, because if she had been drug-free since she was 16, that would mean that she had begun experimenting when she was 7! I asked for clarification, and Barbie said that it was, in fact, true. She credited her husband with helping her get off drugs. Now her only addiction was cigarette smoking.

I asked Barbie whether she remembered her experiences in foster care when she was little, and she said that she did, mentioning the names of her foster parents. When I questioned her about the counseling that her mother had mentioned to the school social worker, Barbie reported that the counselor had told her that everything she said would be confidential but that the counselor then repeated what Barbie had said to her mother and her mother's boyfriend. Barbie felt very betrayed by this, and I explained that counselors are obligated to report it if they believe that a child is being abused. I wasn't sure if this was the case in this situation. Barbie felt that it was wrong for the counselor to tell her that she could trust her, then later to betray this trust.

I also asked if Barbie remembered the First Place School, and she referred to the school social worker there by name. When I inquired whether she had been there long enough to make any friends, she recalled a Chinese boy and walking to the park to go swimming with her school class once a week.

Barbie was one credit short of being able to graduate with her class in Arizona, but she later obtained her GED. When she returned to live with her mother, she held different jobs in fast-food restaurants and in stores. She met her future husband when she was 16, and she said, "He's the best thing that ever happened to me." At another point in the conversation, she said that she was happier now than she had ever been in her life.

Barbie maintained weekly telephone contact with both her sister and her mother. She confirmed that she had never had any contact with grandparents or other relatives. However, she appeared to be making a new life for herself in a new part of the country where she was involved with her husband's family. She was looking forward to the baby's birth.

CONCLUDING COMMENTS

Contracting assumes that a client has the motivation and ability to follow through with an agreed-upon plan. Sometimes a plan that seems logical and feasible on one day can become invalid when the client's circumstances change and the plan becomes unworkable. Therefore, the time frame of contracts with multiproblem clients and families should be short, and there should be frequent monitoring and revisions of goals, where appropriate.

The case of Barbie Smith graphically illustrates the impact of homelessness on school attendance and child development. This population of children clearly requires special services such as those described here. However, the lack of follow-up after a family obtains housing and a child leaves the program can have serious consequences if the child goes for protracted periods of time without schooling. This situation needs more careful monitoring by public assistance programs that provide financial support to families. Computerization should permit tracking of homeless children's school attendance to ensure that such children do not fall between the cracks.

This case is unusual because of the follow-ups over the course of 15 years. One of the usual characteristics of social work practice is that practitioners may never know the outcome in the lives of most of the children they have served. We must take some comfort in the belief that we provided the best service possible during the time we were involved, and that families will be more inclined to find other help when they have had a positive experience with social workers in the past.

DISCUSSION QUESTIONS

1. Discuss the ethical issue involved in trying to broaden a client's views of what he or she needs, as described in the beginning of this chapter. To what extent should the contract reflect the worker's vision about the client's potential for growth and change, and how does this conform to the principle of client self-determination?
2. What intervention(s) do you think would have been appropriate to encourage Barbie's more regular school attendance? If the school social worker suspected that Mrs. Smith had resumed drug use, how might this have been handled?
3. Consider the concepts of "risk" and "resilience" as they apply to Barbie Smith. Suggest some factors that may have contributed to her resilience. What do you predict for her future, and on what do you base your prediction?
4. Discuss the pros and cons of providing a *separate* school program for homeless children. How would you address the important issue of integrating children who have been in a separate program into a regular school program at a later date?

PART III

DIFFERENT METHODS OF HELPING CHILDREN

CHAPTER 6

Helping the Family Help Their Child

A child is born into a family system which ideally tries to support and nourish his or her development. Most families try their best to help their children succeed. However, the stresses of modern life mean that this goal may fall short, thereby leaving children without the strong foundation that will give them the stamina and confidence to learn and try new undertakings. Parents may be working hard to meet the family's financial obligations, and they may lack the energy and time to interact meaningfully with their children. Or an adolescent single-parent mother may find it next to impossible to juggle being in school with being a parent. Children sense their parents' anxiety, and they may withdraw and spend more hours with peers or on line instead of relating to their parents at home. Some children may fall behind in school or become angry and aggressive with peers, or they may withdraw and become isolated. Although the parents certainly are not to blame for their children's problems, their responses are critical in helping or hindering various helping efforts by any practitioners who may become involved.

Families today come in many different sizes and forms. The majority (69%) of children in the United States under the age of 18 live in families with two parents, and about 23% live with a single mother (U.S. Bureau of the Census, 2016). Of the 50.7 million children living with two parents, 47.7 million live with two parents who are married, and the remainder live with two unmarried parents. Other family formats are those consisting of two mothers or two fathers, or with a grandparent or other relative as the main caretaker. When the child develops difficulties that concern the school, the parent(s) will be notified and the social worker will try to set up appointments to explore the problem or to make a referral to an outside practitioner. Some parents may be very cooperative, but others, who are pressured with their own time constraints, may present special challenges in trying to engage them.

This chapter deals with the various options of helping a child through involvement with the child's family. The focus here is not on family therapy per se but rather on *the child*, with acknowledgment that the child's family is a critical resource in helping alleviate any problem. Chapter 7 addresses some methods for working with the child *individually,* although, even when individual therapy is the treatment of choice, most therapists will consult with the parents periodically. The family model that is recommended here is one that integrates child and family treatment (Drewes, Bratton, & Schaefer, 2011; Gil & Selekman, 2015; Schaefer & Carey, 1994). It includes the following options:

- Parent counseling/guidance
- Parent–child sessions
- Sessions with siblings
- Sessions with the entire family

Regardless of the focus of treatment, cultural and ethical considerations must be acknowledged and addressed, and these are discussed in the following section. The different treatment approaches listed above all rest on a foundation of systems theory, which assumes the mutual interacting influences of each member on the others. In addition, "the family is viewed as a transactional system that functions in relation to its broader sociocultural context and evolves over a multigenerational family life cycle" (Walsh, 2012, p. 29). All these approaches to working with the child in a family context emphasize a competency and strength-based perspective, rather than focusing on deficits and pathology, which might have been typical in past years. Ideally the helping efforts will involve an interdisciplinary team, rather than only one practitioner, and the child's "problems" will be analyzed in terms of how the child's and family's strengths can be mobilized to achieve a positive goal.

DIFFERENT LEVELS OF FAMILY INVOLVEMENT

As I emphasize in this book and demonstrate in various examples, work with children should *always* include some sort of involvement with their parents, when parents are living and available. Whether siblings are seen depends on the nature of the presenting problem and on conflicts in relationships that become evident as the work progresses. For example, in previous publications (Webb, 1993, 2002a), I have included several cases involving sibling and family sessions following deaths and parental separation following divorce.

The deployment of one or both parents in the military may call for certain adaptations in interventions with caretakers that are focused on helping children. Sometimes it may be possible to hold a telephone conference call using Skype to include an absent parent in a family session, and when this is not possible, a copy of the deployed parent's photograph in the session can serve to emphasize the parent's ongoing role in his or her child's life. Absent family members, whether deceased, deployed, or divorced, continue to play a symbolic role and to exert influence on the child and the family.

Sometimes it is appropriate for a babysitter or a member of the extended family (e.g., a grandmother) to be included in sessions with the child. Adults who have frequent and significant contact with the child should be invited to present their perspectives on the problem situation. I usually see the entire family together for one or more sessions in the beginning to assess the nature of the family members' interactions and to involve them in thinking about how they might get along better. I refer to myself as a "child and family social worker," thereby indicating to the family my ability to work flexibly with the various family members in different combinations, as well as in a group.

Parent Counseling/Guidance

When a child is being seen on a weekly basis, I try to confer with the parents monthly in "counseling/guidance sessions." The main purpose of these parent meetings is to give and receive feedback about the child's progress. The meetings also offer the worker the opportunity to ask questions about matters the child may have raised, to reinforce a parent's positive efforts with the child, and to support the parent regarding his or her continuing frustrations.

The issue of confidentiality always comes up in family work. Because of my belief that it is important to encourage parent–child communication and to convey the sense that the parent(s), child, and practitioner are all working *together* to try to alleviate the problem situation, I do not want to overvalue the importance of a child's relationship with me and leave a parent feeling like an outsider. Therefore, I share my impressions about the child openly with the parent, and, *without quoting the child verbatim,* I give the parent a sense of the nature of the child's participation in his or her sessions with me. Because this is a two-way street, I also share with the child, discreetly and appropriately, concerns that the parent may have brought to my attention. Sometimes the parent meeting indicates the need for a family session, which I then schedule, after clarifying with the child the purpose and potential positive outcome from such a meeting.

Practitioners in agency practice sometimes encounter parents who are reluctant to come to parent or family meetings. These parents may not be aware that their child has a problem, or they may prefer to let the school or someone else handle it. Often, such parents may be burdened by work and home responsibilities and worries. Their child's difficulty may arouse their anger, and they may resent that yet another demand is now being placed on their time. Practitioners, in turn, sometimes become resentful when parents are unwilling to put the necessary effort into trying to help their own children. *It is the professional's responsibility to reach out and make the extra effort to connect with parents who seem resistant to becoming involved.* Often, doing this requires stretching one's empathic sensitivity, to try to understand and feel what this mother's or father's life must be like. Offering to make a home visit may have a positive effect, as may trying to schedule an appointment for coffee or lunch in a restaurant near a parent's workplace at a time convenient for the parent. A practitioner who sincerely believes in the importance of parents' involvement and backs up this conviction with both words and action has a better chance of engaging parents effectively.

Parent–Child Sessions

Certain circumstances may make it appropriate to see a child together with a parent. First, there may be no choice if the child has separation problems of such severity that he or she cannot tolerate being separated from the parent (usually the mother). Second, it is essential to have the parent present during at least part of the session when a behavior modification program has been set up; the therapist will need to encourage the parent to praise the child for gains or to discuss with both the child and parent certain alterations in the program if the child is not achieving success with it. The use of parent–child sessions together with a behavior modification program is described in greater detail later in this chapter (see the case of Tim).

When a child is experiencing separation anxiety, as in the case of Tammy (Chapter 7), the issue becomes one of helping mother and child learn to separate from each other. The session itself serves as a training opportunity. It is advisable for the practitioner to have a separate session or a telephone conference with the mother before the joint session to coach her in an overall plan for gradual separation and increase her willingness to carry out the plan. Depending on the child's tolerance level and other possible contributing factors (such as the mother's own need to keep the child close), a plan can be established for the mother to sit in the doorway of the playroom, watching but not playing actively with the child. When the child appears to have established an adequate level of comfort with the practitioner, the practitioner may suggest to the mother that she look at an interesting article in a magazine in the waiting room. The mother should then leave without a big goodbye scene, which might raise the child's anxiety again. This planned leavetaking may need to be repeated several times before the child can eventually begin the session in the playroom without the mother. This protocol for gradual separation can also be applied to a day care or nursery school situation in which the child cannot tolerate separation from the mother and, with modification, to bedtime separation problems.

Sessions with Siblings

Sessions with siblings may be appropriate and helpful in cases in which the nature of the presenting problem constitutes a shared family experience—for example, the death of a relative or an upcoming parental divorce (Webb, 1993, 2002a). Such sessions may also be useful when the practitioner becomes aware of intensive sibling conflict while working with one child in the family.

Other children in a family *always* have some reaction to the fact that one of their siblings is in therapy. When the family considers the necessity for treatment as a weakness on the treated child's part, the sibling who is not in treatment may feel superior to the brother or sister who needs individual help. However, sometimes certain privileges accompany therapy, such as additional attention from the parents or a dinosaur sticker or a food snack at the end of a session. This can make the treated child appear to be the recipient of special "goodies" that are not accorded to other siblings in the family.

I try to alert parents to this possible source of strain and suggest that they use the situation to emphasize that each brother and sister is different and that the siblings will all have different positive and negative experiences in their lives. This discussion can prove to be a window into how each child is perceived in the family, as well as how the child in treatment views him- or herself in comparison with the other children.

When siblings are seen together, it is important to model respect for individual difference as a principle of interaction. Certain guidelines and rules need to be made explicit, just as in group or family sessions (see Figure 6.1, later in this chapter). I have found it especially important with siblings to establish the ground rule that differences or arguments that emerge during the session must not continue when the siblings leave the office. They may repeat positive statements about one another, but not negatives.

It is sometimes necessary to separate siblings when they are arguing and unable to take turns speaking and listening to one another. This happened in the case of the Martini sisters, ages 8 and 10 (Webb, 1993, 2002a), whose anger toward each other became excessive and out of control following the closely timed proximity of their parents' separation and their uncle/godfather's death. Unable to express their rage at their grieving parents, they took it out on each other. When I attempted to see them together, the sessions were dominated by arguments, name-calling, destructive putdowns, and some tears of frustration.

Realizing that the joint work was becoming counterproductive, I began splitting the sessions and seeing each girl individually. Prior to doing so, I told the girls that I could see how angry they both were and that they had a right to feel angry, but that I could not let them take their feelings out on each other. I also advised each parent to echo this principle and to separate the girls physically when they fought at home. In individual sessions, one girl drew a frightening werewolf with his teeth bared, and the other pounded, poked, and aggressively rolled out various lumps of clay. After several months of these split sessions, during which each girl was permitted to express her angry feelings symbolically through play, the parents reported noticeably reduced fighting at home, and I resumed some conjoint sessions with them.

Sessions with the Entire Family

The purpose of seeing the entire family together is twofold: (1) to see firsthand how family members relate to one another and (2) to help the family find and use more positive and gratifying ways of relating.

Seeing the Parents First

Whole-family sessions provide wonderful opportunities to observe family members' interactions, but they also can seem very intimidating to the practitioner, who may feel outnumbered and quite uncomfortable in the role of outsider. Hepworth and Larsen (1993) recognize that work with the entire family requires advanced skills; they suggest that students and practitioners with little experience in family work begin by seeing the parents without the children. This permits the practitioner to become familiar with the overall problem situation and to begin establishing an alliance with the parents prior to introducing the children into sessions later.

In Chapter 4, I listed four reasons for seeing parents alone before seeing children: (1) establishing the alliance, (2) obtaining the developmental history, (3) preparing a parent to prepare a child for the first session, and (4) obtaining signed releases. Wachtel (1994) notes another interesting and important advantage of seeing the parents alone first. Wachtel points out that many parents who come for help regarding their children's problems have developed some feelings of resentment toward the children, because their problems appear to expose the parents as "failures." Parents need to "unload" these negative feelings, including their fears that there is something drastically wrong with their children. Obviously, it would be contraindicated for them to do this in the child's presence. Therefore, the cathartic value of having the practitioner listen and respond appropriately to the *parents'* concerns helps strengthen the alliance with them while also permitting the practitioner to offer hope and therapeutic optimism that the situation can improve in time.

The "Joining" Process

When the practitioner meets the entire family together for the first time, it is essential that he or she find ways to "join" (Minuchin, 1974) with the family. "Joining" refers to efforts on the practitioner's part to become accepted and "to establish an alliance with the family as a whole, with the key subsystems, and with each individual" (Chasin & White, 1989, p. 17). It is the process through which the practitioner moves from being an outsider to being an insider. This process relies on the practitioner's individual personality and style, as well as on his or her ability to establish enough of a feeling of comfort and connection with various family members that they will be able to tolerate having a stranger know about aspects of their lives not usually revealed to public scrutiny. Different authors suggest different techniques for joining, including small talk, mimicking the family's affect and style (Hepworth & Larsen, 1993), and commenting on a child's clothing, jewelry, or hairstyle (Chasin & White, 1989). The expectation among certain cultural groups dictates that the professional find a way to engage families through small talk about the weather or recent news reports to establish a degree of ease prior to introducing any topic of concern such as a child's problems (Zayas, Canino, &

Suarez, 2001). As always, the worker must find a way to adapt to the family's expectations as a prelude to establishing the professional relationship.

Setting Ground Rules for Family Sessions

Regardless of the topic of a "joining" conversation, the family session will move inevitably toward dealing with the important matters that are causing concern. Because the family has its own characteristic method of communicating (which may well include members' interrupting, shouting, and insulting one another), it is incumbent upon the practitioner to set ground rules early in the first session, to establish this meeting as different from interactions that occur in the family living room or kitchen. Sometimes, in the middle of a shouting match, I have found it effective to stand up and quietly offer to leave the room, stating that the family members obviously do not need me to carry on their battles. I point out that if they continue to fight in my office the same way they do at home, then they are wasting their money and all our time. This statement can be a prelude to establishing a rule that only one person speaks at a time and that family members may disagree with one another but may not insult other persons or put them down because they have different opinions. Setting such ground rules as these in the first session establishes a climate of safety that models respect for the rights of different individuals to express themselves without being heckled. Figure 6.1 lists some suggested ground rules and guidelines for family sessions.

Some Practical Suggestions for Working with the Entire Family

When the worker has had a preliminary meeting with the parents prior to the first session with the entire family, he or she will have a sense of the parents' personalities, as well as some background information about the various family members. Depending on the nature of the problem and the ages of the children, the practitioner should prepare to have toys or activities that are age appropriate and that will permit the family to interact nonverbally through play, as well as verbally. During the preliminary meeting with the parents, I

FIGURE 6.1. Ground rules and guidelines for family session.

Only *one* person talks at a time.

No insults, cursing, or putdowns.

Disagreements and arguments are not to be continued outside the office.

Children deserve the same respect as do adults.

Everyone has the right to "pass" (i.e., not to answer or speak).

Parents are in charge of setting limits for children.

tell them that we cannot expect their children to sit quietly and talk during the entire family meeting, so I will have some toys and activities for the children. I also tell the parents that I may ask them to participate in playing with their children. I make it clear that, although I will be responsible for providing some play materials, I expect them, as the parents, to remain in charge of their children's behavior. In other words, if the children start whining and arguing, I want them to handle it as they would at home.

Some suggested items for family session activities include paper and markers, puppets, clay, blocks, and selected board and card games. It is important, however, to avoid overstimulating the children through exposure to numerous toys. Because the purpose of the family session is to learn how the family interacts, it is appropriate for the practitioner to take a directive stance—suggesting, for example, that the children draw a picture of their family doing something (i.e., Kinetic Family Drawing; Burns & Kaufman, 1970, 1972). Alternatively, the family may be asked to act out through puppet play something upsetting that happened in the family. The point is that the family session is not a "free play" period; it is a time for understanding and discovering new ways of family interaction. The toys and play activities are used to facilitate this understanding.

Cultural Considerations

In some cultures, children are expected to be "seen but not heard." This view may present a strain between the practitioner's desire to permit the children to "have a voice" and the more traditional belief that "adults know best." For example, in the videotape *Tres Madres,* the family therapist Harry Aponte (1990) conducted a family session with three generations of family members, including the 7-year-old girl who was the "identified patient." The child was rarely invited to participate in the adult conversation, and the tape showed her yawning and looking bored. Aponte clearly viewed the child's problem of sleepwalking as secondary to the girl's mother's unhappiness and inability to function appropriately as a mother. Although this dynamic may indeed have been crucial to understanding the case, I question the need to have the child present during this discussion when she had no part in it. A play therapist, sensitive to the *child's* needs as well as to the mother's, would have provided paper and markers and suggested that the child draw pictures of her bedroom, of where her mother lived and where she lived, and of how she would like to have her family live.

The conclusion that the child's symptom was related to the lack of a strong maternal presence could have also been deduced from a discussion centered on the child's drawings. The difference is that one approach meaningfully includes the child and the other ignores her. When I have presented this example and viewpoint at workshops, however, some participants have responded that both Aponte and this Hispanic family might have been uncomfortable, for cultural reasons, in giving so much attention to a young child (see Zayas et al., 2001, for a discussion of parent–child relationships in mainland Puerto Rican families).

In my own practice with families of different ethnic backgrounds, I have learned to explore the parents' views about child involvement before including children in an entire family session. Some parents accept my offer to help them try a different way of relating to their children through play. However, this may be too difficult for others to attempt; in these situations I try to adapt my work to the reality of the clients' beliefs even when I may disagree with them.

What to Notice in Family Sessions

After a session with the entire family, the practitioner should try to answer the following questions:

1. Who seems to be the dominant parent? Do the children seem to accept parental rules, or do they try to split the parents by encouraging them to disagree?
2. Do parents share in the discipline, or is one or the other targeted for this role?
3. Which parent appears to set the limits for the children? Do the parents seem to agree, or is one more permissive and one more strict?
4. To whom do the children turn for affection and comfort?
5. Are any alliances between the children apparent? How is the symptomatic child treated by the other family members?
6. How does the symptomatic child relate to each parent? Does each parent respond differently to the child?
7. How would the situation have to change for the family to feel better?

In a meeting later with the parents to give and receive feedback, the practitioner will solicit the parents' reactions to the family session and also share some of his or her own impressions. This discussion can result in some important decisions about goals. Another family meeting would be scheduled after the elapse of a period of time during which the parents will have tried to implement changes.

A Note of Clarification

As is evident in the preceding discussion, my view of "working with the family" is not the same as "family therapy" in the sense of seeking to change the family's roles and structure (Minuchin, 1974; Minuchin & Fishman, 1981). Rather, the integrated child and family approach presented in this book focuses on communication patterns and interactions among family members, to help them deal with the presenting problem in a manner that puts them in control of their own behavior. This systems view recognizes that when one person in a family has pain (which may show up in symptoms), all family members feel the pain in some way (Satir, 1983). This integrated child and family approach resembles Satir's (1983) "growth model" of family therapy in its focus on clear communication among family members, which in turn promotes enhanced self-worth in each individual adult and child family member.

ETHICAL CHALLENGES IN FAMILY WORK

Because of its complexity, work with families places extra demands on practitioners, who must strive to be fair, objective, and self-aware even during very intense emotional interactions. The goal of maintaining professional neutrality may be especially difficult when the lives of young children are at stake and the impulse to "rescue" them is ignited in the worker. Often individuals enter the helping professions because of their sincere, altruistic motivation to help people, such as children, who for various reasons cannot help themselves. What is the danger, then, in wanting to "rescue" children? From whom or what are they being rescued? And what will become of them after the rescue?

There is a significant difference between helping and rescuing, because the implication in "rescue" is that the individual is being removed from a dangerous situation. In my opinion, a child-rescuing mentality serves to establish a barrier, rather than a bond, between a practitioner and a parent. When the worker becomes judgmental toward the parent, his or her ability to work effectively with the parent is greatly reduced, and ultimately the child suffers.

Work with children requires the ability to relate to their parents. This relationship, however, inevitably stimulates memories and overtones from a practitioner's *own* family of origin. In supervising child therapists, and in my own work, I have often traced a lack of empathy or other therapeutic impasses to experiences in the practitioner's own family of origin or present family (Webb, 1989). "Countertransference can be triggered by identification with one of the clients, the family, the style of communication, and similar events in the therapist's life" (Miller, 1994, p. 16). Therefore, it is incumbent on practitioners working with families to be self-aware and to receive regular supervision or consultation to help them recognize areas of possible identification with the families with whom they are working.

Efforts to help children without attention to helping their families are shortsighted and will have limited impact. Admittedly, trying to empower a family to help itself may seem more formidable than spending time individually with a child. However, more attention must be focused on this essential larger task if we are truly to integrate child and family helping.

Confidentiality is another thorny issue that frequently comes up in the context of family work. I have noted in Chapter 2 that children really do not have the legal right to confidentiality with respect to their parents, whose status affords them power to demand that a child reveal certain matters or who may require that a child's medical (counseling) records be revealed to them. When these matters come under dispute, the court may appoint a guardian *ad litem* to represent the child's best interests, but even then the child's position may be ambiguous and conflicted if he or she is caught between the demands of two hostile parents in a divorce proceeding. This situation is discussed more fully in Chapter 11.

Consistently in this book, I present the position that confidentiality between parent and child is neither feasible nor in the child's best interests. I argue for open communication between parent and child to increase their understanding of each other's needs and feelings. When the child and parent treat each other with respect, confidentiality will not be a concern. Practitioners must consistently help families work toward this goal.

INTEGRATING CHILD AND FAMILY THERAPY IN WORK WITH (OR DEALING WITH) ATTENTION DEFICIT/HYPERACTIVITY DISORDER AND CHILDHOOD GENDER IDENTITY ISSUES

The remainder of the chapter focuses on helping children and their families deal with two different problem situations in which involvement of *both* the child and the family is critical to bring about some improvement. The two conditions are attention-deficit/hyperactivity disorder (ADHD) and gender identity issues. Although the child is designated as the "identified patient" in both circumstances, involvement of the family is essential to help motivate and encourage the child to persevere with the short- and long-term treatment goals and to achieve a positive sense of identity. Both childhood conditions are considered serious, requiring lifelong attention and commitment for successful outcome.

Attention-Deficit/Hyperactivity Disorder

A diagnosis of ADHD usually follows some years of the parents' increasing awareness and growing concern about their child's difficulties in following instructions, very high energy level, and constant distractibility. This disorder is more common in boys than in girls and is found in approximately 6.8% of children (Nigg & Nikolas, 2008). The onset of the hyperactive behaviors usually occurs before the age of 3, but many children do not come to professional attention until around age 7, when they cannot meet the additional demands placed on them in school.

ADHD is a biologically or constitutionally based disability of unclear etiology. According to DSM-5 (American Psychiatric Association, 2013), the characteristics of children with ADHD include two different groups of behavior: (1) *symptoms of inattention and disorganization* (e.g., easy distractibility, forgetfulness, lack of follow-through, difficulty organizing tasks and activities, and careless mistakes) and/or (2) *symptoms of hyperactivity–impulsivity* (e.g., fidgeting, excessive talking, seemingly "motor-driven" activity, interrupting others, blurting out answers, and difficulty taking turns). A formal diagnosis of ADHD requires at least 6 out of 9 possible behavioral characteristics in one of these two subgroups (or 12 out of the total of 18 in both) "that have persisted for at least 6 months to a degree that is inconsistent with developmental level and negatively impacts directly on social and academic/occupational activities" (American Psychiatric Association, 2013, p. 59).

Social workers who want to recommend a reference to help parents understand this condition can suggest Russell Barkley's numerous books on the topic (2006, 2013, 2014). Barkley's books on this topic would also be helpful for practitioners who want to learn more about this condition (Barkley, 2006; Barkley, Robin, & Benton, 2014). Other useful references are Pelham and Fabiano (2008) and Pelham, Guaggy, Greiner, Fabiano, and Waschbusch (2017). Palombo (2002, p. 144) describes the situation as follows:

> The profile of an individual child's neuropsychological strengths and weaknesses is analogous to the topography of a landscape. For some, the terrain is fairly flat; that is, their competencies are evenly distributed. Other children's profiles look like a terrain filled with prominent peaks. These children are gifted in multiple areas. Yet the valleys between the ridges indicate that their gifts are rarely uniformly distributed across the entire terrain. Gifted children may also have learning disorders (Vail, 1989). For children with learning disorders the terrain is highly variable. There are peaks and valleys that are notable for the contrast they present. The valleys between the peaks are much deeper than one would expect, indicating a great disparity between the areas of strength and those of weakness.

Obviously, these differences create great uncertainty for parents and for teachers who find it difficult to understand and accept how a child's behavior can vary so greatly. See Dane (1990) for more discussion on this topic.

Different Helping Approaches

A multimodal approach is most effective in helping children with ADHD and their families. Specific interventions include psychostimulant medication, usually methylphenidate (Ritalin); behavior management skills training for the children's parents and teachers; cognitive, supportive, and play therapy to enable the children to develop self-esteem; and supportive counseling for parents. Several of these methods were employed in the case of Tim (see the next section). Mash and Terdal (1997, p. 111) state that there is overwhelming evidence for the efficacy of stimulant drugs in conjunction with behavioral interventions in the treatment of children with ADHD. Both procedures require family support, as demonstrated in Tim's case.

Family Considerations

The impact of living with a "hyped-up" child with many distractible and agitated behaviors cannot be minimized. Children with ADHD do not slow down, and even when watching television they may bounce on the couch, poke or tickle a sibling, and/or laugh raucously and fall on the floor. Bernier and Siegel (1994, p. 146) state that "the child's noncompliant, disruptive behavior contributes to chronic stress in parents, which in turn produces unproductive parenting behaviors that exacerbate the ADHD symptoms." The cycle of negative parent–child interactions that often characterizes a family with a child who has ADHD results in fewer gratifications in the parental role and reduced parental self-esteem. These factors in turn sometimes precipitate or aggravate parental problems, such as depression (Bernier & Siegel, 1994).

A focus on the parents and the family system, therefore, is essential when working with a child with ADHD. If the practitioner can effectively support the parents, this may help to prevent a negative cycle of behaviors that could become worse as the child gets older (Hallowell & Ratey, 1994). The case discussion that follows illustrates some cognitive-behavioral approaches in work with a 7-year-old boy with ADHD and his family.

The Case of Tim, Age 7: Helping a Child with ADHD and His Family

FAMILY INFORMATION

Mother	Kathy Marino, age 35, nursery school teacher.
Father	Tony Marino, age 37, music store owner. Plays in band several nights a week and on weekends.
Sister	Chris, age 3, attends nursery school (but not in Mrs. Marino's class).
Child client	Tim, age 7, second grade; plays hockey and soccer. ADHD diagnosed at end of first grade.
Paternal grandparents	In their 60s, babysit two or three times per month.
Maternal grandparents	In their 60s, live out of state.
Maternal uncle	Age 38, lives out of state; had ADHD.
Son of uncle	Age 10, has ADHD; on Ritalin.

The Marinos are a Caucasian Catholic family of Italian descent.

PRESENTING PROBLEM

The parents sought help because of Tim's recent diagnosis of ADHD. The school had wanted to retain Tim at the end of first grade, and the parents, who disagreed, had had Tim tested and put on Ritalin. They were concerned about how to handle this situation with him. The mother also wanted guidance as to how to manage Tim's difficult behavior at home.

ASSESSMENT AND PLAN FOR INTERVENTION

I saw the parents for an initial meeting, followed by three play assessment sessions with Tim. I requested and received the report from the psychologist, who stated that Tim's "principal dysfunction appears to be in the inattention component, somewhat less in the impulsive component, and even less in the hyperactive factor." (The hyperactive and impulsive components are now combined into one symptom group in DSM-5.) The psychologist recommended Ritalin, tutorial assistance, parent counseling, and cognitive-behavioral therapy for Tim.

My evaluation, which I shared with the parents in the feedback session, was that I found Tim to be a charming, very likable child who demonstrated in the sessions with me many of the characteristics of ADHD that would probably cause him difficulty in school. Specifically, I was concerned about the rushed, slapdash manner in which Tim made several drawings, without apparent care as to details (see Figures 6.2 and 6.3). The figure of the person (Figure 6.2) was very distorted, with enormous arms, and none of the figures in the family drawing (Figure 6.3) had hands or feet. These drawings were immature for a 7-year-old.

Moreover, in playing some board games with Tim, I noticed that he had a great deal of difficulty waiting for his turn and following rules, and I wondered how this might affect his social interactions. Curiously, when I asked Tim about friends, he was not able to remember any of their names. Tim also

FIGURE 6.2. Tim's Draw-A-Person.

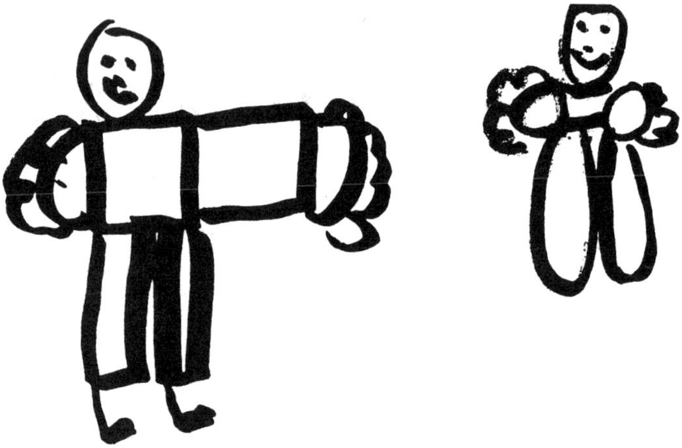

FIGURE 6.3. Tim's Draw-A-Family.

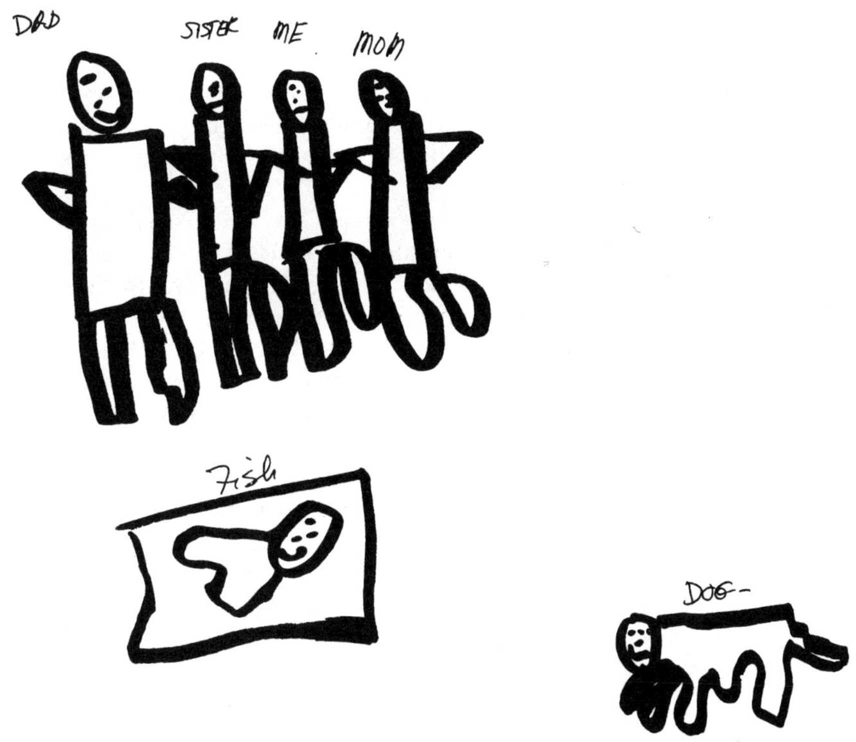

seemed to have a very distorted concept of numbers, telling me that his mother was 103 years old and that there were 93 children in his class at school!

The parents, especially Mrs. Marino, were very open about feeling "overwhelmed" by Tim. He was going to begin Ritalin soon, but even if it helped, they wanted some assistance in learning how to manage him. Because of Mr. Marino's long work hours, the mother often felt unsupported and unable to endure Tim's constant talking, night fears, and excessive demands in the evenings. We agreed on a plan for parent counseling, some mother–child sessions, and some work with Tim alone.

INTERVENTIONS

Sessions with Tim. My first goal was to establish a positive relationship with this boy, something that had already begun during the assessment phase. I had referred several times to the fact that I helped children and families with their troubles and worries. When Tim could not think of any worries, I let him know that his mother had told me that she lost her temper and yelled at him sometimes. He acknowledged that this happened but seemed incapable of recalling an example of when this happened or of thinking about what might help.

Sessions with Tim and His Mother. I suggested to Tim that we invite his mom into the session, and together the three of us would come up with some techniques to use when they were beginning to lose control, so they wouldn't end up screaming at each other.

I asked them to think of a signal they could give each other that would mean they had to stop talking and separate for a while. They came up with a hand movement across the mouth, which was supposed to signify "Zip your lip." Mrs. Marino was afraid that Tim would try to use this every time she told him to do something he didn't want to do, so I emphasized that this was meant *only* to keep them from screaming at each other. The next week, both Tim and his mother were happy to report that the signal had worked. There had been less negative interaction between them.

Mrs. Marino next wanted to figure out a way for Tim to be able to spend some time alone. She stated that he usually hung around her every minute when she was home and that she needed some quiet time to herself. I asked Tim to think of some things he could do by himself in his room. With Mrs. Marino's help, we made a list. Realizing that Tim would need an incentive to carry out these solitary behaviors, I introduced a graph and suggested a star system for every day Tim succeeded in staying by himself for 10 minutes and, if he got at least four stars, a reward at the end of the week. Tim became very animated as he thought about the rewards he would want, and he finally settled on a computer game, which he would be able to "earn" at the end of a month.

The concrete nature of the graph and the stars proved to be an excellent technique for motivating Tim, although there were some disagreements about whether time spent playing with his sister would count and whether he had to check with his mother *before* spending the time alone, as he sometimes would claim that he had completed a 10-minute period when his mother was not even home or aware of his behavior. Tim wanted to put more stars on the graph than he had earned, but his mother, with my support, was able to set appropriate limits. At the end of the month Tim earned his reward and immediately *asked* to start a new graph. (See Figure 6.4 for Tim's first graph.)

Another control technique that was useful for Tim was to have him construct a stop sign out of construction paper and hang it up in his room. With his mother, we talked about Tim's need to "slow down." His teacher had written this on his report card, and I thought that a tangible, visible reminder might be useful, as this had been effective with the graph. I also began to use some verbal directives during play sessions, when Tim appeared to be rushing. I would say to him, "You're going too fast. Close your eyes and imagine the stop sign. Count to five; then you can open your eyes and proceed *slowly*."

FIGURE 6.4. Tim's weekly graph for the first month of the graph/star system intervention.

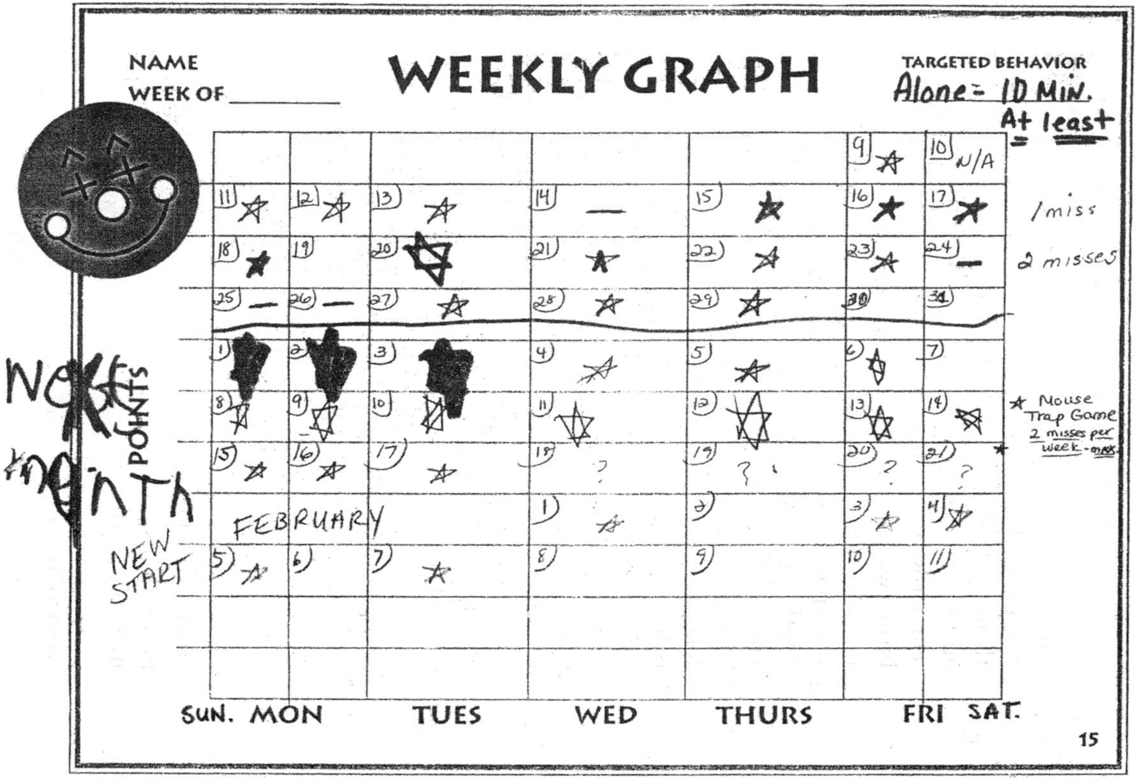

Parent Counseling. The parents had a good understanding of the biological component of ADHD, so it was not necessary for me to educate them about that. Nonetheless, Mr. Marino was not entirely happy with the idea of giving Tim a pill to help him concentrate better. He was afraid that this might mean that Tim would stop trying to help himself. I used the example of wearing glasses to help see better; this improves the focus, but it doesn't change the person's basic vision. Similarly, Ritalin does not change the underlying neurological condition, but it gives an immediate benefit for the person's ability to concentrate.

In discussing the graph with Mr. and Mrs. Marino, I emphasized that it motivated Tim because it gave him an immediate reinforcement that he knew would "pay off" later. I emphasized that it was very important for them to give Tim consistent praise whenever he behaved appropriately. I stated that the stars, for now, were an additional reinforcement but that the most important thing was for them to praise Tim when he showed control. Because it was not possible to know exactly how much Tim really *could* control his behavior even when he tried, it was necessary to set small, reasonable goals that he could achieve, so that neither he nor they would become frustrated. I pointed out that this was why I had suggested a 10-minute period of solitary play, rather than 30 minutes. I suggested that after consistent success with one goal, they could extend it in small increments, such as trying a 15-minute period after Tim demonstrated success with the 10-minute period.

Tracking Progress

I followed this child and family on a weekly basis over a school year, with several breaks because of holiday vacation periods. There was steady improvement in the mother–child relationship, to the point at which Tim no longer wanted his mother present during his sessions. His mother also confirmed during the parent sessions that she was feeling much better and that the tension between her and Tim had diminished substantially. I believe that this improvement was the result of several factors working together for this child's benefit:

1. *The medication,* which Tim took on school days and which improved his ability to concentrate and complete his schoolwork.

2. The various *behavioral methods* geared toward helping Tim control his own behavior and the tangible rewards he received when he succeeded.

3. The *increase in Tim's self-esteem,* which resulted from his having success experiences and receiving positive reinforcement from his parents.

4. The *parents' ability to work together* and support each other. In the parent meetings, Mr. Marino became more aware of his wife's need for

additional support in managing Tim. Mornings were especially difficult for her: She had to get to her job on time, and Tim was often noisy and resistant to getting dressed, which added to her stress. Although Mr. Marino had trouble getting up because he worked late in the evenings, the couple worked out a tradeoff of days on which each parent would be responsible for Tim in the mornings, and this relieved Mrs. Marino from feeling that she had to manage him entirely alone every day.

I planned to follow up with this family periodically, but I did not anticipate that they would need ongoing weekly meetings because they achieved such impressive gains in a relatively short time.

DISCUSSION

This case demonstrates how a child and family under the stress of a recent ADHD diagnosis can be helped effectively. The Marinos seemed to feel unable to function well despite their many strengths and areas of achievement. The interventions helped them to assume control of their lives once again and to feel better about one another, which inevitably led to improved parenting.

The specific behavioral interventions demonstrated in this case that are applicable to other children with ADHD and their families are listed in Figure 6.5. The members of this family were remarkable in their ability to help themselves once some limited guidance was offered to them. Many families will require longer and more extensive help. However, the principle of supporting the parents so that they can be more effective in supporting their own children is the key to working with families of children who have ADHD.

I did not contact Tim's teacher to collaborate with her, because Mrs. Marino assured me that the school was also employing behavior modification

FIGURE 6.5. Selected interventions for children with ADHD.

- Hand signal to stop arguing
- Graph and star system, charting one goal
- Solitary time/quiet time for parent and child separation
- List of solitary activities for child
- Stop sign (construction, display, and discussion)
- Tangible, agreed-upon reward for achieving goal
- Parents' use of praise to reinforce positive behavior
- Play therapy to promote and enhance Tim's self-esteem

techniques with him, and her descriptions of his teacher's approach seemed appropriate to me.

There probably will not be a true "termination" in this case, as ADHD typically continues at least until adolescence and sometimes into adulthood. It is important for the parents to know that they can contact me in the future, depending on their perceived need.

Update on Tim, Age 14

Tim and his mother came for one follow-up session at my request. He was a good-looking adolescent with close-cropped hair and a friendly manner. He spoke openly about his difficulty with his schoolwork, and he accepted without complaint the fact that he goes to the resource room 2 days a week for tutoring. He is passing all his classes in the C range, with an occasional D. He says that he does not like school, but he likes to be with his friends and have fun.

He has taken Ritalin and more recently Concerta to help him control his distractibility. He takes the medications only for school. He has achieved considerable success in hockey; he is on a varsity team and is a high-scoring valuable player. Tim's family supports his interest and attends all his games. Tim is very sociable, and his life revolves around ice hockey and his team. When I asked him about his plans after he graduates from high school, Tim said he might like to be a sports trainer.

In summary, this young man appeared to be doing well, despite his ongoing disability. He has good support from his family and school and appears to have good self-esteem related to his strong achievement in hockey.

Childhood Identity Issues: The Transgender Child

Modern society is beginning to acknowledge that children's biological/physical identity may not conform to their psychological/emotional selves (Goldman, 2008; National Geographic, 2017). Detailed personal accounts have been published in reputable newspapers about children who are uncomfortable with the gender into which they were born and the resulting turmoil this issue brings to their families who may feel shame or stigma associated with their children's insistence on being identified as a different gender (Jones, 2017; Peachman, 2017). Some families learn to accept this reality, whereas others cannot understand, refuse to acknowledge their child's insistence, and respond with punishment. Examples are given that illustrate the children's dilemmas and their families' divergent responses.

It is important to distinguish between gay and lesbian youth and those who are transgender. The transgender status involves drastic changes in appearance that may be difficult for families to tolerate and accept. The following definitions from Goldman (2008, pp. 24–26) clarify the terminology that describes different forms of gender identity:

- A *gay male* is a male with a homosexual attraction to another male.
- A *lesbian* is a female with a homosexual attraction to another female.
- *Transgender* refers to individuals whose gender identity or expression is different from their physical anatomy.
- *Transsexual* refers to transgender persons who identify with the opposite gender and who may seek gender reassignment surgery and/or hormones to become more like the gender with which they identify.

Goldman emphasizes the strong desire of the transgender male or female to be perceived by others as the gender with which they feel they identify. Some may become depressed and even suicidal when their perceived identity is not recognized as genuine by others (Jones, 2017).

DSM-5 (American Psychiatric Association, 2013) defines *gender dysphoria* in children as a condition demonstrating a "marked incongruence between one's experienced/expressed gender [i.e., the desired gender] and assigned gender [i.e., the gender at birth], of at least 6 months' duration, as manifested by at least six [out of eight criteria]" (p. 452). The first (mandatory) requirement involves a strong desire to be of the other gender or an insistence that he or she *is* the other gender. Other criteria involve a preference for to cross-dressing, paying with toys or games/activities of the other gender, and having playmates of the other gender, with a strong dislike for one's own sexual anatomy and a desire to have the secondary sex characteristics of the other gender. To conform to the diagnosis, all these conditions must be associated with clinically significant distress or impairment in school and other areas of functioning. The fact that gender dysphoria is a recognized psychiatric diagnosis may help some parents realize that their child has a bona fide condition that others share, and this recognition may result in their less likely minimization of the child's stated preferences in the future. Although gender dysphoria is relatively rare, occurring in less than 1% of the population, according to Brown (2014), it has nonetheless received growing public attention because of the difficulties associated with it.

Like gender-dysphoric youth, gay and lesbian young people who self-identify about their gender identity in their midteens may have had an internal sense about their orientations at much younger ages. The prejudice and stigma associated with homosexuality can cause youth to feel anxious and reluctant about openly admitting to their feelings about their sexual preferences. However, there is a growing trend toward greater acceptance as education and awareness about these issues has gradually increased, and as some public figures have openly revealed their own changed sexual identities.

The previous discussion emphasized how transgender youth often feel strongly that they were born in the "wrong bodies." The examples below illustrate the many stresses for young children who declare their transgender status and the varying responses to this in the child's family, from acceptance to denial.

The Case of a Resistant Mother Who Learned to Love Her Son

This heartfelt account of a transgender son was published in *The New York Times* (Jones, 2017). In the article, titled "How My Mom Learned to Love Her Son," the author, Tennessee Jones, reviews the numerous tragic events in his childhood, when he was a female with a strong desire to become male. When Tennessee was about age 9, he (then "she") remembers his mother beating him severely on several Sundays when he didn't want to wear a dress to church; Tennessee attempted to defend himself by saying that God was more concerned with someone's spirit than with his or her appearance, but his mother was unable to acknowledge her daughter's persistent desire to be a male. Tennessee came out about his male gender identity at age 17. Following that admission, one teacher told him that he would be going to hell, another warned him never to enter her classroom again, and the school administrator told Tennessee that he made him sick to his stomach (p. 9). At age 24, the anatomically female Tennessee had his breasts removed, and 4 years later had a complete hysterectomy. His mother had begged him not to "destroy parts of [his] body" under the "'delusion' that [he] was a man." Because of his mother's strong resistance, he decided not to have any further contact with his mother until after the surgeries were completed. In a strange twist of fate, 5 years later his mother was diagnosed with cancer of the uterus, and she contacted her then son to seek his advice about details of the operation based on his own experience. Over these shared experiences, the mother and son reconciled and engaged in some deep discussions and discoveries about each of their own past histories and feelings about one another and the gender issue.

The article clearly conveys the author's strong conviction that gender is immutable and how he felt absolutely compelled to make the transition into his "true" male self. He refers to friends who committed suicide and to the fact that many people hate trans people. The statistics indicate that about 40% of transgender people report having attempted suicide (Peachman, 2017). Depression is common, as is the scorn and hostility of many in and outside the family. In the case here, the author reports feeling rejected when he noticed that his mother had no photos of him as a child posted on her walls because she did not want to be questioned about the daughter who no longer existed. Thus the mother's acceptance of her daughter's transgender status is by no means complete, and the son continues to regret his mother's negative response.

A Family's Positive Response to Raising a Transgender Child

A different reaction by a different family regarding their transgender child was also published in *The New York Times* in January 2017. The experiences reported (by Peachman, 2017) might be viewed as ideal, because the parents openly accept their 4-year-old son's gender dysphoria and desire to be considered a girl. Despite the parents' support of their preschooler's gender identity, it is probable that many problems will inevitably arise in the future as this young child grows older.

Although anatomically male, this 4-year-old consistently pretended to be a female and wanted to dress up in princess costumes. He told his mother emphatically that he was not a boy, but "a girl in my heart and my brain." The parents had noticed that whenever their son would dress as he wished—in female clothes—he would become a much happier child.

After consulting with mental health practitioners and gender experts, the parents became convinced that their son was not just going through a phase. They permitted him to choose a new female name, and then they sent out a group email message announcing that their 4-year-old son would be starting prekindergarten that year as a girl named Ellie. They are participating in a TransYouth Study Project, the first large-scale national longitudinal study to examine the development of transgender and gender-nonconforming children. Although this family has received support from their community, they are aware that other families in similar situations may receive hate mail and death threats. They realize that there may be struggles ahead, such as about bathroom rights, but at this point their child currently is very happy as a girl and looking forward to being in prekindergarten.

Discussion

The cases in this chapter clearly emphasize the pivotal role of families in helping their children cope with biological conditions that negatively affect their lives. In the case of the boy with ADHD, the role of the social worker was critical in helping the boy learn to accept and adapt to the reality of his condition, as well as in helping his parents learn some methods to cope with their frustrations about their son's hyperactivity and to help the boy achieve some control over his behavior.

The role of a social worker in helping gender-dysphoric youth was not mentioned in either of the published cases reported here, so we must project our own versions of how a social worker might have assisted either family. In the first case, the school was unanimously negative about Tennessee's transgender status, as was the mother. It is unfortunate that the 9-year-old child had to cope alone with his situation, but he was able to persevere with his gender change at a later age. We do not know any details about his education or career after graduation. Hopefully, he did have some positive contact with helping professionals who validated his strong feelings and supported his choice for gender change.

In the case with the positive family, it is likely that the honeymoon will not last forever, and it is probable that the child will encounter numerous problems as she grows up and her identity change becomes known to her peers. Often such children are bullied or ostracized, and it will be important for the growing child to develop some contacts with other transgender girls such as herself so she will not feel isolated and depressed. Fortunately, she and her family are part of a research study where such contacts may be possible. Although the numbers of transgender youth are relatively low, many adolescents self-identify as gay or lesbian, and society is becoming gradually more open. Social work practitioners have an important role in creating a climate of acceptance in schools, recreational groups, and all locations in which young people interact.

CONCLUDING COMMENTS

This chapter has reviewed various ways of working with families to help their children. Although some practitioners follow a child-centered approach and others focus primarily on the family, I prefer an integrated child and family model because it offers the flexibility to tailor the helping method to the specific needs of each case situation.

It is assumed in this integrated approach that the practitioner will *always* involve the parents. We have discussed the different helping approaches that may be appropriate, such as parent counseling, working with the parent and child together, sibling sessions, and sessions with the entire family. Different members or subsets of the family may be seen, depending on the circumstances.

This work places special demands on the practitioner, who must endeavor to remain objective and try to understand the problem situation from the different perspectives of various family members. Ethical considerations surrounding confidentiality and cultural differences between clients and the practitioner require careful self-monitoring and regular supervision and consultation.

The strength of the family becomes the practitioner's ally once the helping relationship has been forged and mutual goals have been established. When the case involves a child with ADHD or gender identity issues, certain guidelines can help the family offer appropriate support to the child, once the parents feel that they are supported and respected by the worker.

DISCUSSION QUESTIONS AND ROLE-PLAY EXERCISES

1. How can a practitioner prepare to meet with an entire family for the first time? What information is essential to ensure the success of the meeting, and how can the practitioner best obtain this? Role-play the first 5 minutes of a family meeting with the Marino family.
2. If children become silly and out of control during a family session, what kind of response from the worker is appropriate and helpful? If the parents are unable to control the children, what options does the practitioner have?
3. Discuss how the child's therapist can effectively involve resistant parents in the treatment of their children. How can the therapist manage his or her own feelings of resentment toward the parents for their lack of involvement?
4. How should the practitioner respond when a child with ADHD and his or her family do not experience success in using a hand signal or the graph? If the parents want to punish the child, should the worker suggest another alternative? Discuss both in terms of whether the worker *should* intervene and, if he or she does so, what form the intervention might take. Role-play some different alternatives.
5. Make a list of potential positive reinforcements for a child whose parents cannot afford costly incentives, such as computer games and bicycles. How does the worker respond to the parent who thinks that offering rewards is "just bribery"?

CHAPTER 7

Individual Play Therapy with the Child

Play therapy is the preferred method for a social worker or other clinician to assist a child in dealing with his or her "problems" or anxieties. Because children have limited verbal abilities, we cannot expect them to adapt to our adult style of communication. Therefore, the social worker must "meet the (child) client where he or she is"—namely, on the level of *nonverbal* communication. It has been said that play is the child's work, so the therapist's work involves communicating with the child through the use of play in order to engage him or her. This applies primarily to children up to about 12 years of age, although play therapy has been used effectively with adolescents and even adults.

Many schools of social work do not teach the use of "play therapy" methods, which require specialized training on a post-master's level. I founded, directed, and taught in a post-master's certificate program in child and adolescent therapy at a university for more than 20 years, and I concur that play therapists require advanced training and supervision to understand all the nuances and symbolism of children's play. Nonetheless, I also know that numerous social workers in child welfare agencies and in schools and family agencies are confronted daily with children who desperately need assistance with their anxieties. Often a trained play therapist is not available to help these children, and their cases have been assigned to "regular" social workers. Because of this indisputable fact of life, I believe that it is incumbent for all social workers who deal with children to have some knowledge about play therapy, together with the courage to use it to the best of their ability for the benefit of their child clients. Hopefully, these workers will be able to receive supervision from someone who is trained and experienced, either in their agency or in the community. The Association for Play Therapy (APT) has a list of registered play therapy supervisors (RPT-S) in all states. This book is dedicated to the principle of ongoing learning; assisting children with their various difficulties can serve as a worthy helping experience, both for the child client and the social worker/play therapist. Of course, it will be beneficial to all if social workers decide to obtain more advanced instruction and experience in play therapy on a post-master's-degree level. Meanwhile, I hope that this chapter will introduce the field in a manner that will be useful and interesting to social workers, even as it will be a helpful resource for the benefit of their child clients.

In play therapy, the social worker or counselor uses the child's language of play as the primary helping method, with the amount of verbal communication dependent on the child's age and inclination to talk. When the child *can* talk, the worker or therapist talks with him or her, but usually the child is more comfortable and fluent in the language of play, so the therapist must accept the challenge of "speaking" and responding to the child through the child's symbolic language. Thompson and Rudolph (1992) state that in play therapy "the assumption is that children will translate their imagination into symbolic play action rather than words" (p. 197). Numerous examples in this book illustrate play communication with child clients.

Because this chapter focuses on one-to-one counseling with the child, it covers some of the basic techniques and approaches used in play therapy, distinguishing between directive and nondirective methods and between open-ended and planned short-term treatment of children. To illustrate the blend of nonverbal and verbal helping methods in work with an older child with verbal ability, a case is presented in which cognitive-behavioral methods combined with parental support helped a 10-year-old girl gain control over her sleep disturbance. The literature on the use of cognitive-behavioral play therapy has grown tremendously since I worked with this case, in which I used some of the methods described by Kendall (2000). Readers who want more information about using cognitive-behavioral methods for a variety of problem situations may consult Friedberg, McClure, and Garcia (2014) and Cohen, Mannarino, and Deblinger (2017).

INDIVIDUAL VERSUS FAMILY INTERVENTIONS

As stated repeatedly in this book, helping a child *always* includes work with the parents or caretakers and other significant family members. It also frequently involves contacts with teachers, the family physician or pediatrician, and other professionals who have had contact with the child and who have relevant information to share. Although this chapter focuses on one-to-one intervention with the child, this work *never* occurs in isolation and often (as in the cases to be discussed) entails tandem work with the parents. When the clinical social worker or counselor has established a cooperative relationship with the parents and has formulated a plan for individual work with the child following the series of assessment interviews, he or she then proceeds to work with the child in separate sessions. Parental contact then typically occurs monthly, sometimes with the child included in the parent sessions.

RATIONALE FOR WORKING SEPARATELY WITH THE CHILD

Like adults, children experience anxiety, which can arise from both internal and external sources. Defensive responses (i.e., defense mechanisms) can effectively ward off anxiety (Freud, 1937). However, when the defenses are immature or inadequate—as is true for many children—the anxiety may be converted to symptoms that "bind" the anxiety, but at a cost that interferes with day-to-day functioning.

The Case of Anna, Age 5: Posttraumatic Anxiety Disorder

An example of such anxiety can be seen in the case of Anna, age 5, who developed excessive clinging to her mother during the month following a fire that destroyed the family's apartment in the middle of the night. Although Anna could ride the school bus and attend school as usual, when she was in her new home she could not tolerate having her mother out of her sight. She followed her mother into the bathroom and from room to room in the family's new three-bedroom apartment. Anna's symptoms of clinging were specific to the home situation, indicating that the fire had destroyed her sense of safety and ability to play by herself or with friends in the apartment after school. When she was in her mother's presence, Anna felt secure. However, her need to keep in her mother's proximity interfered with her age-appropriate task of developing increased autonomy and peer relations. Anna's symptoms decreased after several play therapy sessions in which I directed her to draw pictures of the fire and of her favorite stuffed animal that perished in the blaze. On one of her pictures she dictated to me a "goodbye message" to her toy bunny, which was lost in the fire, and this activity seemed to help provide some closure and alleviated her symptoms. The use of drawings to help "debrief" children following traumatic experiences is discussed more fully in Chapters 12 and 14. The next case illustrates the use of puppets in individual work with a child.

The Case of Tammy, Age 4: Play Therapy and Parent Counseling

Tammy, age 4, was very fearful about having her mother leave her at nursery school. Her mother gave Tammy a picture of the two of them together, which Tammy carried in a little purse attached to her waist. Whenever she missed her mother, she could look at the photo. This "concrete" method of keeping her mother close worked successfully, until the day another child started crying. The teacher took that child on her lap, trying to console her. Tammy began sobbing and crying for her mother and could not be comforted by any of the adults present in the classroom. They had to call her mother to come pick her up. The next morning, when it was time to leave for school, Tammy said she had a stomachache. She began crying and subsequently vomited. This "symptomatic behavior," fueled by anxiety, lasted only until Tammy's mother, thinking that the child might have a virus, permitted Tammy to remain home; the stomachache anxiety disappeared as soon as the separation from the mother was no longer threatened. This behavior was repeated for several days, and although the mother recognized the meaning of Tammy's symptoms, she did not know how to cope with her daughter's separation fears. During the assessment phase, it became apparent to the social worker that the mother was quite depressed over her inability to become pregnant. Tammy's age-appropriate separation concerns were thus magnified because of the child's worry and confusion about her mother's sadness.

This case was successfully treated through parent counseling and individual play therapy sessions with Tammy. Tammy's fears had escalated to the point at which work with the mother alone was not sufficient to reassure the child that it would be safe for her to spend a few hours each day away from home, playing with peers. In play therapy sessions, Tammy played out her mother's concerns about becoming pregnant through her choice of a spider puppet who laid "thousands and thousands of eggs." It was evident that Tammy understood her mother's wish to get pregnant, even though the mother denied her daughter's knowledge of this. In directed play therapy, I took the role of a honeybee puppet who offered to babysit for the spider's children, so the mother spider could go shopping and buy food for her hungry spider babies. Tammy and I (as the spider and bee) played repeatedly the "goodbye"/leavetaking of the mother spider and her subsequent return to her children. During the mother's absence, I (as the babysitting bee) encouraged the spider children to have a good time playing and enjoying themselves. In effect, I gave both mother and child permission to pursue their own developmental needs. After less than 3 months, Tammy's separation fears at nursery school had totally abated. About a year later, the mother and Tammy came back to show off Tammy's new baby sister!

This example demonstrates the necessary tandem work with *both* the child and the parent to relieve the child's symptoms. Individual work with either the mother or the child would have been insufficient. Although counseling the mother to reassure her child that she (the mother) was "all right" was an essential part of treatment, it is unlikely that this reassurance alone would have diminished Tammy's anxiety, which seemed rooted in her conflict about whether to be a "big girl" or whether to remain "Mommy's baby." Individual work with the child moved things along more rapidly than would have occurred if I had intervened only with the mother. Through play communication, Tammy received the message that it was all right to play and have fun with peers in her mother's absence. The work with the mother emphasized my encouragement that she could "let Tammy go," even as the mother spider left her children safely in the care of the babysitting bee.

Situations Calling for One-to-One Interventions with the Child

When a child has developed symptoms, or when the child's behavior is so extreme as to interfere with his or her ability to interact with others and to proceed with age-appropriate social and cognitive tasks, then individual work is necessary to alleviate the child's anxiety and/or to help the child modify the behavior that is interfering with the normal push toward growth.

Other situations in which individual work with a child is recommended include instances in which the child has been abused, neglected, or abandoned by a parent. Children in these situations will benefit from the opportunity to express their confusion, rage, and neediness with a play therapist or social worker who validates their feelings and gives them the implicit message that what happened was not their fault. These communications often occur through the metaphor of play, with emotions expressed by puppets or doll figures. It is tricky work for the play therapist to confirm such a child's feelings without "blaming" the abusive or neglectful parent. The child needs to feel that the parent loves him or her, despite the hurtful behavior. The social worker or play therapist working with a child in this type of situation usually benefits from an opportunity to deal with his or her *own* feelings in supervision, as the tendency of the worker to join with the child and "blame" the parent for the child's difficulties must be recognized and held in check.

Sessions with a child alone also serve an important function when the child has low self-esteem because of a physical or cognitive disability. A one-to-one relationship with an adult strongly benefits the disabled child, who comes to feel valued as a person despite the disability. Of course, in such a situation the social worker is simultaneously counseling the parents to ensure that they are also attempting to enhance the child's deflated self-esteem. However, children sometimes discount their parents' attempts to praise them, whereas they can more easily accept an expression of genuine positive regard from an unrelated adult.

Yet another circumstance that merits one-to-one intervention with a child is exposure to traumatic events. When children have witnessed or been victims of violence, they require prompt "debriefing" to avert later development of symptoms. This debriefing gives them the opportunity to reenact in play what they witnessed or experienced in real life; it thus gives them a sense of control over a situation in which they were helpless. This controlled repetition puts distance between the frightening event and the present circumstances. The role of the social worker supports and emphasizes a child's survival of such a frightening experience and his or her present safety.

Thus children in a variety of situations gain from a one-to-one helping relationship with a social worker or other clinician who is dedicated to understanding and spending time to help them. When the opportunity for individual play sessions is presented in a thoughtful and appealing manner, most children flourish through the experience once they get to know the play therapist and understand the special opportunity for self-expression that the play therapy sessions provide.

However, the fact that something helps does not necessarily argue for its universal application. The realities of economic and time constraints may prevent many families from committing themselves to bringing children for unlimited play therapy appointments, unless the children's symptoms urgently motivate them to seek help. Almost always, the parents will also be expected to attend some counseling or family therapy sessions, so seeking help for children may result in a major commitment of time and resources that is difficult for many families. Because of these realities, time-limited contracts that are problem-focused are generally better understood and accepted by parents than are treatment goals geared to more general and vague objectives, such as "improved self-esteem." Parents who are from non-European Anglo backgrounds may not understand the concept of mental health services and will require sensitive counseling regarding their child's needs and potential benefit from therapy. My edited book *Culturally Diverse Parent–Child and Family Relationships* (Webb, 2001) provides guidance for practitioners who are working with families from different cultural backgrounds.

In summary, children with the following types of presenting problems will benefit from one-to-one sessions with a play therapist (in addition to whatever intervention may be occurring simultaneously with their parents and/or families):

1. *Children whose anxiety has escalated to the point at which they are not functioning appropriately at home or at school.* They may have developed symptoms, the course of their normal development may have been arrested, and/or they may appear to be "stuck."

2. *Children who have been abused, neglected, and/or abandoned.* As noted, children need to express their confusion, rage, and other feelings about why this happened to them; they also need to understand that it was not their fault. Because their ability to trust adults may be impaired, work with these children may require more time than work with children whose development has not been so seriously compromised.

3. *Children with disabilities that engender feelings of low self-esteem.* Often these children are painfully aware that they are "different" from their peers, and this difference may cause them pain and anger. Work with these children proceeds well when the social worker or counselor can identify some genuinely likable qualities and/or talents in which the youngsters can begin to take some pride. These children's ability to accept themselves as persons with disabilities frequently follows the experience of mourning (through play therapy) for the qualities or abilities they never had.

4. *Children who have been traumatized.* Depending on the circumstances, individual play therapy may be a valuable option, in addition to group and/or family approaches. The more violent the trauma, the more likely it is that victims will require individual intervention. Ideally, this should be offered *before* the emergence of symptoms, as a preventive strategy.

5. *Children who show signs of gender confusion.* This may be manifested in preferred forms of dress, in friendships, and in choice of activities. Often parents and other adults may press these children to conform to their biological gender and this can make the children very anxious. Situations such as these will require both individual and family counseling to safeguard the child's emotional and physical needs.

SELECTED PLAY THERAPY TECHNIQUES

It is ironic that many social work students have contact with young children during their internships and are expected to interact helpfully with them, yet their coursework may not have prepared them in even the most basic play therapy techniques appropriate for work with their child clients. A few years ago I sent a survey to all baccalaureate and master's programs in social work to learn details about curriculum content related to direct intervention with children. Although 48 out of 84 returned responses from BSW programs indicated that their courses contained content related to providing services for *children,* half (24) of the respondents stated that they did not think there was a need to teach *play therapy* content in their curricula. The reasons given for this were the beliefs that play therapy content is "too specialized" and "not relevant to the work of BSW practitioners." The two negative responses out of a total of 48 from the MSW programs stated that (1) their curriculum was not "therapy-oriented" and (2) that their curriculum was based on a "family systems" model.

Although I do agree that play therapy is a specialized field, I nonetheless argue that social workers at *all* levels can and should be able to use some basic play therapy techniques in their work with children. Generic practitioners need this knowledge and skill just as clinical specialists do, and, clearly, familiarity with play therapy techniques is essential for social workers using a family systems perspective.

Terminology

Let us not be afraid of the word "therapy." I suspect that some of the negative responses in the survey about including play therapy in the social work curriculum reflect a backlash against the medical (clinical treatment) model and a preference to cast social work in a broad context that sees the individual in terms of family and social influences. Although I share a wide view of social workers' professional identity, I do not exclude the concept of therapy as a legitimate helping method *within social work* for individuals (of any age) who are in pain and need of service. The dictionary lists "care" as a synonym for "therapy."

What Is Play Therapy?

The term "play therapy" refers to helping interventions with children that employ *play* techniques within the context of a helping relationship. Clinicians who refer to themselves as "play therapists" come from many disciplines in addition to social work, and all have had specialized training and supervision on an advanced level. The list of child-related professional organizations in the Appendices includes the Association for Play Therapy, which regulates post-master's-degree training in this field. Some social workers may wish to obtain this advanced training. However, social workers at all levels can learn to utilize selected play therapy techniques in their work with child clients.

The choice of specific activities will vary according to the child's age and responsiveness to different options; therefore, each social worker's office should contain a range of play materials from which the worker and the child can make selections. (See Figure 3.3 for a list of basic supplies.) The following subsections discuss selected basic play therapy techniques and necessary supplies.

Play Therapy Materials

Figure 3.3 and Table 4.1 list play therapy equipment that I recommend for *every* social worker's office. Even a worker specializing in gerontology may be called upon, for example, to intervene with a school-age grandchild of a terminally ill woman being transferred to hospice care. Providing this child with some drawing paper and markers and suggesting that she draw her happiest memory about "Gramma" will not only occupy the child and permit the worker to speak with the child's mother about necessary plans for convening the family but will also serve an anticipatory grieving function for the child and the mother, who can recognize in the picture a concrete portrayal of the grandmother's significant role in the family. The grandchild can communicate her feelings through concrete images rather than in words, because young children have limited abilities to express emotions in language.

Art/Drawing

In my experience, plain white paper, colored paper, and colored markers are the most useful of all play therapy supplies. Children as young as 3 and as old as 18 can express themselves meaningfully through art and drawings, especially when the play therapist or social worker makes it clear that "drawing here is not like drawing in school; you don't have to be good at it to be able to show how you feel." Furthermore, family members can work on drawings or collages together, when given the opportunity and encouragement to express themselves in this manner.

Chapter 4 discussed how the Draw-A-Person and the Draw-A-Family tasks can provide useful information in assessing how a child sees himself or herself and his or her family. I usually keep these drawings in a special folder with the child's name on it, so the child and I can examine them together at different points in our work. I often ask the child to repeat both these drawings after several months to note any changes over the course of time.

When the child refuses to draw or says that he or she can't draw, the "squiggle game" (Winnicott, 1971a, 1971b) almost invariably intrigues the child even as it loosens up his or her inhibitions. In this game, which is essentially a technique of communication through drawings, the child and worker or therapist take turns closing their eyes and then making some kind of "scribble/squiggle" line on the paper, which the other person then has to turn into a figure or object. Each drawing receives a name, and after several have been completed, the child is asked to pick his or her favorite and make up a story about it. An example of the use of this method with a 9-year-old girl whose friend had died tragically can be found in Webb (1993, 2001). This child, who could not bear to talk about her dead friend, made up a "squiggle story" that was replete with danger and threatening death themes. See Di Leo (1973), Oster and Gould (1987), Rubin (1984), and Malchiodi (1998, 2006, 2011) for guidance in understanding and interpreting children's drawings.

Clay and Play-Doh

Also of compelling appeal across the age span, modeling materials allow a child to create something completely original. Play-Doh is soft and malleable and thus more appropriate for use with the preschool child; modeling clay is stiffer and requires some manual strength to mold into shapes, therefore making it more suitable for school-age children. In a video demonstration of play therapy techniques (Webb, 1994b, 2006a), a 4-year-old child who was completely uninterested in drawing enthusiastically created dragons and monsters with Play-Doh, thereby suggesting some of his own fears about uncontrolled aggression. On the same video, a 12-year-old girl created a sun with clay as she reflected on how her earlier therapy using clay had helped her gain control over her anger. See Oaklander (1988) for specific suggestions about using clay in group, family, and individual work with children.

Dolls/Puppets

Miniature, bendable family dolls readily lend themselves to reenactment of scenes from a child's family. Preschoolers eagerly engage in this type of play, which can be facilitated through the use of dollhouse furniture representing the kitchen and bedroom(s). These supplies can be stored in a small container, such as a lunch bag or satchel. I mention this to emphasize that the minimum supplies for play therapy are easily portable and do not require extensive storage space. A fancy dollhouse, for example, is neither necessary nor appropriate, as many children live in small apartments, whereas the typical dollhouse represents a suburban upper-middle-class home. Children are very creative about adapting objects in the office to their play needs (e.g., using tissues for blankets or a turned-over bowl for a kitchen table). *A worker does not need to offer elaborate play materials to engage a child in play activities.*

Animal and insect puppets appeal to boys and latency-age children, who may believe that dolls are "sissy" and only for girls or younger children. Woltmann (1951/1964) suggests that the selection of puppets should provide the child with the opportunity to express a variety of emotions. For example, an alligator puppet will almost always call forth aggressive, biting play, whereas a rabbit or duck is more "neutral." Assuming that the child and the worker/therapist can each hold two puppets at a time, Woltmann suggests (as a minimum) that the choices available to the child should include two neutral and two aggressive puppets. My own preference is to offer a choice of at least six puppets, so that the child who may not wish to select aggressive puppets will not be forced to do so. Again, I stress that hand puppets are neither heavy nor bulky and can be easily stored in a desk drawer with other play therapy supplies. Often it is possible to find small finger puppets representing insects or animals. When several hand and finger puppets of the same type are used in combination, they often become a "family," and the child may act out some interesting family dynamics using the finger puppets as the children and the larger hand puppets as the parents.

Card and Board Games

Since the publication of *Game Play* (Schaefer & Reid, 1986, 2001), there has been growing awareness of the usefulness of board games with latency-age children in therapy. There has also been a virtual flooding of the market with "therapeutic" board games. Schaefer and Reid (2001) have pointed out the numerous ways in which child therapists can help children while playing board games with them. This understanding is crucial to knowing the difference between just playing with a child and playing *therapeutically* with a child. In numerous workshops on play therapy across the country, I have been asked, "How can playing checkers or Monopoly with a child be therapeutic?" My answer is that unless the worker or therapist has a purpose in mind and responds consistently to the child during the play according to this purpose, the playing of a game may *not* be therapeutic (apart from the opportunity it provides to build a relationship with the child). For example, it can help the child to point out to him or her during the play that he or she seems to have trouble following the rules and that this must cause problems when he or she plays with other children. The therapist can then offer to help the child slow down and wait for his or her turn, so that he or she can "be a better player."

Because I am focusing on *basic* play therapy techniques and the necessary supplies for these, I limit my recommendations here to two games that I have found especially useful in work with elementary school-age children: the Talking, Feeling, and Doing Game (available on Amazon) and the card game Feelings Playing Cards (also available from Amazon). (See websites for suppliers of play resources and materials in the Appendices.) These games have certain features that make them attractive to school-age children. In common with commercial board games, they feature the possibility of winning (and losing), and this characteristic enables a worker/therapist to see and talk with a child about how he or she wins or loses during daily activities. In contrast to commercial board games, however, these therapeutic games require a discussion of feelings as an integral part of playing. They give the worker/therapist the opportunity to model "feeling" responses that the child may initially consider inappropriate. For example, when a card in a game asks, "What is the worst thing that someone can say to someone else?" and the therapist responds, "That you are stupid," the child learns that talking about embarrassing issues is all right. Chips are awarded for each response, further motivating the child to respond to each question.

USING THE CHILD'S PLAY THERAPEUTICALLY

Playing therapeutically with a child takes training, experience, and the special ability to relate to the child both playfully and with respect. It is not my intention to suggest that simply by acquiring some play materials, a worker can then, as if by magic, successfully carry out play therapy. In fact, having the necessary supplies is only the beginning of a process that will take hours of persistent relearning of the language of play and struggling to communicate through this symbolic language. We all knew this language as children ourselves, so using it as adults requires the ability to tap into old understandings from our childhoods.

At first, the work feels awkward and confusing. Social workers with many years of experience have said to me, "At least when I speak to adults, I usually know that they understand me; with children, it can be very puzzling. How do I know that I am playing helpfully or therapeutically with a child?"

This is, of course, the $64,000 question. We do *not* know initially whether our work with children is helpful. We do know that it will not harm children to spend time with adults who are interested in them. Just as in adult therapy, the *relationship* is the key to being helpful, not whether a worker invariably makes the "right" response. And progress takes time, whether with adults or with children. When supervising therapists who are doubtful about the effectiveness of their work with children, I often find myself relying on the phrase "Trust the process; it may take time."

Evidence-Based Considerations

An entire issue of the *International Journal of Play Therapy* (January 2010) focuses on the future direction of play therapy research. Two articles debate whether and to what extent play therapy methods have a valid evidence base (Phillips, 2010; Baggerly & Bratton, 2010). This matter is still controversial, but it is clear that an increasing body of research testifies as to the strength of play therapy methods, especially for children facing medical procedures (Li, Lopez, & Lee, 2007), in filial therapy (Landreth & Bratton, 2006) and in parent–child interaction therapy (Reddy et al., 2005). See Baggerly et al. (2010) for a review of evidence-based research as applied to play therapy.

LETTING THE CHILD DIRECT THE PLAY

As an experienced play therapist, I feel comfortable asking a child what he or she wants me to do (or say). Letting the child direct the play can reveal far more than a response that *I* might guess to be appropriate. I have also found that when the child continues to play a specific game or repeats a story theme (whether or not I immediately understand the underlying meaning of the play), it often serves a purpose for the child. Usually, by reflecting about the *themes* of the child's play retrospectively over several sessions, I begin to comprehend its significance. For example, a child therapist in supervision commented that her 5-year-old child client repeatedly set up a play situation in which the therapist was "in jail" because she had done something "bad." The therapist felt trapped, did not understand why the child kept repeating this play, and did not know what to say or do to help the child. I asked the therapist to think about what this play theme might mean in terms of the child's life. Her parents had recently divorced, and, although she said this was better because "now they pay more attention to me when I am with them," the child says she doesn't have any idea why they divorced. When the therapist asked her to make a guess, the child said, "Someone must have done something very, very bad." In her play, the child's concrete thinking was struggling to figure this out.

Ultimately, improvement of the problem or the symptoms suggests that something beneficial has happened. Occasionally, a parent credits the child's play therapy. However, this evaluation (no matter how flattering) cannot be accepted as the *exclusive* reason for change. The parent or parents have also been interacting with the child in a different way based on parent counseling or family therapy, and it is important that the worker or therapist attribute some of the child's improvement to the changes in the *family*. Almost always, progress is multidetermined.

Steps in Play Therapy Interactions with the Child

Play therapy with a child can be divided into the following phases:

1. Establishing the relationship with the child.
2. Observing and listening to the child.
3. Identifying themes in the child's play.
4. Formulating a dynamic understanding about the child (the assessment).
5. Responding to the child in a play context according to this understanding.
6. Setting goals to help relieve the child's presenting problem.

These phases of child therapy may overlap. They are listed in order of both occurrence and difficulty, which explains why some workers who are new to working with children may be unable to respond using a child's play language, despite their ability to relate well to young clients. A *therapeutic* response within a child's play language requires that the worker understand first what the child is communicating and then how this communication reflects interactions and/or feelings from the child's life. Sometimes the connection between the symbolic play and the child's life is obvious, but just as often it is not. The ability to connect the symbol to the child's life requires many hours of supervised practice experience with children. For example, probably most readers instinctively understood the underlying meaning of Tammy's selection of the spider puppet who laid "thousands and thousands of eggs." This could be viewed as the child's wish for her mother to have many babies. My quick response to the child's play scenario followed from the dynamic understanding that Tammy was afraid to leave her mother because her mother was sad (because she couldn't make any more babies) and needed her to help her feel better; furthermore, I believed that Tammy needed practice in saying goodbye to her mother and permission to have fun in her mother's absence. This dynamic understanding formed the basis for my assumption in suggesting and playing the role of the babysitting bee who could encourage the little spiders to play and have fun in their mother's absence.

When this kind of connection is not readily apparent, it is important for the worker to be able to tolerate ambiguity and to exercise patience while letting the helping process evolve. Not knowing is all right and is well tolerated by children (who often feel baffled themselves in trying to understand their world). It is perfectly acceptable for the therapist to ask clarifying questions to the child (within in the language of play). For example, the therapist who didn't understand why her child client repeatedly put her in prison could have said to the child: "I don't know why I am in prison. Tell me what I did that was bad."

When the child has been given the explanation of who the worker is ("someone who helps children and parents with their troubles and worries") and how the child and worker will interact ("sometimes we talk, and sometimes we play"), then the child is free to begin revealing his or her concerns to the worker/therapist. Incidentally, social workers should avoid using the term "working" in referring to their interactions with children. Talking and playing do not qualify as "work" in a child's *literal* understanding of the word, and if a worker says that he or she is going to be "working" with a child, the child may become confused about what to expect.

DIFFERENT CHILD THERAPY APPROACHES

Brief Historical Synopsis

The practice of child therapy has been in existence since the 1930s and 1940s, when Melanie Klein (1937) and Anna Freud (1946/1968), working separately, adapted methods of adult psychoanalysis to child analysis. Despite disagreements between these two child therapists about certain theoretical and practice issues in work with children, both therapists agreed about the importance of the therapeutic relationship with the child, and they both relied on play as the primary method of therapeutic communication with children.

In the more than 80 years since the beginnings of child therapy, many variations have evolved. Social workers, counselors, psychologists, psychiatrists, and others have developed a wide range of therapeutic interventions. In fact, Kazdin (1988) lists more than 230 "alternative psychosocial treatments" for children and adolescents—a number that seems mind-boggling, even allowing for his inclusion of group and family interventions. Kazdin's list contains some treatments with similar names, suggesting overlap among various approaches; it also includes activities such as yoga and sports groups (not considered therapy in the usual sense), as well as some discrete play therapy *techniques,* such as Winnicott's "squiggle game" and the Talking, Feeling, and Doing Game. It is important to note that these games are always used in combination with other helping methods and cannot therefore be considered as integrated psychosocial treatment methods. Thus Kazdin's list of alternative "treatments" must be viewed with great reservations in regard to the total number. Even with these reservations, however, it *is* evident that there has been a proliferation of treatment approaches geared to children. No longer are most methods guided primarily by the theoretical underpinnings of psychoanalysis; instead, various behavioral, cognitive, and client-centered therapeutic models have been adapted from adult treatment approaches to serve the purposes of child therapy. Four major approaches utilized by contemporary child therapists are (1) client-centered (child-centered) treatment, (2) psychodynamic child therapy, (3) cognitive-behavioral treatment, and (4) integrated child therapy.

Client-Centered or Child-Centered Therapy

The basic tenets of the client-centered approach with children, as described by Axline (1947), are as follows:

- Establishment of a warm rapport with the child.
- Empathic understanding and respect for the child's ability to solve his or her own problems.
- A nondirective stance on the part of the therapist, who lets the child lead the way without directing the child in any manner, for as long as the child needs treatment.

In *Dibs: In Search of Self,* Axline (1964) demonstrated the child-centered approach, using play therapy with a 5-year-old boy who was on the verge of residential placement because of his mutism and his teachers' inability to have any helpful interactions with him. Dibs flourished in nondirective play therapy with Axline, in which he developed and achieved his exceptional potential, in large measure because of Axline's ability to convey her genuine positive regard for him.

The child-centered approach has changed very little since its inception in the 1940s, with Axline's (1947) text continuing to be "the single best guide for client-centered psychotherapy with children" (Johnson, Rasbury, & Siegel, 1986, p. 130). Other past and current therapists following the child-centered model include Moustakas (1959) and Landreth (2002a, 2002b, 2012).

In summary, child-centered therapy is permissive, nondirective, and open-ended. Because it proceeds at the child's pace, it tends to be long term. It focuses on the person of the child, not on the child's problem. Its emphasis on the child's potential for growth is very appealing to social workers and others who wish to focus on clients' strengths rather than on pathology. These positive factors must be balanced against the realities of parents' ability to pay for long-term therapy and/or on the limits established by insurance companies about the acceptable length of treatment.

Psychodynamic Child Therapy

Over the years, what began as child psychoanalysis has evolved into a less intensive, more practical approach to working with children—one that still recognizes the existence and power of instincts and conflicts in motivating behavior but that now tends to focus on problems in the child's present life rather than on the child's internal intrapsychic world. Because it is assumed that a child's behaviors and symptoms reflect complex, unconsciously determined meanings, therapy with the child relies on a thorough assessment to facilitate the therapist's understanding of the child's unconscious motivations, fantasies, impulses, and conflicts as reflected in his or her play. The therapist may utilize aspects of the relationship to make interpretations about the child's wishes and fears with respect to meaningful and significant relationships in the child's past and present life (Brandell, 2002; Chethik, 2000; LeVine & Sallee, 1992).

Although therapists differ in the specifics of their approaches, psychodynamic child therapy tends to be more directive than child-centered therapy.

Especially when it is geared toward helping a child who has been traumatized, it may be focused and of relatively short duration (Terr, 1983, 1989). Using a psychodynamic framework of understanding, the therapist engaged in crisis intervention helps the traumatized child reconstruct the traumatic experience so that the child can gain mastery over the trauma, acknowledge that he or she has survived, and realize that the trauma belongs in the past. To bring about this transformation requires a high level of direction on the part of the therapist, who may provide specific toys to facilitate the play reenactment. This form of crisis therapy has been helpful for child victims of sexual and cult abuse, in addition to children who have witnessed violence and atrocities and who may be showing symptoms of PTSD. Bevin (1999), Strand (1999), and James (1989) provide examples of therapy with traumatized children that utilize crisis intervention reconstructive techniques. This work is stressful and demands a high level of skill. An evidence-based approach can be found in the trauma-focused cognitive-behavioral therapy model (TF-CBT; Cohen, Mannarino, & Deblinger, 2012, 2017), which is discussed further in Chapter 15. *Therapists should not engage in this type of work without special training and supervision.*

In summary, psychodynamic child therapy focuses on helping the child cope with his or her everyday life and with the problems that result in disturbing symptoms. It relies on an in-depth understanding of the child's history and present circumstances in order to make connections in play and/or in words that will relieve the child's anxieties and open up new possibilities to the child. When used in crisis intervention, this form of therapy is very directive. Concurrent parent counseling is an essential component of the one-to-one work with the child.

Cognitive-Behavioral Treatment of Children

In contrast to child-centered or psychodynamic therapy, cognitive-behavioral therapy (CBT) focuses on the child's thoughts (cognitions) and behaviors, rather than the child's feelings. There are many different forms of CBT, all of which employ learning principles in attempting to alter dysfunctional behavior. After a careful assessment of the presenting problem and of the environmental and/or cognitive antecedents of the problematic behavior, an individual treatment program is tailored to the specific needs and situation of the individual child and family. When the therapist finds that the child's maladaptive thoughts are leading to maladaptive behavior, then the intervention emphasizes helping the child change his or her negative thoughts through self-instructional training, sometimes referred to as "self-talk." When environmental factors appear to be contributing to the persistence of a behavior pattern, then the intervention will target these reinforcing environmental responses through various techniques, such as positive reinforcement of desired behaviors, negative consequences or punishment to encourage behavioral change, and the use of tokens (Friedberg et al., 2009; LeVine & Sallee, 1992; Kendall, 2000, 2006, 2012).

Because children are so dependent on the significant others in their environments, parents and teachers are often enlisted to help with children's behavior modification plans. According to Johnson et al. (1986), "the success of behavioral procedures is often highly dependent on the direct participation of significant members of the child's environment in the treatment program" (p. 184). In the TF-CBT model, parents are viewed as essential sources of support for children, and separate sessions are arranged for them prior to eventual parent–child sessions at the point when the child is able to verbally discuss the traumatic experience with the parent. The collaboration of a 10-year-old girl and her parents in a cognitive-behavioral treatment approach is described in the case of Linda, in the following section.

Synthesis of Approaches: Integrated Child Therapy

It is possible and useful to combine therapeutic approaches when this seems indicated by the circumstances of the particular case. Wachtel (1994) recommends an integrated treatment approach that employs a combination of systemic, psychodynamic, and behavioral interventions simultaneously. Wachtel (1994, pp. 201–202) states:

> We do not wait until all systematic issues are resolved before attending to the psychodynamic aspect of the problem, nor do we attempt to fully resolve psychodynamic or systemic issues before introducing behavioral interventions. Instead, *psychodynamic and systemic understandings of the problem go hand in hand with behavioral methods targeted at the symptomatic behavior.* (emphasis added)

Drewes and colleagues (2011) have edited a book that demonstrates the many ways that an eclectic approach can effectively integrate more than one perspective in treating children. This philosophy recognizes that models of practice often overlap and that the experienced practitioner learns to adapt practice to the client's needs rather than vice versa.

THE CASE OF LINDA, AGE 10: PARENT AND CHILD COGNITIVE-BEHAVIORAL APPROACHES

Family Information

Mother	Ann, age 34, buyer for department store.
Father	Jim, age 35, architect in building firm; recovering alcoholic (12 years).
Child client	Linda, age 10, fifth grade; on gymnastics team.
Sister	Amanda, age 8, third grade; very artistic.

Linda's godfather	Robert, age 35, former restaurant manager; recovering alcoholic (14 years).
Linda's godmother	Terry, age 34, secretary.
Robert and Terry's children	Susan, age 6, and Brian, age 4.

Linda was young Brian's godmother, and Linda and Amanda referred to Robert and Terry as "Aunt" and "Uncle." Robert was Jim's Alcoholics Anonymous sponsor; they generally attended meetings together three times per week. Ann had attended Al-Anon in the past (sometimes with Terry), and the girls had attended a group for children of alcoholics (Unicorn) several years earlier. At the time of intake, Ann was engaged in her own therapy, as was Jim.

This was a Catholic family of European cultural background. The family members observed major milestones, such as First Communion, according to the expected practice in their religion, but they did not attend church regularly.

Presenting Problem

Upon the recommendation of her pediatrician, Ann consulted me because of her concern about Linda's sleep problem of 2 months' duration. Linda was waking every night in the middle of the night because of bad dreams about robbers; she would turn on all the lights in the house and then come into her parents' bedroom and stand by their bed until one of them awoke and returned with her to her bedroom.

The parents reported that Linda's sleep difficulty had begun during the family's vacation with Robert and Terry and their children. Linda had awakened in the middle of the night and become panic-stricken when she mistakenly thought a "robber" was kidnapping her godson, Brian. Actually Robert was carrying his son to the bathroom, but in a strange location and in the dark, Linda was disoriented and terrified. She had to spend that night sleeping in the room with her parents, and she had continued to awaken every night since then. The parents were at first sympathetic, assuming that Linda's problem would subside spontaneously, but they were now becoming tired, annoyed, and concerned about Linda's behavior.

Assessment

I saw the parents once so that I could obtain their view of the problem and learn about Linda's developmental history and the family background. I then saw Linda for two assessment sessions in which we discussed the problem and several possible ways to deal with it.

In the meeting with the parents, I learned that Linda was functioning on a very high level in school and with peers. She was an excellent student and an enthusiastic member of the school gymnastics team. She had slept in her own room since age 2 and had not had separation problems; however, the mother considered Linda somewhat anxious and intense and thought that she put a lot of pressure on herself to succeed. Through the years Linda had expressed some fears at night related to bad dreams, but she was easily consoled, and the parents had not been concerned until this current nightly problem. The father said he had recently lost patience with Linda, yelled at her, and shaken her when she woke him up in the middle of the night. Both parents were firm in feeling that "this just cannot continue."

In the two assessment sessions with Linda, I tried to understand the reason for the persistence of this problem. Linda said that she woke up because of a dream that a robber was going to "get" her. When this happened, she would get up and put on all the lights in her room, the hall, and the bathroom. Then she would walk into her parents' bedroom and stand by their bed until one of them woke up. She would tell them she had a bad dream, and then either her mother or her father would take her back to her room, reassuring her that it was only a dream and that she was all right.

Because of Linda's age, the work with her combined talking and some play (drawing). During Linda's discussion with me, I asked her to sketch a floor plan of her house and her bedroom so I could get a better picture of her family situation (see Figures 7.1 and 7.2). I also wanted her to draw her dream, and I asked her to draw it in two different ways: the dream she was having now, and the dream she would have later when she was no longer waking up with the bad dream. Figure 7.3 depicts Linda's two dreams, in a "before" (i.e., current) version, with the alarm clock registering 2:00 and a male figure saying, "I'm going to get you"; the "after" dream shows her lying in bed asleep while having a happy dream of going down a slide and saying, "Whee!" I also asked Linda to draw a picture of herself showing how she would look after she had a good night's sleep without waking up. She drew a figure with a smile, saying "Rise and shine," with the alarm clock indicating 7:00 A.M. (Figure 7.4).

In asking for the "after" drawings, I was deliberately conveying the positive suggestion to Linda that her bad dreams would end and that she would feel better as a result. I also made several references to how brave she must be to be able to perform back flips on the balance beam in gymnastics. I wanted to emphasize Linda's strengths in a manner that would help her feel confident and assured that she could successfully master her nighttime fears.

Knowing that it was developmentally unusual for a 10-year-old to be going into her parents' bedroom every night, and also having heard from the father than his patience was wearing thin, I made the decision to begin work immediately on extinguishing this behavior of Linda's. I tried to make this behavior seem inappropriate (ego-dystonic) to Linda by saying to her in a sympathetic tone, "It must be *very* embarrassing for a 10-year-old to have to go to her parents at night! I know that many 4- and 5-year-olds do this, but it certainly is not what most 10-year-olds want to do. We need to think together

FIGURE 7.1. Floor plan of Linda's house.

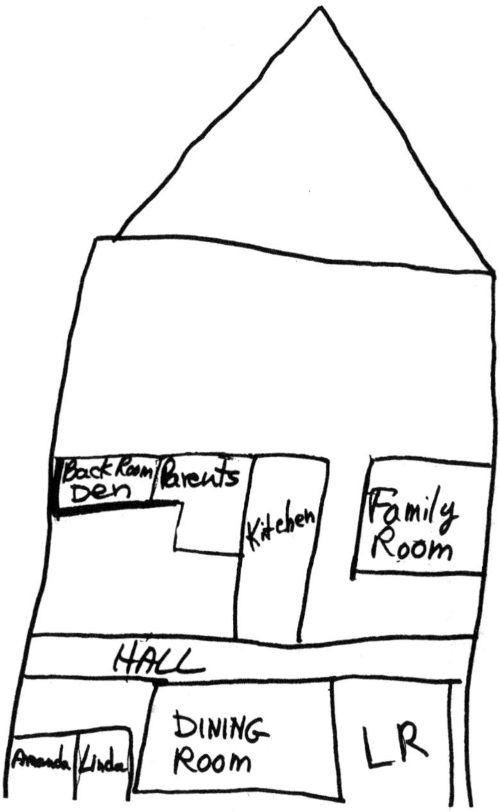

about what you can do for *yourself* when you wake up to help you feel better." I then involved Linda in making a list of substitute behaviors, such as listening to her Walkman radio, drawing, writing in her diary, and so forth. A family meeting was planned for the next week to talk about some of the ways Linda's parents could help her, as well as to obtain everyone's input and agreement to a behavior modification plan.

Family Meeting

The meeting was attended by Linda and her parents. I began by stating a common purpose—that of our working together to help Linda get control over her "nighttime problem." Everyone wanted relief in this situation, and each would have a part in helping.

First, we agreed that Linda was old enough to take care of herself at night without involving her parents. She couldn't control her dreams or the fact

FIGURE 7.2. Floor plan of Linda's bedroom.

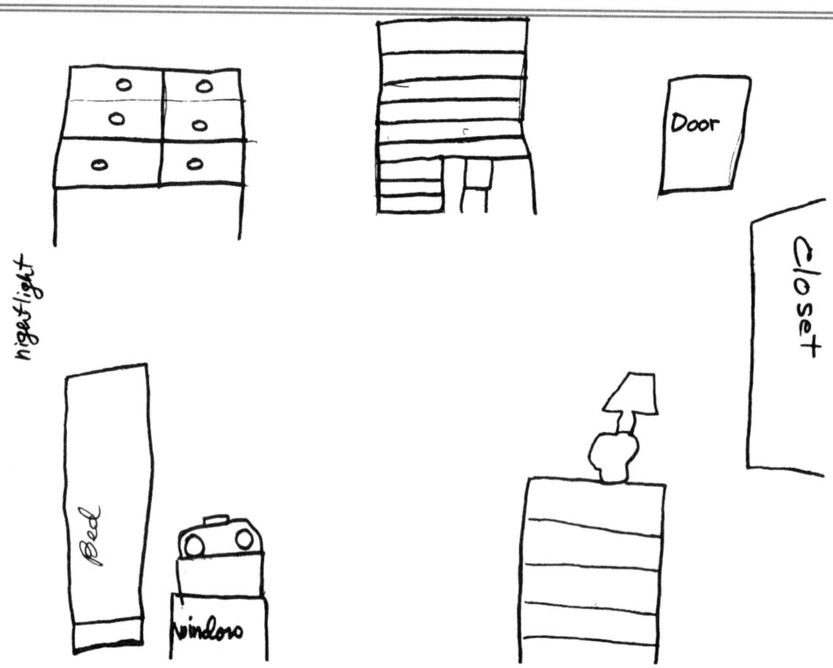

that she woke up, but there was no need for her to go into her parents' room and wake them up. I encouraged Linda to tell her parents that she would not disturb them but that she wanted their permission to put on the lights when she woke up. I suggested that the parents close their door so the lights would not disturb them.

I mentioned that Linda was going to try hard to control her anxiety and that we needed to figure out a way to reward her, because this might take a lot of effort. Together we decided on a time frame for successful completion of the desired behavior (Christmas, which was 6 weeks away) and a reward for succeeding. Linda said she wanted some new bookshelves and some drapes for her room and that she was hoping for a bicycle for Christmas. I suggested that we set up a token system of rewards, with the drapes to come after 2 successful weeks, the bookshelves after 4 weeks, and the bicycle after 6 weeks. I also suggested a gradual tapering of the lights at night: the first week, Linda would be permitted to put on as many lights as she wanted; the second week, all the lights in her *own* room; the third week, only her bedside lamp; and after a month, only a flashlight. The family was enthusiastic about the plan, although the father wanted to know how they would handle slipups. I suggested that if the problem returned for more than 2 nights out of 7, the reward system should slow down accordingly. I also planned to see Linda every week and wanted her to report her progress to me.

FIGURE 7.3. Linda's drawings of her "before" and "after" dreams.

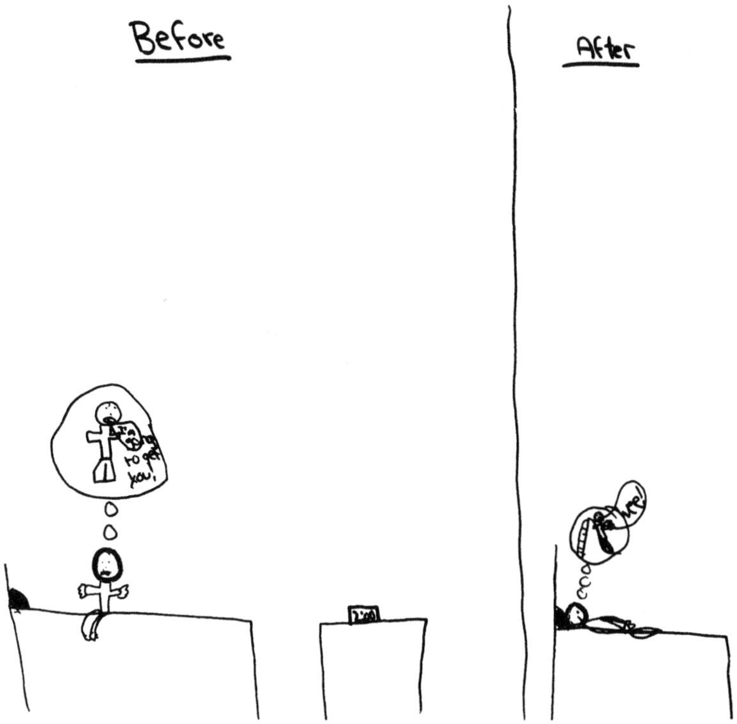

FIGURE 7.4. Linda's "good night's sleep" drawing.

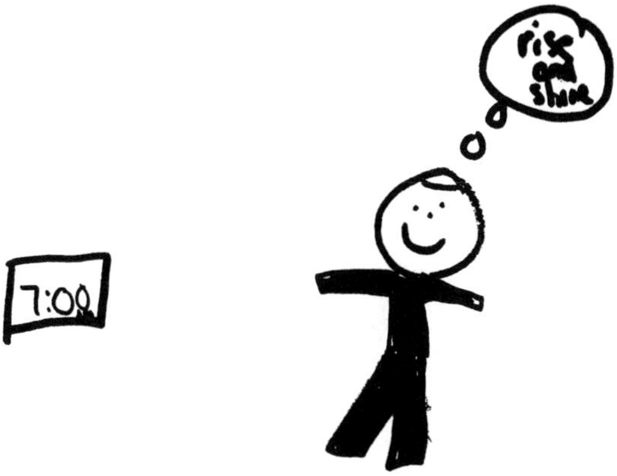

Treatment Summary

Complete symptom alleviation occurred within 3 weeks, and Linda was sleeping through the night with no more bad dreams. Two weeks after the family session, Linda had to cancel her appointment because she had hurt her foot in gymnastics. The pediatrician was giving her anti-inflammatory medication and wanted her to stay off the foot for 3 days. During our phone conversation, I asked Linda how she was doing at night. She said that she was still waking every night, but she just turned on her bedroom light and then went right back to sleep. I suggested that perhaps the medication would cause her to sleep through the entire night (positive suggestion). The next week Linda reported that she was now sleeping through the night. I kept in contact with the parents to ensure that they would carry through with the agreed-upon rewards. During the gradual tapering of sessions on a monthly basis after Christmas, Linda experienced no further nighttime difficulty.

Discussion

The rapid improvement in this case could be attributed to several factors. First, I framed Linda's behavior in a way that was distasteful to her by suggesting that it was typical of younger children; second, her parents removed whatever secondary gratification Linda may have derived from receiving their attention in the middle of the night and instead rewarded her for her strengths (bravery). A third factor may have been the implicit message to Linda that her parents were serious about wanting her to manage her own anxieties. The short-term time frame (6 weeks) was appealing and manageable to all.

It is obvious that this situation required simultaneous involvement of both the child and the parents in a mutually agreed-upon plan. My role as the therapist was that of catalyst and facilitator. In retrospect, the improvement may seem "too good to be true." I took a risk in suggesting that such a rapid change of behavior could occur. I based this on my knowledge of child development (i.e., most 10-year-olds do not have bad dreams that cause them to go into their parents' bedroom for help), as well as the indications from this girl's developmental history that her development had been proceeding normally until this unusual event. It is fortunate that the parents sought help before the problem escalated and a spiral of negative interaction was set into motion.

CONCLUDING COMMENTS

One-to-one work with the child gives the social worker an opportunity to know the child in a different manner than is possible when the child is seen together with the parents. When the worker encourages the child to play and conveys to the child that he or she will help through *both* playing and talking, the worker relieves the child of the obligation to communicate in the adult's verbal mode. Meeting the child on his or her level respects the child's individuality in a way that is unusual in child–adult relationships.

In one-to-one work, the therapist/worker uses play to interact with the child for the purpose of understanding and helping. This conforms to the commitment of the social work profession to meet clients at the level at which the clients are comfortable. Therefore, *all* social workers must be prepared to use play in their interactions with children.

DISCUSSION QUESTIONS

1. Discuss the dynamics of the separation problem as depicted in the case of Tammy. Why was it necessary to see *both* mother and child in order to resolve this problem? If you were the social worker, what information and advice would you give to Tammy's teacher about managing Tammy's separation difficulties?
2. Why is it important for family therapists to be familiar with play therapy techniques? Give an example of a case in which it might be appropriate to use play techniques in a family session. How can the family therapist go about implementing this?
3. Imagine that you are working with a child who has very low self-esteem because of physical and cognitive disabilities. How might the treatment of this child differ, depending on whether you were to follow a child-centered, a psychodynamic, or a cognitive-behavioral approach?
4. Discuss the reasons for using play in work with children under 12 years of age. How can social workers become more comfortable in using play techniques?

CHAPTER 8

Group Work with Children

Many children feel more comfortable interacting with a social worker or counselor in the company of other children than in a one-to-one counseling situation (Nisivoccia & Lynn, 2007; Schiffer, 1984). Whereas the prospect of working with six to eight children at the same time may challenge or even intimidate the counselor or social worker, the group format has the opposite effect on the child group members, who experience mutual support and energy according to the "strength in numbers" principle. The group situation, in comparison with one-to-one counseling, gives a child greater freedom to speak and participate when he or she feels inclined to do so, as other members share the spotlight and can fill an uncomfortable silence. Of course, most children do not choose the helping methods through which adults offer them assistance. Even children who feel distressed and worried about some aspects of their lives usually have no idea about either who can help or what means are available for doing so. When such children find themselves in a group with peers who have similar worries, they feel a sense of relief that they are not the only ones and are hopeful about the prospect of peer understanding and support.

RATIONALE FOR THE USE OF GROUPS

Children live and must be able to function as social beings. Their initial experience in their family group gradually broadens to include peer relationships when they enter day care or preschool and eventually formal schooling. Some children, in addition, are exposed to group programs in religious settings, and others benefit from participation in recreational groups (e.g., Boy or Girl Scouts and team sports). Indeed, whether or not they are involved in other group activities, school-age children typically and spontaneously form their own neighborhood cliques, "gangs," and clubs (Malekoff, 2002; Sarnoff,

1976; Aronson, 2017). In fact, Davies (2011) points out that school-age children define themselves in terms of their group membership, not just as individuals.

Children's intrinsic need for belonging and peer acceptance attests to the importance of group experience for their developing sense of personal identity. It is therefore quite logical to employ a group format to help, treat, or counsel children who are experiencing personal, emotional, or behavioral difficulties that interfere with their optimal functioning.

A helping/counseling/therapy group provides children with a social experience in a safe, nurturing environment that encourages emotional expression and problem solving in the process of demonstrating different individual styles of interacting and coping with common problems. Depending on the type of group and its composition, each member will inevitably be exposed to a variety of responses beyond his or her individual repertoire. Therefore, a counseling group constitutes a learning experience, in addition to providing support and acceptance.

There is general agreement about the rationale for treating children in groups. Different group workers (Ceballo, 2000; Connors, Schamess, & Strieder, 1997; Haen, 2017) have described these as the curative elements of peer interaction, the validation of personal experiences, the recognition of universal reactions, and the positive perception of the leader's therapeutic role. Nisivoccia and Lynn (2007) further specify that the group breaks the isolation of individual members, deals with the taboo of shame, raises self-esteem, helps children learn to respect limits, and enhances their ability to relate to others.

The power of the group to promote behavior change can be far greater than generally occurs in individual treatment because of the members' strong desire for peer acceptance. Peer pressure becomes a strong force in middle childhood because children are afraid of being rejected, excluded, or viewed as inadequate by their peers (Davies, 2011). A structured group involving both activity and verbal interaction can, through the influence of the peer culture, assist the children with their individual problems and growth needs (Kolodny & Garland, 1984; Nisivoccia & Lynn, 2007; Diamond, Gans, & Mortola, 2017). During the beginning phases of the group, the leader may ensure protection for the shy, tentative individual who fears exposure, but the balance soon shifts in the form of group pressure on individual members to take risks and make changes in their usual ways of relating. Ideally, groups combine both acceptance and confrontation, serving as a behind-the-scenes cheering squad for individual members.

DIFFERENT TYPES OF GROUPS FOR CHILDREN

There is a tendency among some group workers to distinguish between "therapy groups" and "activity groups," with those preferring the latter indicating that they do not want to "pathologize" children's behavior by indicating that they need "therapy" (Malekoff, 2002). On the other hand, professionals with mental health backgrounds consider "therapy" as a positive, not a negative, term. When, for example, children have been sexually abused, group therapy is generally considered the treatment of choice (Pelcovitz, 1999; Finkelhor & Berliner, 1995). An antimedical bias, as discussed in Chapter 4, should not lead to rejection of appropriate *group therapy* treatment when this is indicated by the nature of the child's experiences and behavioral responses.

However, services for children, whether in the form of therapy groups or activity groups, should occur in a format that is developmentally appropriate. This means that with young children the use of activities may be essential to supplement verbal discussions and meet the children's needs for concrete representations of their experiences. Activities provide opportunities for socialization and ego development and therefore contribute to a "therapeutic" outcome. For example, a group of children in foster care were guided over several weeks in a project called "Write Your Own Life Story/Picture Autobiography" (Brandler & Roman, 1991). The structured drawing and personal storytelling became "a tool to address the terrible grief these youngsters [felt] about the loss of family" (Brandler & Roman, 1991, p. 128). Hence, an activity can become therapeutic, even as the "therapy" involves an activity; the distinction between "therapy groups" and "activity groups" overlooks the basic interrelationship between the two in work with children.

According to Davis (2011), the following three types of groups are typical in schools, and it seems clear that this categorization can apply to all children's groups. The three categories are as follows:

1. *Remedial groups* (referred to as "task groups" by Fineran, Nitza, & Patterson, 2017): focus on work tasks and improving specific skills.
2. *Supportive groups* (referred to as "counseling groups" by Fineran et al., 2017): provide emotional/psychological counseling.
3. *Psychoeducational groups:* focus on specific issues.

In addition to the three types of groups above, Fineran et al. (2017) include psychotherapy groups, which have the goal of eliciting change from its members through the process of personality change.

Remedial groups can include those that deal with anger management, stress management, or study skills, to name a few. Examples of supportive groups could be those addressing grief and loss, bullying, changing families, or ADHD. Examples of groups that focus on psychoeducation would be those that deal with peer relationships, adoptive or foster children, or disaster/crisis responses. All these groups include counseling sessions that are time limited, with pupils who have been prescreened by the leader and whose parents have given permission for their child to attend. Psychotherapy groups offer support while encouraging individual personality change in a safe environment. Examples of different types of groups are given later in the chapter.

Historical Overview of Group Work with Children

Reviews of the development of group psychotherapy with children can be found in Johnson et al. (1986), and in Aronson (2017), from which the following discussion is loosely drawn. In the early 1930s, activity groups were initiated at the Madelyn Borg Child Guidance Institute in New York as an adjunct to individual therapy for children who appeared to require socialization experience. Over a period of 8 years, Samuel Slavson (1943) studied and worked with more than 750 children in 55 separate group treatment programs. He stated that

> in group therapy, we work with children who are directly rejected by parents, family, school, street gangs and community center. . . . They are either excessively aggressive or excessively withdrawn; obsessed with great fears or guilt; they overcompensate . . . by nonsocial or antisocial behavior. . . . What a child needs in such circumstances is a haven of relief, a sanctuary where these distressing, threatening, and hostile pressures can be removed and relief supplied. (pp. 2–3)

The appropriate treatment environment, according to Slavson, is a permissive, noncontrolling setting that provides children the opportunity to express their thoughts and feelings through play and action. The role of the therapist, in Slavson's model, is nondirective or client-centered, although grounded in psychoanalytic theory.

Adaptations of Slavson's "activity group therapy" were developed by Redl (1944), Axline (1947), and Ginott (1961) in approaches that stressed ego development through play activities and personal accomplishments. Axline and Ginott employed nondirective methods in which the therapists verbalized and reflected the children's feelings as they emerged in the context of play.

Because the nondirective and noninterpretative format of activity group therapy requires some capacity on the part of the children for self-regulation and emotional control, Slavson later developed a more structured and interpretation-oriented group for disturbed children who needed and benefited from external control and guidance from the therapist. This modified approach, called "activity–interview group psychotherapy," was pilot tested with latency-age children and subsequently adapted for use with prelatency and early-latency-age children in the 1950s by Slavson and Schiffer (1975). Activity group therapy as practiced by Slavson has now been replaced by problem-focused, short-term, and highly structured groups (Schamess, personal communication, August 13, 2010).

Behavioral group treatment models emerged in the 1960s as an alternative to psychodynamic and client-centered approaches (Rose, 1967). Focusing on behavior rather than personality as the target of change, behavioral group therapy is highly structured, with specific tasks and goals set for the members. Learning and reinforcement principles, such as behavioral contracting, rehearsal, extinction, modeling, and systematic desensitization techniques, help children to acquire skills in making friends, reducing their aggression and anxiety, and learning about the impact of their behavior on others (Rose, 1972; Bloomquist, 1996). Later versions of this behavioral model are found in various CBT interventions, such as those for children with ADHD (Reddy, 2010) and in family-based group CBT interventions for childhood anxiety (Pahl & Barrett, 2010).

Current Wide Range of Children's Groups

In the second decade of the 21st century, we find a veritable plethora of groups for children. These vary according to the nature of the problem situation, the children's developmental stage, and the philosophy and theoretical stance of the helping personnel regarding the appropriate type of intervention.

Numerous group models target children who have experienced loss, either through parental divorce (Kalter & Schreier, 1994; McGonagle, 1989; Dyson, 2015) or through the death of a family member, teacher, or close friend (Bullock, 2007; Griffin, 2010; Schuurman & DeCristofaro, 2007, 2015). Group work has been used with children in families with HIV/AIDS (Dane, 2002; deRidder, 1999), with siblings of handicapped children (Block & Margolis, with 1986), residents of a shelter for battered women and their children (Roberts & Roberts, 1990), and for children in residential settings (Creeden & Haen, 2017). The literature also includes accounts of school-based support groups for children of cancer patients (Call, 1990; Goodman, 2007), activity groups for children who have witnessed violence (Nisivoccia & Lynn, 1999, 2007), and crisis "debriefing" groups for children in shelters following a natural disaster (Baggerly, 2007; Hoffman & Rogers, 1991) or following school shootings (Miller, 2012). Most of these groups employ a structured, time-limited format, as do groups for children with a variety of problems discussed by Rose (1998) and Gallo-Lopez (2006). The use of play therapy in groups is discussed by Sweeney and Homeyer (2000), Reddy (2010), and Kestly (2010).

Numerous accounts discuss using cognitive and behavioral methods in groups with children. Examples of these include a play group for a 5-year-old boy who had difficulty with peer relationships (Boulanger & Langevin, 1992), a skills training approach in working with depressed children (Stark, Rafaelle, & Reysa, 1994) and with children who have social skills deficits (Schaefer, Jacobsen, & Ghahramanlou, 2000; Reddy, 2010; Hariton, 2017), and cognitive-behavioral group therapy for children with anxiety and phobic disorders (Ginsburg, Silverman, & Kurtines, 1995; Pahl & Barrett, 2010; Friedberg et al., 2017). With such groups being so ubiquitous, one might ask whether there are any situations in which the referral of a child to a group would be contraindicated. This question is discussed further in the next section.

An Integrated Model for Children's Groups

As previously mentioned, there has been and still is some disagreement in the helping professions between practitioners who provide group therapy—focused on helping individuals within a group format (termed the "remedial" model; Papell & Rothman, 1966; Vinter, 1959)—and other practitioners who focus on the group as an entity unto itself, believing that the individuals in such a group benefit both through providing assistance to others and through receiving support from the other group members (the "mutual aid" model; Schwartz, 1977; Gitterman & Shulman, 1986; Shulman, 1984, 1999, 2006). For reasons related to children's immature development and special need for adult protection and guidance, neither model in its pure form seems apt for application to children. Rather, I recommend an approach that integrates elements of both models. Children will not participate in a counseling group (even when they are required to do so) unless they find it enjoyable, interesting, or otherwise appealing. They are social beings, however, and once they begin participating in a group, most benefit greatly from the feeling of acceptance that emerges from the experience of group membership.

Perhaps a new model of social group work merits consideration for use with children. I suggest that we refer to this model as the "integrated model." With the dual goals of helping each child group member toward greater appreciation of individual and group (social) awareness, this approach would meet the children on their level (by providing activities) and at the same time would increase their sense of self-esteem through the experience of group sharing, acceptance, and bonding. The definition of group work formulated by the American Association of Group Work in 1948 seems especially applicable to work with children within an integrated framework just described: "Group Work is a method by which . . . both group interaction and program activities contribute to the growth of the individual, and the achievement of socially desirable goals" (quoted in Sullivan, 1952, p. 420).

There seems to be a growing recognition of the importance of group work with children. Work with children is different from work with adults, and it does not conform to structures adapted for adults. Group work with children is a promising and rewarding field of practice for social workers. The discussion and case examples in this chapter and elsewhere in this book attest to the viability and versatility of this helping method.

CONSIDERATIONS IN PLANNING A GROUP FOR CHILDREN

Group Composition: Prescreening to Determine Membership

In planning a group for children, the following factors must be weighed in a preliminary interview with each child in order to determine the child's suitability for placement in the group:

- The focus and purpose of the group
  - Type of problem situation
- The optimal degree of homogeneity and size considerations
  - Ages and gender of members
  - Child's level of maturity and attention span
- Contraindications for group membership

The Focus and Purpose of the Group

The worker who is planning a group tries to be certain that a given child will fit in so that the group will be beneficial to him or her. Sometimes referrals come from well-meaning teachers or school personnel who do not understand the complexities of forming a group that will meet the needs of all its members. For example, a child from a family with divorced parents might not be a suitable group candidate when he or she had witnessed numerous episodes of family violence. Because the violence takes precedence over the breakup of the marriage, if possible such a child would be more appropriately placed in a group with other children who have similar experiences. The following section presents specifics about the process of group formation.

The Optimal Degree of Homogeneity and Size Considerations

Because each child deserves the opportunity to participate in the group, the leader(s) must weigh all factors impinging on the comfort level of the members. Usually, the degree of homogeneity based on the nature of the problem situation provides a unifying bond, referred to by Schwartz and Zalba (1971) as "the common ground." For example, a child who has HIV may feel tremendous support in a group of peers with the same diagnosis, and the mixing of genders in such a group would not be contraindicated because the significance of the diagnosis outweighs the possible importance of gender commonality. On the other hand, a mixed-gender group would not be appropriate for children who have been sexually abused and whose discussion might be constricted in the presence of members of the opposite sex. In the first group session of a witness-to-violence group, the leader stated that each girl there had "witnessed something terrible and may have some feelings about it" (Nisivoccia & Lynn, 2007, p. 303). This statement helped establish the common ground.

According to the "Noah's Ark" principle (i.e., two by two), each child in a group should share certain identifying characteristics with at least one other group member. Thus it is not advisable to put a single boy in a group with all girls or a single white child in a group with all black children. Children have a need to belong and to fit in, and because they tend to think concretely, they pay close attention to physical characteristics.

Kindergarten or first-grade children, who often have difficulty focusing for longer than 20 or 30 minutes at a time, probably would do better in a group limited to three or four children. Thompson and Rudolph (1992) and

Johnson et al. (1986) recommend that the age range and/or grade span among child group members not exceed 1–2 years.

Contraindications for Group Membership

The leader(s) must consider the personality attributes of prospective members to form a balanced group. Children who present in an extreme way—for example, as excessively self-absorbed, domineering, or unable to give attention to the concerns of peers—probably would be ostracized by a group, with negative consequences for both the individuals and the group as a whole. Yalom (1985) cautions against admitting a potentially "deviant" member into a group because of probable negative responses that will be detrimental to all. In situations in which a leader questions whether a prospective group member will "fit," better results may be obtained through arranging a period of individual counseling for the child rather than risking the possible demoralizing experience of rejection by the group. Of course, it might be argued that a "misfit" desperately needs socialization experience. However, a period of individual counseling might help such an individual to reach a point at which group contact would be beneficial.

In addition, group membership may be contraindicated when an individual has been exposed to a stigmatizing or traumatic event that may be difficult for the prospective member to discuss with others or that may be too horrific for children in general to hear. In the witness-to-violence group, all members had observed disturbing events, so it was possible for them to support one another. However, it would not be appropriate to put a child who had seen a parent murdered in a divorce group with children who had witnessed milder forms of parental conflict. Also, the child who has been bereaved by suicide usually benefits from individual, rather than group, therapy, as does the child who has been a victim of a traumatic experience (Eth & Pynoos, 1985). When a child has symptoms of PTSD, the usual treatment protocol includes guided reenactment of the trauma at the child's pace, facilitated on an individual basis with a trained therapist (Bevin, 1999; Cohen et al., 2012). However, when a group of children (e.g., a school class or club group) has undergone the same traumatic experience (e.g., a natural or human-made disaster), a crisis debriefing group soon after the event is helpful and can serve a preventive intervention purpose. Crisis intervention group debriefing is discussed more fully later in this chapter.

Group Format and Structure

Open-Ended or Time-Limited

A major consideration regarding the structure of the group is whether it will be open-ended or time-limited. An open-ended group is ongoing and permits members to remain as long as they perceive the need to do so. When old members withdraw from the group, new individuals are added; this permits more seasoned members to orient, and serve as role models for, the newer members. An example of this type of group is the Alcoholics Anonymous model for children living in substance-abusing families, the membership in which may change from week to week, although some members may attend indefinitely as a core group. Other groups targeted for these children follow a structured approach, using a curriculum within an 8- or 12-week format, while the group membership remains constant. This model is discussed more fully in Chapter 13.

Either the open-ended or the time-limited group format can be useful, depending on the purpose for which the group is being formed. Because children's sense of time is guided by school semesters, vacations, and holidays, a time-limited framework can conform naturally to their lives. A 12-week group, for example, can be completed between Labor Day and the Christmas vacation. If the group will be repeated during the spring semester, some of the same children may choose to enroll again. In this situation, the leader(s) should evaluate in advance whether to extend a reenrollment offer to previous group members. Sometimes there are more children than can be accommodated in the available groups, and "triage" decisions must be made to ensure that all children who need service receive it.

Length of Group Meetings

The optimal length of the group meetings also needs to be determined, with practical matters usually dictating these decisions. When a group meets during school, for example, the length of the class period determines the length of the meeting. However, if the group meets after school, meeting length can be determined by the age of the members and the size of the group, allowing the amount of time needed to ensure members' full participation. In general, the larger the group and the older the members, the longer the meeting time. For a group of older (11- and 12-year-old) children involved in a structured activity, 1½ hours would be the suggested time period, whereas a 20-minute group meeting may be appropriate for a group of 5- and 6-year-old children.

Frequency of Meetings

The frequency depends on the setting and the purpose of the group. In residential settings and hospitals, group meetings may be convened daily or several times a week. Outpatient settings, such as clinics, community recreational settings, and schools, more typically hold group meetings on a weekly basis.

Leadership Considerations

The question of whether to have a single group leader or coleaders deserves reflection, although in many settings coleadership is not an option because of limited staff availability. There are many advantages to coleadership, especially when one leader is male and the other female, as this arrangement simulates parental roles and provides the opportunity for role modeling. Coleadership also permits the leaders to share impressions about the group, as well as to divide responsibilities for collaborating with other professionals involved with the children, for keeping records, and for maintaining contacts with the parents or guardians, according to the expectations created and agreements made when the group was initiated.

However, coleadership can become a problem if the leaders become competitive with each other, cannot agree about goals, or cannot work comfortably together because of personality or philosophical differences. These possibilities need to be discussed prior to the beginning of the group, so that another leadership plan can be implemented if they cannot be resolved.

When a leader works alone, it is important that he or she receive supervision, because the process of reviewing the group's progress and impasses will assist the leader in maintaining the necessary degree of objectivity. The leader will also benefit from systematic thinking about the nature of his or her leadership role with the group.

Necessary Ground Rules for Children's Groups

In order for a children's group to function effectively, the children must understand the expectations involved in membership. Often part of the first group meeting is devoted to the establishment of rules, which the children are invited to draft for themselves with the leader's assistance. A basic expectation relates to attendance. Children are urged to attend every session, and if they disagree or disapprove of something that happens in the group, they are advised to bring it up at the time. Some group leaders ask children to sign a contract in the first session, agreeing to come for the planned number of group meetings.

Kalter and Schreier (1994) mention these other typical rules in children's groups:

1. Listening (i.e., only one person talks at a time)
2. Right to pass (i.e., members have no obligation to speak or respond)
3. No putdowns (i.e., there is to be no teasing or name-calling)
4. Confidentiality (i.e., members can report outside the group only what they and the leaders have said in the group, not what other group members have said)

The Importance of Confidentiality

Probably no issue is more critical than confidentiality. Children may not understand the rationale for keeping what is discussed by others private, and even if they do understand, they may not have the self-control to maintain the promised confidence. Some group leaders use a "confidentiality contract" to emphasize the importance of this issue (Stark et al., 1994). Figure 8.1 illustrates such a contract.

FIGURE 8.1. A sample confidentiality contract.

CONFIDENTIALITY CONTRACT

It is important for me to respect the rights of others to confidentiality, just as I want them to respect *my* right to confidentiality.

I hereby promise not to tell ANYONE outside the group what any other group member says during our meetings.

WHAT IS SAID IN THE GROUP MUST **STAY IN THE GROUP**.

This promise lasts even after the group is over.

Name ______________________________ Date ________________

The limits and conditions on the worker's promise of confidentiality should be mentioned in the initial group meeting during the orientation discussion of group members' responsibilities to one another and to the group. Specifically, the worker or counselor states that there are three circumstances in which he or she will be obligated by law to reveal what members say in the group. These are situations in which members (1) discuss their intent to hurt themselves (2) discuss their intent to hurt others, or (3) disclose that someone is hurting them.

In situations in which the leader is obliged to break confidence and report a member's disclosure of physical or sexual abuse, serious repercussions can arise for the continuation of the group, because members may no longer feel that the group is a safe place. This also tends to be true in family and individual treatment. The matter of confidentiality continuing even after death has been litigated in court (National Association of Social Workers, 1994).

GROUP PLAY INTERVENTIONS FOR CHILDREN WITH ADHD: AN EXAMPLE OF A REMEDIAL SKILLS-BASED GROUP

Because ADHD is one of the most common childhood disorders, mental health and school professionals need to understand its characteristics and be able to employ methods to help children deal with its troublesome symptoms. The brief summary here is taken from Reddy (2010), in which several developmentally appropriate games (DAGs) are used in a group format with the goal of enhancing social skills, controlling impulses, and alleviating anger/stress difficulties in children with this diagnosis. The games are an integral part of a group training program that runs for 10 sessions with up to 15 people (children and adults) involved. This behavior management approach monitors and reinforces positive behaviors with stickers and a point system to motivate children to follow directions; to use words, not behaviors, to express feelings; and to control their hands, feet, and mouths. Selected games (such as Bean Bag Toss, when a child misses his or her throw into a bucket) involve a frustrating situation in which the child is encouraged and guided to use anger management strategies to cope with his or her frustration. The program can be implemented by teachers and professionals who have received training in using it.

Other DAGs are described by Reddy (2010) and Reddy and Alperin (2017). Games of this type have been shown in research studies to improve the social skills, self-concept, and visual–motor skills of participating students more than other, traditional school-based games.

BANANA SPLITS GROUPS FOR CHILDREN OF DIVORCE: AN EXAMPLE OF A SUPPORTIVE SCHOOL-BASED GROUP

Banana Splits groups are school-based peer support groups created for school personnel to use with children affected by divorce (McGonagle, 1978/1989). The manual states: "Banana Splits is a group for any kid whose family structure has changed. Living with a single parent, a stepparent, a grandparent, all are valid prerequisites for membership" (1978/1989, p. 3). It is a comprehensive program that originated in a single school and that has, over the course of a decade, spread to many states. These groups are still being offered in schools decades after they originated. Readers who wish to obtain the training manual can consult *www.counselorresources.com*. The manual includes curriculum guidance for conducting groups in elementary schools and secondary schools and for parent groups and staff development. The program philosophy is based on the triad of the home, school, and child, recognizing that children in divorcing families respond to multiple stresses related to the changes in their lives and that these stresses can affect their school performance over many years. Therefore, students are urged to attend the group during a 3-year time frame, and they are welcome to return at any time in the future when a change, such as a parent's remarriage, threatens their stability.

The groups provide peer support for students who are all confronting similar problems, such as divided loyalties, visitation, and future or current parental remarriage and adjustment to a stepparent and stepsiblings. Permission is obtained from the custodial parents for their children to participate in this group, and parents are encouraged to contact the group leader with any related concerns and to attend periodic parent educational/discussion groups.

The recommended frequency and time of group meetings in the elementary school is biweekly during the students' 30-minute lunch period. The recommended number of children in the group should be no more than 10. The meetings consist of a combination of activities and discussion.

Initially, each child draws and colors a banana, which he or she then attaches to a paper palm tree after writing his or her name on it. The name "Banana Split" was chosen because of the positive associations to ice cream and to the reality that divorce involves a "split" in the family.

Selected activities for the elementary group include the following, chosen at the leader's discretion:

- *Graffiti wall.* The leader invites the students to write, on a paper-covered wall, their thoughts about the split or some problems that need to be solved, and/or to write answers to problems written by others. No names are ever used, and the paper is displayed for about 6 weeks. (See Figure 8.2 for an example of a graffiti wall.)
- *Pizza pie.* Students are given two drawings with large circles, each representing a pizza. One page is labeled "The Pieces in My Happy Pie." Students are instructed to divide each "pizza" into slices and label each slice with something that makes them happy. Then the same exercise is repeated with the "Sad Pizza Pie."
- *Drawing exercises.* Drawings that depict children in difficult and/or ambiguous situations serve as the focus for small-group discussions. The pictures (given to each student to color) include different scenes, such as a child in court, a child whose braided hair is being pulled by a man and a woman on either side of her (see Figure 8.3), a child sitting at a school desk looking very tuned out and preoccupied, a child writing a letter that starts "Dear Mom," and a child carrying his own suitcases and walking toward an airplane.

The discussion manual lists suggested questions for the leader to ask about the subject of each picture. The students may then be invited to write their answers to the questions on a "private" paper. Then group members discuss the drawing and share their feelings.

Many activities associated with holidays or other special occasions are included in the manual. One involves holding an end-of-the-year picnic at which pizza is served and the children make their own banana splits. The school social worker/counselor/psychologist also writes a letter to the parents to invite them to an end-of-the-year coffee and dessert meeting to discuss the group.

The Banana Splits program sounds very impressive and seems to hold great potential for helping children, parents, and school personnel understand and cope with the family changes that result from divorce. Logistically, however, I think that many schools would find it difficult to implement the program because of the large numbers of children in "split" families and the realities

FIGURE 8.2. Example of comments elementary students wrote on the graffiti wall. Used with permission of Interact.

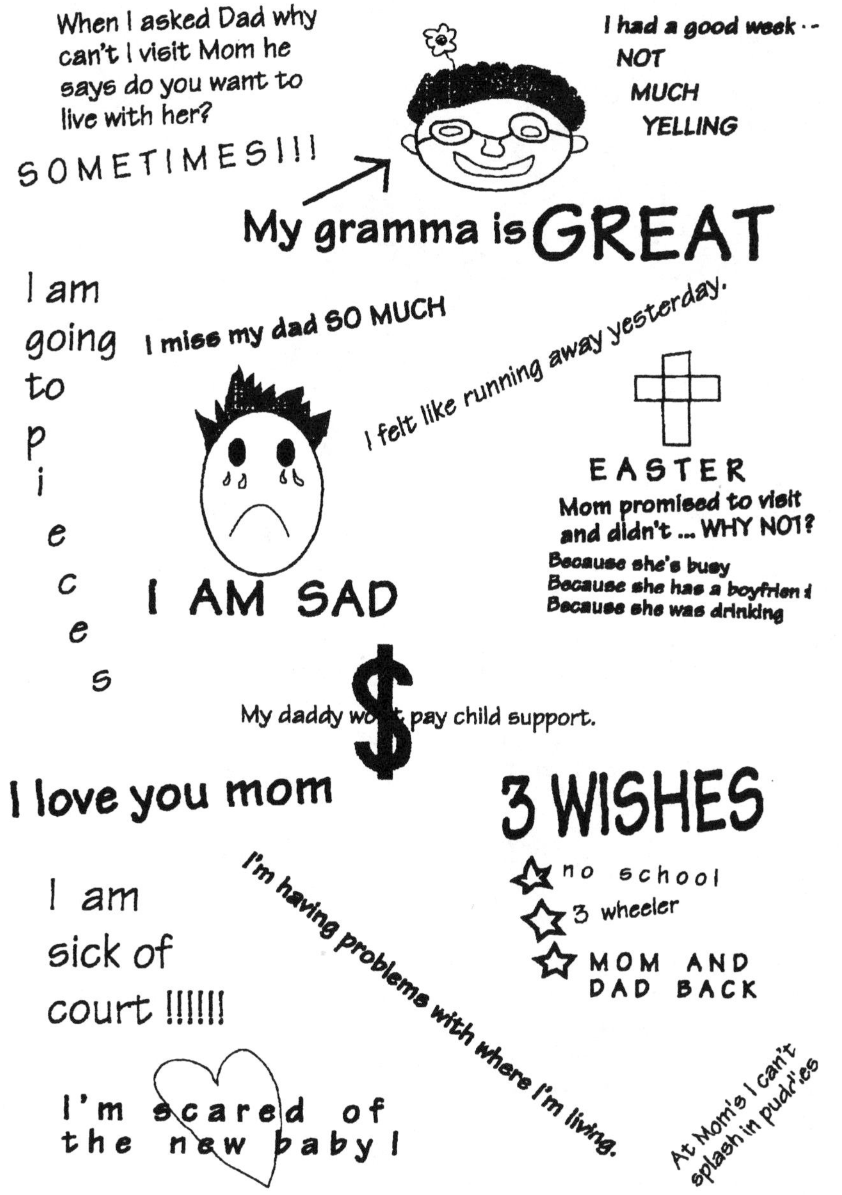

FIGURE 8.3. "Push-me–pull-you" drawing for use in a Banana Splits group. Used by permission of Interact.

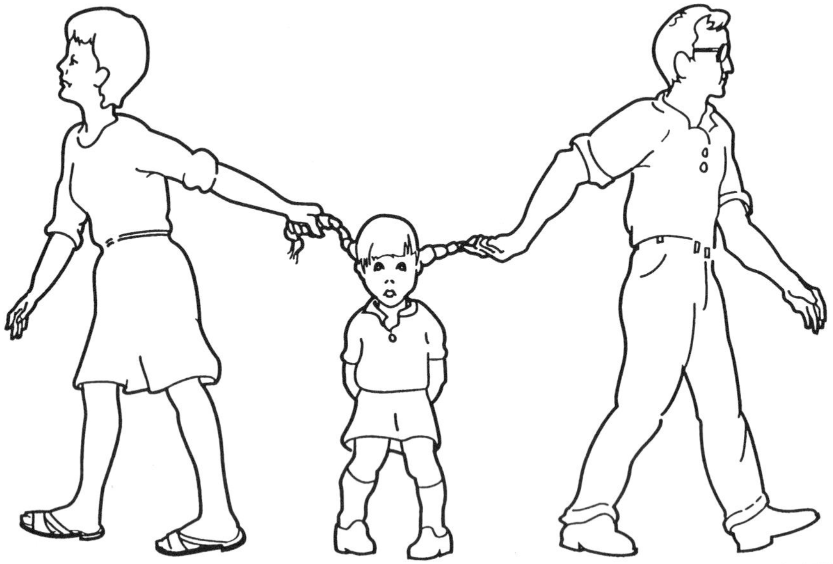

of other demands on the time of school professionals. Graduate interns certainly could lead some of the groups, providing they are supervised. Another possibility is to train volunteers to offer this service just as hospice uses nonprofessional staff to run many of their groups and provide associated services. Children clearly stand to benefit from this validating and supportive program.

CRISIS INTERVENTION GROUPS FOLLOWING DISASTERS: AN EXAMPLE OF A PSYCHOEDUCATIONAL GROUP

Both natural and human-made disasters (e.g., explosions; bus, airplane, and train crashes; terrorist attacks; random shootings) occur with distressing frequency and unpredictability in our world. The normal responses to such abnormal events include a range of anxiety reactions related to stress and associated with the perceived threat to one's personal and physical safety. Children, like adults, experience fear and anxiety when they witness unthinkable events such as the collapse of a building, the flooding of their home and community, or the random shooting of classmates on their school playground. Following crisis events such as these, children may develop moderate to severe symptoms depending on their developmental level, past experiences, and emotional and physical health, as well as the responses of parents to the crisis (Vogel & Vernberg, 1993, as reported in Baggerly & Salloum, 2010). For example, one study found that 55% of elementary school children showed moderate to severe symptoms 3 months after Hurricane Andrew (Vernberg, La Greca, Silverman, & Prinstein, 1996). Sometimes, cultural factors such as reluctance to admit feelings of helplessness and terror may prevent the honest sharing of feelings and lead to repression and avoidance of seeking help (Kotani, Nakamura, Hashimoto, & Hanai, 2017).

Our growing knowledge about the impact of trauma on the lives of children (and adults) has led to intervention models both for the immediate impact phase and for short- and long-term recovery phases (La Greca, 2008; Blaustein, & Kinniburgh, 2019). Due to space constraints, this chapter focuses only on crisis intervention for survivors in the immediate impact phase. Readers who want information regarding treatment approaches in the later phases may consult Cohen et al. (2017).

Crisis Debriefing Groups

When a community or group of individuals has experienced a crisis, the initial method of intervention is to conduct a crisis debriefing group. The group format permits individuals to offer support to one another, even as they identify reactions in other survivors that are similar to their own. This type of group tends to be quite large and usually includes an educational component often referred to as "psychological first aid" (Baggerly, 2007; National Center for PTSD, 2005). The intent of this intervention is to inform victims of the crisis about typical responses to crisis events, the average duration of anxiety responses, and where to obtain help if symptoms persist longer than expected. Baggerly (2007) lists seven objectives for disaster responses focused on children that incorporate play therapy techniques, using a protocol set up by the National Center for PTSD (2005). These objectives are as follows:

1. Normalize symptoms.
2. Manage hyperarousal.
3. Manage intrusive reexperiencing.
4. Increase accurate cognitions.
5. Increase effective coping.
6. Seek social support.
7. Foster hope.

Examples of how these goals were achieved by the team of play therapists who went to Sri Lanka and Thailand following the tsunami in 2004 are given in Baggerly (2007). The next section further elaborates on group goals in helping children after a crisis.

Tasks in a Crisis Group for Children

In any crisis situation, rumors abound. Children are particularly vulnerable to anxiety related to incorrect information or a lack of information, and adults may unwisely seek to "protect" them by withholding information. Furthermore, children trying to understand puzzling events will often create their own explanations of why something happened and who was to blame. When children have experienced a frightening event together, it is advisable to convene them as a group to talk about, or "debrief," each child's experience of what happened. Clearly, the first task of the leader in such a crisis group is to give information. In language appropriate to the age of the individuals, they should be told about what happened and about the efforts to help survivors like themselves. This corresponds with the fourth objective above.

A second step in crisis intervention groups with children is to encourage each child to tell his or her own story, giving details and providing vivid descriptions. The leader should ask for specifics related to the individual's perceptions through all five senses. In other words, the child should be asked about what he or she heard, smelled, felt, and tasted during the crisis experience, in addition to describing his or her visual memories. Traumatologists (e.g., van der Kolk, 1987; Eth & Pynoos, 1985; Lindy, 1986) have learned that the detailed and timely recall of traumatic memories helps in the prevention of PTSD. Because children have limited ability to articulate their experiences in words, drawing and play activities can be utilized to assist them in externalizing their feelings about traumatic events. An excellent video illustrating school-based interventions with children following earthquakes is available from the Federal Emergency Management Agency (1991). This tape demonstrates a classroom debriefing that includes drawing activities in addition to class discussion. Figure 8.4 shows a sample drawing made by a child in a debriefing session following an earthquake.

The individual storytelling and the drawings provide the leader of the crisis group with the opportunity to universalize and normalize reactions to the crisis, so that group members do not feel peculiar or stigmatized because of the nature of their feelings (first objective above). Sometimes parents and other adults unwisely minimize children's feelings, thereby depriving them of the opportunity for validation that occurs in a debriefing group. This validation is supportive and helps children put the frightening experience in the past so that they can move on with their lives. When children appear to be extremely upset by the experience, the crisis group can teach relaxation methods to help them learn to manage their hyperarousal (second objective) and to manage any intrusive reexperiencing of the event (third objective).

A final task of the crisis group is to help the children identify the strengths resulting from their having survived the experience. Implicit in the circumstances of both natural and human-made disasters is a sense of helplessness. Although it would be unrealistic to assure children that they can survive all future disasters, it is helpful to assist them in identifying what they have learned from this experience and even to indicate ways in which they may feel stronger and better prepared to meet frightening experiences in the future (seventh objective; foster hope).

FIGURE 8.4. Child's drawing in a debriefing group following an earthquake. Drawing courtesy Katharyn E. K. Ross, National Center for Earthquake Engineering Research, State University of New York College at Buffalo. Used with permission.

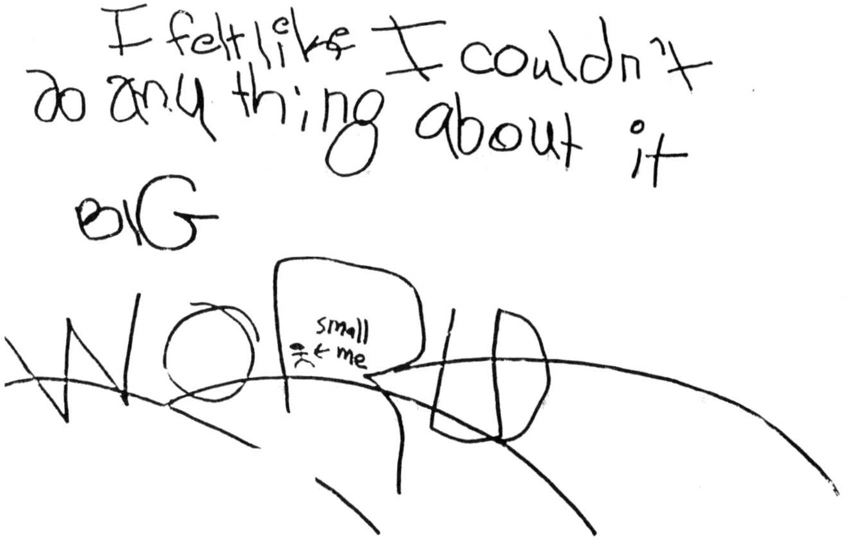

In summary, the following tasks guide the work of leaders in crisis debriefing groups with children:

1. Give information about the crisis in language comprehensible to the children.
2. Encourage detailed recounting of the crisis experience by each group member.
3. Universalize and normalize personal reactions to the crisis.
4. Identify strengths and new coping abilities gained as a result of the crisis experience.
5. Refer individual children who are having difficulties to a mental health specialist for more specialized assistance.

Case Example 1: The World Trade Center Bombing, February 26, 1993

In two previous publications (Webb, 1994a, 2004), I analyzed and made recommendations regarding the intervention of a school-based crisis team following the February 1993 terrorist attack on the World Trade Center in New York City, during which 17 kindergarten children and their teachers were trapped in an elevator for 5 hours. This example offers readers the opportunity to analyze the intervention of a crisis team in an unforeseen situation in which a group of children was frightened and the adults were not able to comfort them, as no one knew the circumstances of the crisis event until it was over.

I was not a member of that crisis team, but I read numerous accounts of their interventions and spoke to various school personnel who were involved in the aftermath of this crisis. For the purposes of this chapter, I invite the reader to apply the principles of crisis debriefing to this event.

The facts of the situation are as follows. The children, from nearby Brooklyn, were on a school-sponsored field trip to the second-tallest building in the world; they had enjoyed the view from the observation deck on the 107th floor and eaten lunch. As they were descending in the elevator, preparing to take the bus trip back to their school, the elevator suddenly stopped between the 36th and 34th floors. No one in the elevator knew that there had been a bomb blast; however, the lights and ventilation went off, and the children could smell smoke. There was no communication between the elevator and the outside world for several hours. On the eventual rescue and safe return of the children to their school many hours later, the bus was greeted by camera crews and the crisis team carrying balloons. Several parents were described as "hysterical," and most parents preferred to take their children immediately to the safety of home for the weekend rather than accept the invitation of the crisis team to attend a group meeting when they descended from the bus. Only a few families attended this first debriefing session.

The next involvement of the crisis team took place in the kindergarten classroom the following Monday morning (the bombing had occurred on Friday). According to oral reports and the accounts of teaching personnel, the team members spent approximately half a day in the classroom; they engaged the children in play activities, using blocks and other play materials to reenact the explosion in the building, which had been repeatedly portrayed on TV over the weekend. The crisis team also encouraged the children to draw pictures of their experiences.

Was this intervention sufficient to relieve the tension and fears these children may have experienced during their 5-hour ordeal of being trapped in a dark, hot elevator? For some children it may have been, as we know that simple exposure to a traumatic event does not automatically result in traumatization for all individuals. In fact, the available research indicates that "even after extreme trauma . . . only approximately 40% of an exposed population develop Posttraumatic Stress Disorder" (McFarlane, 1990, p. 74). However, there is no way to distinguish those who are vulnerable from those who are not, so a group crisis debriefing intervention targeted to the entire exposed population is the most prudent response, as it offers the best means of preventing severe reactions later.

Ideally, such an intervention should involve every child in a verbal and play reenactment of what he or she experienced. We do not know about the specific meaning of a crisis to each individual involved until we ask and listen. Because young children's verbal abilities are limited, play approaches (together with verbal inquiries) are necessary. Let us consider what could have been done in this case, using the five tasks described above as a guide.

1. *Give information about the crisis.* In this event, as in many crisis situations, there was a lot of confusion about what actually happened and who was to blame. In trying to explain these circumstances to 5-year-olds, a simple statement such as "Something very serious happened, and we don't know yet who or what caused it" would have conformed to the truth; it would also have permitted a reassuring follow-up about the fact that they were safe now and the police would take charge of the situation. Such an explanation, in language children can understand, permits the children to leave the matter in adult hands so that they themselves can proceed with their lives.

2. *Encourage detailed recounting of the crisis.* Each of the 17 children should have been given the opportunity to describe what he or she experienced. Although it would not have been feasible for each 5-year-old to listen to the accounts of 16 other children, it would have been possible to divide the group in half, so that each child would have heard about the experiences of 7 or 8 other children. In view of the children's young ages, their accounts would probably have been rather brief; nonetheless, they would have offered a trained observer an insight into the degree of each child's perceived stress in this situation. Children appearing to be seriously stressed could have been identified for further follow-up on an individual basis. This conforms to the fifth task of making referrals for those children who seemed extremely upset.

3. *Universalize and normalize personal reactions.* After several children had expressed their feelings, either verbally or through drawings or play, the leader could have begun to draw parallels (where appropriate) and to ask whether others felt the same way. Even when expressed feelings were not shared, the leader could have validated each child's individual experience.

4. *Identify strengths and new coping abilities.* The sense of helplessness and dependence on adults typical of young children may have helped these kindergarteners. Whereas with older children the ability to control their anxiety might have been most important, the younger children in this situation who were able to lie down on the floor (at the adult's instructions) and go to sleep may have fared better than some others who tuned in to the anxiety of the adults and began to cry for their mothers and experience somatic reactions. The crisis group leader would have needed to emphasize that all the children survived a difficult situation, even those who were very worried. Feelings of gratitude about being rescued and the experience of cooperating with

the rescue personnel would have helped restore a sense of security to these young children.

5. *Refer children who require more assistance.* Although the methods described here will help most children return to their former level of functioning after a brief period of anxiety following a crisis, some children will not restabilize and will require more individual attention. These children should be referred to a mental health specialist for a complete evaluation. Often the crisis situation serves as a "last straw" that tips the balance of a child with a precarious adjustment, and the referral can serve to help this child not only with the immediate concerns related to the crisis but also with his or her underlying issues.

Case Example 2: The World Trade Center Attack, September 11, 2001

It is chilling to face the reality that terrorism has increased so significantly since the first World Trade Center bombing in 1993. The truck bombing of the Alfred P. Murrah Federal Building in Oklahoma City killed 168 people and injured more than 500 others (Kight, 1998), and the four plane crashes on September 11, 2001, killed almost 3,000 and affected millions of citizens who watched the events unfold on television and who joined in the national grieving process.

After September 11, I developed a new tripartite formulation for the assessment of the traumatically bereaved child (Webb, 2002b), specifying factors that are particularly compelling for traumatically bereaved children following terrorist attacks. Included are the following, which are fully discussed in *Helping Bereaved Children* (Webb, 2002a, 2010):

- Extent of violence/trauma/death (including degree of destruction and proximity to the event)
- Degree of life threat
- Solitary versus shared experience
- Loss of a family member (typically a parent)
- Loss of a predictable future

To what extent can crisis or bereavement groups help children who have experienced traumatic grief under these unique circumstances? Do the guidelines I reviewed earlier in this chapter apply in a crisis of this magnitude?

Because I lived in the Greater New York suburbs at the time of September 11, 2001, I know that there was a great lag in the implementation of bereavement services by various agencies. Initially, this was understandable, as families were not ready to grieve because they were still focused on the identification of remains and hoping for a miracle.

Certainly, the first guideline, "give information about the crisis," was operative here insofar as the families needed to know if their loved ones had been found. Information was very slow in coming, which added to the stress, to the continuation of hope, and to feelings of denial about the death and postponement of funerals and memorial services.

The second task, "encourage detailed recounting of the crisis," was not appropriate due to the traumatic nature of the deaths and the probable mutilation of the bodies. Developmental factors would affect children's ability to comprehend or accurately envision the nature of the deaths. Many children and adults saw bloodied people running from the scene in television playbacks. Some schools, in well-meaning efforts to help, encouraged children to draw or write about what they saw, and several children drew pictures of the falling bodies of people who chose to jump rather than to wait for certain death in the raging fires. We do not know whether children who drew these pictures and wrote stories or poems about the event were traumatized or relieved by doing so.

The third task, "universalize and normalize individual reactions," certainly is relevant here. Parents and children need to be informed that some of their reactions, such as sleep difficulties, are related to their traumatic bereavement. Information about PTSD helps older children and parents understand some of their symptoms. However, many children, even those who attended bereavement groups, could not bear to talk about their losses until after the 6-month anniversary (Hartley, 2004). So the timing of normalization has to occur in synchrony with the children's readiness to share some of their reactions.

The fourth task, "identify strengths and new coping abilities," also is time sensitive. It is difficult for people to comprehend that they might gain strength through surviving a loss of this magnitude. Most would rather turn back the clock and resume their previous lives. Many would resent anyone suggesting that they will "grow" from the experience, and this abstract idea would be lost on most children.

However, the outpouring of gifts and offers to help in the form of teddy bears and other toys probably *did* have an effect on many children, who may have marveled that people they did not know from all parts of the country and the world tried to help them.

CONCLUDING COMMENTS

This chapter, emphasizing the wide applicability of group work with children, recommends a helping approach that combines play and art activities as a means of furthering communication with young clients. The group modality appeals to youngsters, who benefit from the sense of belonging and peer support intrinsic to an effective group. In group work with children, activities are considered as therapeutic tools, so the distinction that is sometimes made between "activity groups" and "therapy groups" does not apply. Instead, I have proposed an integrated model that joins both approaches.

It is important for the success of a group that the leader or leaders plan its composition and involve the members in adopting certain guiding principles that will assure each person confidentiality and respect. When these procedures are followed, the group can result not only in improved social interactions but also in increased feelings of self-esteem among individual members.

The special circumstances and guidelines for conducting crisis debriefing groups have been presented. Unlike other groups, which require prior screening of members, a crisis group consists of all individuals who shared a traumatic event. Timely and detailed attention to the emotional state of each individual helps prevent future possible symptom development, even as it helps group members realize that many of their feelings are shared by others. Bereavement groups with traumatically bereaved children must respect their varying abilities to deal with their painful traumatic memories. Accepting the support of others can help them heal, even as they can gradually reach out to other group members.

I hope that this chapter will encourage more social workers to use groups with children and will thereby reduce the neglect of this helpful modality in work with young clients.

DISCUSSION QUESTIONS AND ROLE-PLAY EXERCISE

1. Review some of the advantages of group interventions for children. What is the appropriate manner for preparing a child to enter a group?
2. Imagine that in a group for children with divorced parents, the male and female leaders disagree about the issue of visitation with the noncustodial parent. Consider the ideal way for the leaders to resolve their differences and speculate about the possible repercussions in the group if the matter remains unresolved.
3. How would you begin a group composed of 6- to 8-year-old children with parents who died in a traumatic explosion? Role-play what you would say and how you might deal with the silence of children who cannot talk about the death because it is too painful.
4. Identify a crisis event involving a group of children that was reported in the news media. Outline a model preventive intervention approach that would utilize group debriefing with the child survivors.

CHAPTER 9

School-Based Interventions

Next to the family, the school is probably the biggest influence on a child's life. In fact, because the school assumes responsibility for students during the time the children are on the school premises (i.e., the majority of children's waking hours), the school's role has been described as *in loco parentis*—"in place of the parents" (Allen-Meares, Washington, & Welsh, 2000). This shared responsibility for the well-being of the dependent child makes the liaison between school and home both logical and essential.

SCHOOL–HOME–COMMUNITY PARTNERSHIPS

In addition to the natural link between school and home, an even broader liaison exists between the school and community agencies. This reciprocal community–school relationship includes, on the one hand, school-initiated efforts to involve the community in matters related to children's safety and well-being and, on the other hand, the community's vested interest in obtaining the school's participation and involvement in projects outside the school that have an impact on children. Examples of the former efforts are school-initiated programs that link latchkey children with senior citizens, so that these children have regular, planned telephone contacts with adults after school. Conversely, examples of programs initiated in the community and later implemented in the schools are the Good-Touch/Bad-Touch curriculum (*www.goodtouchbadtouch.com*) and the Child Lures Prevention program (*https://childluresprevention.com*), which were developed because of community concern about sexual abuse of children.

Thus school-based interventions necessarily include work with the community and with parents, in addition to individual and group work with children. Helping children through school-based interventions includes work "from the outside in" (collaboration initiated by professionals outside the school system), as well as work "from the inside out" (efforts initiated in the school and reaching out into the family and community).

"From the Outside In": Essential Communication with the School

Any effort to help a child must *always* consider the nature of the child's functioning in the school environment. Because learning requires mental energy, a kindergarten child's preoccupation with her mother's impending surgery, for example, may cause the child to have trouble concentrating and to appear "spacey" to the teacher. (See Chapter 12 for details about such a case.) Ideally, the medical social worker, knowing that the mother has a young child, would obtain the mother's written permission to contact school personnel to inform appropriate persons about the impending surgery and hospitalization. This information would serve to alert school personnel and facilitate interventions for predictable changes in the child's behavior related to her worries about her mother and for her adaptation to the substitute caregiving she would receive in her mother's absence. Referral to the school social worker would ensure that the child would receive support during this difficult period.

As a matter of privacy and confidentiality (Family Educational Rights and Privacy Act (FERPA; 20 U.S.C. §1232g 34CFR Part 99), school personnel are required to secure written parent permission before discussing information about any student in their district. Similarly, professional helpers in the community who are working with a family in distress should *routinely* ask for written permission to contact the school for information about the child's past and current functioning. Sometimes parents (and even professionals) do not perceive the need for this contact, especially in situations that may appear to be non-school-related (e.g., following a death or some other traumatic family event, such as a house fire). However, professionals in the community should point out to parents the relationship between a child's emotional state and his or her ability to concentrate and learn. In addition, parents need to understand that when *they* are worried, the child usually intuits the parents' concerns, even in the absence of direct information. When social workers in family and child welfare agencies, hospitals, and emergency crisis clinics inform school personnel about a child's exposure to an upsetting event, this not only helps with the current situation but may also pay future dividends by building rapport with relevant school staff members that will expedite referrals and facilitate future collaboration about this and other cases.

ADDITIONAL "OUTSIDE" INFLUENCES ON THE SCHOOL: LEGISLATION

Because most schools receive their funding from federal, state, and local appropriations, the services offered to children depend on the availability of resources and the legislation governing specific programs. The establishment of these programs, in turn, affects the role of the school social worker. Hancock (1982, p. 41), in a statement as true today as it was 36 years ago, summarizes the significance of legislation on school social work practice as follows:

> School social work practice is affected by federal and state legislation, as well as by the resultant school district policies and procedures. School social workers must become familiar with current laws relating to education and be alert to new legislation. The effectiveness of school social work practice can be greatly diminished by the failure to acquire basic knowledge of legislation pertaining to education and keep abreast of new developments. It is also essential to be thoroughly acquainted with the policies of the school and sensitive to the need for changes in policy.

Reviews of legislation that influence services to children in schools appear in Openshaw (2008), Allen-Meares (2007), and the National Dissemination Center for Children with Disabilities (NICHCY; 2010). The present discussion focuses on specific laws that have a direct impact on the practice of school social workers:

1. *The Education for All Handicapped Children Act* (Public Law 94-142, 1975) was amended and revised in 1990 by the Individuals with Disabilities Education Act (IDEA; Public Law 101-476) and in 2004 by the Individuals with Disabilities Education Improvement Act (IDEA 2004; Public Law 108-446).

2. *The Every Student Succeeds Act* (ESSA, 2015) updates and revises some of the changes from the No Child Left Behind federal law of 2002. It still holds states responsible for making schools accountable and provides a flexible framework, allowing each state to set its own goals for student achievement within the federal guidelines. The law requires annual testing in reading and math in grades 3–8, and children must also be tested in science once in elementary school, middle school, and high school students with individualized education plans (IEPs) or 504 plans can get accommodations on all annual tests. States can choose the tests they use; however, only 1% of students can be given alternative tests. ESSA's academic standards allow states to adopt challenging standards in reading, math, and science without the oversight of the federal government. Accountability measures require states to consider more than just test scores on school evaluations.

It is the responsibility of the states to set achievement targets for students and high standards for students who are farthest behind, such as those in special education. Schools that are struggling to meet these standards will be given federal help on an improvement plan and extra funding (The Understood Team, 2017, p. 1). States must report findings by subgroups, such as special education, minorities, and poverty, and "if a state identifies a school or subgroup as struggling, it must tell parents" (The Understood Team, 2017, p. 1).

ESSA has a federal grant for $160 million for state and local schools to develop literacy skills and evidence-based instruction in literacy, writing, and phonological awareness (The Understood Team, 2017). Under ESSA, states are encouraged to expand personalized learning and utilize ESSA's Universal Design for Learning (UDL). It requires states to have parental and family input during the creation of the state plan and allows states to have their own opt-out laws if parents do not want their children to take standardized tests (The Understood Team, 2017).

Proficiency means that the child is performing at average grade level. All children in the school must meet the adequate yearly progress (AYP) requirements, or the school will fail. If a school fails or falls below the AYP standards, parents and students can choose which school the student will attend in the school district (Heath, 2004) or, if they live in the following states, receive federal vouchers to attend a school of the student's choice: Arizona, Colorado, Florida, Georgia, Indiana, Louisiana, Maine, Ohio, Oklahoma, Utah, Vermont, Wisconsin, and the District of Columbia.

The Education for All Handicapped Children Act, passed in 1975 with no expiration date, guaranteed all children with disabilities between the ages of 3 and 21 the right to a "free appropriate public education" (FAPE) in the "least restrictive environment" (LRE). This landmark legislation requires that an IEP be developed for every child with a disability found to be eligible for special education services and that the IEP specify all the educational and related services to be provided.

The Education for All Handicapped Children Act was amended by IDEA in 1990, with added provisions for assistance to states in developing early intervention services for infants and toddlers with disabilities and their families; the amended law also clarified discipline procedures for students eligible for special education services and provided continued assurance for the education of children and youth with disabilities from birth to age 21. Under this law, the school social worker's involvement includes providing functional behavioral assessment (FBA) assistance (including data obtained from observing the child and information about the child's social development history). Through procedural safeguards, the law ensures that parents participate in the evaluation process, placement discussions and decisions, and educational programming development, and the school social worker often plays an important role in helping to educate parents about the benefits of available services, as well as encouraging their participation throughout the IEP process. The LRE principle emphasizes the expectation that an eligible student's educational placement should be made as close as possible to that of typically developing peers, unless his or her disability and/or learning needs require a more restrictive placement.

IDEA 2004 and the 2006 amendments, with ongoing policy interpretations (Zirkel, 2017), continue to protect the education of all children with disabilities, while also addressing (1) the needs of students who move between agencies within a school year; (2) the circumstances for IEP team participants to be excused from IEP team meetings; (3) invitations to IEP team meetings for agency representatives who are responsible for providing or paying for transition services; (4) obtaining parental consent for initial assessments and reevaluations; and (5) the time lines for conducting initial evaluations for special education services. The current law specifies that these services are to be provided by qualified social workers, psychologists, guidance counselors, or other qualified school district and/or agency personnel (Newton-Logston & Armstrong, 1993, p. 187; NICHCY, 2010).

When IDEA 2004 was signed into law, it required that all education personnel look at poorly performing learners in a systematic manner to assess, analyze, and intervene early to separate those students who need some brief assistance and skill building from those who require long-term individualized attention to succeed in the general curriculum (Harader & Fullwood, 2010). This process involves three tiers and is called response to intervention (RTI).

When students are identified as "at risk" in relation to content area and/or social failure, individual or small-group interventions are implemented in the classroom, After a student has been identified at Tier 1 and interventions (e.g., classroom modifications, small-group instruction, alternative teaching models) are not successful, the student will then move through each successive tier (Tiers 2 and 3) until he or she is successful (Mellard, 2005). Tier 2 interventions maintain systematic and continuous monitoring of student progress (e.g., curriculum-based measurement with an "authentic" assessment that involves giving the student a task to perform and using a rubric to evaluate the performance). In addition, there is monitoring of instructional activities targeted specifically to the students' deficit areas (e.g., problem-solving strategies, specific academic and behavioral difficulties). At the Tier 3 level, interventions are specific to the student's unique deficits and learning needs or style and include individual intensive instruction, typically in a one-on-one learning situation. If, at the end of Tier 3, the student is still unsuccessful, he or she will be referred for formal eligibility evaluation under the requirements of IDEA 2004 (Fuchs, Mock, Morgan, & Young, 2003; Harader & Fullwood, 2010; Kovaleski, 2003; National Research Center on Learning Disabilities, 2006).

A referral to the IEP team results in a comprehensive, full individual evaluation by a school-based team of specialists who gather and review extensive information regarding the child's present level of performance in the areas of academic achievement, learning characteristics, hearing and vision, communication, health, social and physical development, and management needs (New York State Department of Education, 2002a; NICHCY, 2010). Table 9.1 lists and defines disability categories according to the latest federal regulations. A full discussion of each of these disabilities is beyond the scope of this chapter; however, Beauchaine and Hinshaw (2008) and Mash and Barkley (2014)

TABLE 9.1. Classifications of Disabilities

Classification	Definition of the disability
Autism	A developmental disability that significantly affects verbal and nonverbal communication and social interaction. It is generally evident before age 3. Other characteristics often associated with autism are engagement in repetitive activities and stereotyped movements, resistance to environmental change or change in daily routines, and unusual responses to sensory experiences.
Child with a disability	A child evaluated and determined to be eligible for special education placement and related services needs to be shown to have one of the following disabilities: mental retardation, a hearing impairment (including deafness), a speech or language impairment, a visual impairment (including blindness), a serious emotional disturbance (referred to in this part as "emotional disturbance"), an orthopedic impairment, autism, traumatic brain injury, another health impairment, a specific learning disability, deaf-blindness, or multiple disabilities.
Deafness	A hearing impairment so severe that it prevents the processing of linguistic information through hearing, with or without amplification.
Deaf-blindness	Concomitant hearing and visual impairments that cause such severe communication and other developmental and educational problems that the student cannot be accommodated in special education programs solely for either deaf or blind students.
Developmental delay	A disability in child ages 3–9 (or any subset of that age range, including ages 3–5) who is experiencing developmental delays, as defined by the State and as measured by appropriate diagnostic instruments and procedures, in one or more of the following areas: physical development, cognitive development, communication development, social or emotional development, or adaptive development; and who, by reason thereof, needs special education and related services.
Emotional disturbance	A condition that is demonstrated in difficulties in school that cannot be explained by intellectual, sensory, or health factors. Over a long period of time, the student is usually unable to build satisfactory relationships, may be generally unhappy, may develop physical symptoms or have fears associated with his or her school experience, or may demonstrate inappropriate behaviors or feelings. It is a condition characterized by one or more of the following characteristics over a long period of time and to a marked degree, adversely affecting a child's educational performance: (1) an inability to learn that cannot be explained by intellectual, sensory, or health factors; (2) an inability to build or maintain satisfactory interpersonal relationships with peers and teachers; (3) inappropriate types of behavior or feelings under normal circumstances; (4) a general pervasive mood of unhappiness or depression; (5) a tendency to develop physical symptoms or fears associated with personal or school problems. Emotional disturbance includes schizophrenia. The term does not apply to children who are socially maladjusted, unless it is determined that they have an emotional disturbance.

(continued)

TABLE 9.1. *(continued)*

Classification	Definition of the disability
Hearing impairment	Impairment in hearing, whether permanent or fluctuating, that adversely affects a student's educational performance.
Learning disability	A disorder in one or more of the basic processes involved in understanding or using spoken or written language. A child who is learning-disabled has difficulty listening, thinking, speaking, reading, writing, or doing arithmetic. This child's disability results in a severe discrepancy between his or her ability and achievement. A learning disability is not primarily due to a physical, mental, or emotional disability or to environmental, cultural, or economic disadvantage.
Mental retardation	Significantly subaverage general intellectual functioning that exists concurrently with deficits in adaptive behavior. This condition adversely affects a child's educational performance.
Multiple disabilities	Concomitant impairments that result in multisensory or motor deficiencies and developmental lags in the cognitive, affective, or psychomotor areas. The combination of these disabilities causes educational problems that cannot be accommodated through a special education program designed solely for one of the disabilities.
Orthopedic impairment	A severe orthopedic impairment that adversely affects the child's educational performance. Included are the impairments caused by congenital anomalies, impairments caused by disease, and impairments from other causes (e.g., cerebral palsy, amputation, and fractures or burns that cause contractures).
Other health impairment	Having limited strength, vitality, or alertness due to chronic or acute health problems that adversely affect educational performance. These problems may include a heart condition, tuberculosis, rheumatic fever, nephritis, asthma, sickle cell anemia, Tourette syndrome, hemophilia, epilepsy, lead poisoning, leukemia, or diabetes.
Speech impairment	A communication disorder such as stuttering, impaired articulation, a language impairment, or a voice disorder that adversely affects a child's educational performance.
Traumatic brain injury	An acquired injury to the brain due to open or closed head injuries caused by an external physical force or by medical conditions such as encephalitis, stroke, aneurysm, anoxia, or brain tumors. The injuries result in mild to severe impairments in one or more areas, including cognition, language, memory, attention, reasoning, abstract thinking, problem solving, sensory/perceptual and motor abilities, psychosocial behavior, physical functions, information processing, and speech. The term does not include congenital injuries or impairments caused by birth trauma.
Visual impairment	An impairment to vision that, even with correction, adversely affects educational performance.

Note. Based on the Individuals with Disabilities Education Act (IDEA; 2006).

provide a complete review of child psychopathology, including chapters on behavior disorders, various emotional disturbances of childhood, and learning disorders. A section on children with special needs and a case example involving a child with autism appear later in this chapter.

This legislation has caused social workers to assume a visible and important role as case managers in the schools of many states. It was very significant to the field of social work that Congress specifically mentioned the tasks and services social workers would perform when this legislation was passed (Allen-Meares et al., 2000; Openshaw, 2008). Social workers may coordinate an array of interdisciplinary school personnel in developing the IEP for each student identified for special education services. They may also prepare the social history, ensure that all relevant information is considered in formulating goals, and assist in including the parents as equal partners in the educational planning for their child. The recommendations of an IEP for an identified child are discussed more fully later in this chapter.

OVERVIEW OF THE ROLE OF THE SCHOOL SOCIAL WORKER

"From the Inside Out": Working within the School

Social workers have provided school-based services since the turn of the 20th century, when they were called "visiting teachers" because they made home visits to help orient immigrant families to U.S. culture and the role of the school (Costin, 1969, 1987; Allen-Meares et al., 2000; Allen-Meares, 2007). The nature of the school social worker's role has varied since then, with emphasis shifting from providing casework services to the individual child to focusing on the problem rather than on the person to the more recent conceptualization of facilitating home–school–community collaboration (Franklin, 2000). The current role of the school social worker requires adaptability and skills for all levels of practice—micro, mezzo, and macro. As Openshaw (2008, p. 2) states:

> The school social work role varies from school to school and from school district to school district. Some school districts employ school social workers to serve multiple schools or to work with a single broad population. Other districts assign the social worker to a single school or a narrow population. . . . The diversity of the social worker's roles creates a wide variety of functions and responsibilities for school social workers.

The NASW has identified important guidelines for the delivery of social work services in schools, including standards for practice, professional preparation and development, and administrative structure and support. These guidelines are set forth in the *NASW Standards for School Social Work Services*, which were adopted in 1978 and revised in 1992, 2002, 2012, and 2017 (National Association of Social Workers, 2017). "School social workers should be aware that they may be held accountable under these standards whether they are members of NASW or not" (Openshaw, 2008, pp. 2–3).

Costin (1987) identified the following roles and tasks as being included in the parameters of the school social worker's role, and these remain valid 30 years later:

- Identification of children in need
- Extending services to pupils
- Working with school personnel
- Educational planning for disabled children
- Working with parents
- Community services

Additional responsibilities in today's world often include responding to violence and tragedy after a critical incident occurs (Miller, 2003). This may involve setting up and conducting *debriefing groups* in which participants can discuss and gain perspective about what happened, thereby reducing stress and enhancing coping. School social workers may be members of a crisis team whose role is to assess the need for intervention, and then to implement the agreed-upon plan (Miller, 2003). It is important for schools to be prepared in advance for possible incidents of violence, and social workers can play an important role in planning appropriate interventions.

These important responsibilities are carried out within a "host" setting in which social work is *not* the dominant discipline. Because the main purpose of the schools is education, social workers in school settings must help fulfill this educational purpose. Many years ago Hepworth and Larsen (1982, p. 283) specified that the goals of the school social worker

> center upon helping pupils attain a sense of competence, [and] a readiness for continued learning. . . . Increasingly, the focus of school social work is on cognitive areas—learning, thinking, and problem-solving—as well as the traditional areas of concern, i.e., relationships, emotions, motivation, and personality.

In order to facilitate the child's learning, the school social worker serves as a liaison *within* the school system between the children and the school staff and *outside* the school system with the parents and community personnel. This role may include, but is not limited to, the following tasks:

- Collecting information about a child for a social history.
    - Conferring with teachers, school nurses, and other staff members about methods for helping a child.
- Planning meetings for parents, with speakers and discussions focusing on such topics as child behavior, parenting techniques, and relevant community concerns.

- Working with community agencies to establish Big Brother/Big Sister connections for children in need.
- Collaborating with foster care, family, welfare, probation, and other social service agencies involved with the child and family.

According to Franklin (2000), the school social worker's very diverse roles encompass consultation, facilitation, collaboration, education, mediation, advocacy, and intervention. Readers who want a comprehensive presentation of the history and scope of school social work services may consult Allen-Meares (2007) and Openshaw (2008). The case of Pedro, later in this chapter, involves a young child with complicated and difficult behavioral symptoms finally diagnosed as autism. The case demonstrates how a school social worker helped 7-year-old Pedro and his family receive needed special education services.

Necessary Knowledge and Skills

The multidimensional role of school social workers requires both generic and specialized knowledge and skills. The *generic* base of knowledge and skills includes the ability to do the following:

- Think systemically.
- Formulate a comprehensive biopsychosocial assessment.
- Appreciate ethnic diversity and its effects on children's socialization.
- Establish and maintain relationships with parents and with personnel relevant to the work with a child.
- Help all parties formulate specific goals related to the child's needs.
- Link the family system to community resources.
- Monitor the progress and involvement of the child and others with respect to the goals.

The core of *specialized* knowledge required for competent practice as a school social worker includes the following:

- An understanding of special education and its related laws.
- Knowledge about children's rights and parents' rights.
- The ability to work on a team and to communicate and collaborate effectively with professionals who are not social workers.
- The ability to work within the bureaucratic structure of the school system.
- The ability to implement cognitive-behavioral treatment with children, families, and teachers.
- An understanding of the impact of physical, sexual, and emotional abuse and neglect on a child and how to respond appropriately when children are affected by these and other traumatic situations.

- An awareness of the pervasiveness of bullying and an ability to employ various methods for dealing with the repercussions of this.
- The ability to provide therapeutic intervention with children and families in both one-to-one and group formats.
- The ability to apply crisis intervention methods appropriately, including being able to conduct debriefing groups after school incidents such as shootings and a suicide.
- Understand when to utilize appropriate community agencies in a crisis emergency.

The school social workers I have interviewed about the nature of their role emphasize being able to "think on their feet" and to respond quickly and directly as central to competent practice in schools. For example, a teacher in the cafeteria may make an unexpected request for help, or a fight may break out in a corridor that demands prompt intervention by the social worker, who just happens to be in the vicinity. Ginsburg (1989, p. 87) states that "the school social worker should not be hiding in an office. Rather, it is important to be visible and aware of the school's agenda and of what is happening there."

In 1992, NASW developed a School Social Work Specialist (SSWS) credential and administered its first exam for the credential. Many states offer a school social work credential, but it is not required to practice as a school social worker. As noted above, the 2012 *NASW Standards for School Social Work Services* establish national guidelines for school social workers.

ISSUES IN INTERPROFESSIONAL COLLABORATION

Teamwork

Social work with children *always* involves interactions with family members, as well as with others who know the child and may be able to offer a perspective that enriches the worker's solitary view. Teamwork is fundamental in providing services to the child in the school. The members of the team vary in different settings but often include the school psychologist, the child's general education teacher and/or special education teacher, a principal, and a specialized therapist, in addition to the child's parents.

The Case of Johnny, Age 5

Johnny was referred to the social worker when the child's general education kindergarten teacher became concerned about his short attention span, aggression toward other children, and impatience at having to take turns on the playground equipment during recess. The teacher asked the social worker to contact the parents to see whether family stress might be contributing to the child's difficulties. In discussions with the child's mother, the school social worker obtained written permission to observe the child in the classroom. She also gleaned important information about the family. The parents were actively seeking to adopt a baby; in fact, they had recently left Johnny abruptly to go to a hospital in another state, where a prospective adoptee had just been born. When the birth mother changed her mind, the parents returned home and told Johnny that "the mother decided to keep the baby." Johnny, who knew that he himself had been adopted, became very confused about this sequence of events, as well as about his mother's sadness, irritability, and repeated statements about wanting to "get another baby sooner or later."

Several joint counseling sessions with Johnny, the social worker, and his mother provided the opportunity to reassure Johnny that his adoptive parents loved him very much and would never give *him* up, as he had begun to fear. It also permitted both Johnny and his mother to voice their mutual wish to have a little baby in the house, so Johnny could experience being "a big brother." Finally, the mother (with the social worker's guidance) reassured Johnny that if she and his father had to go away again to try to adopt another baby, they would tell Johnny first and say goodbye, even if it was in the middle of the night.

This short-term, school-based intervention brought dramatic improvement in Johnny's peer interactions in school. His ability to focus on his learning also improved, because he was no longer worried about his mother and father's sudden disappearance and about being displaced by a new baby. This example portrays not only successful RTI Tier 1 intervention (i.e., short-term family counseling, anxiety management instruction) but also collaboration between the social worker and the teacher in the ideal situation—one in which the professionals work together to understand the child's problem and in which the parent openly shares the family's concerns with the school social worker. Unfortunately, this ideal state of trust, communication, and cooperation does not always exist.

Ethical Dilemmas: Who Is the "Client"?

Social workers are sometimes uncomfortable with team participation because of the implicit expectation that they share information about families with the other team members. In fact, social workers may feel caught in an ethical bind about disclosing information that was given to them in confidence. Garrett (1994) points out that school social workers may have difficulty determining who the client is, as the school, the child, and the family all have a stake in the designated problem situation. Whereas the NASW code of ethics states that "social workers [should] respect and promote the rights of clients to self-determination" (National Association of Social Workers, 1996, Section 1:02), the application of this principle in school settings requires a concept of "client" that encompasses the triangle of child, family, and school. Even with this conceptualization, however, the social worker may think it unnecessary and inappropriate to divulge to a child's teacher all the intimate details of the parents' marriage and other sensitive family matters.

Professional discretion regarding sharing of information with other members of the school team, in my opinion, must be guided by the best interests of the child and by what will best serve the child's learning experience. Therefore, it may be unnecessary for a teacher to know about a mother's substance abuse background when the mother is in recovery. However, it may be helpful for the teacher to know that this child's working mother leaves her in the care of a babysitter in the evening, as the teacher has noticed that the child yawns a lot and seems tired in school. It is important for the teacher to communicate with the mother that her child seems tired so that the mother will be able to impress on the child's sitter the need for a regular, specific bedtime.

Parents are often concerned about the nature of the information in their children's school records. As already discussed in Chapter 2, the federal Family Educational Rights and Privacy Act (Public Law 93-380, 1974) gives parents the right to inspect their children's school records and dispute any information that they feel is inaccurate. Therefore, all school personnel should be both accurate and discreet regarding the information they write in the record. As parents are increasingly encouraged to take an active role in their children's educational planning, school personnel must continue to view parents as partners.

Interprofessional Communication

Because education professionals with different backgrounds and training must work together as interdisciplinary teams on behalf of the students in their schools, it is essential that these professionals understand enough about one another's respective areas of specialization to communicate effectively. For example, the school social worker needs sufficient knowledge about educational and psychological tests to comprehend their significance in the school psychologist's reports. Similarly, the school social worker should understand the possible contributions of the special education teacher, the speech therapist, and the physical therapist in assisting children with disabilities; they also need to be knowledgeable about the various medications prescribed to alleviate a child's symptoms, especially when fearful parents may ask whether the medications are harmful and if they could cause addiction.

Few school social workers are knowledgeable about the assessment and appropriate intervention for *all* disabling conditions, necessitating interprofessional collaboration, cooperation, and communication. However, school social workers who work with children with special learning needs inherently build the knowledge base and skills that allow them to communicate effectively with colleagues and parents about the disabling conditions and recommended educational interventions by using a team service approach.

Because this team approach is inherent in school social work practice, there can be no sense of personal "ownership" of any case; rather, there must be a sharing of responsibility. School social workers need to understand the essential elements of membership in interdisciplinary teams, which requires (1) interdependence among team members, (2) the ability to practice independently and take on new tasks as necessary, (3) flexibility, (4) collective ownership of goals, and (5) the ability to reflect on processes (Bronstein, 2003).

Working with School Administrators

The role of the building administrator (e.g., school principal, dean of students) has been compared to that of a captain of a ship, insofar as he or she has ultimate responsibility for what happens in the vessel or school building. Parents, the school board, and the community expect the building administrator to be in charge and knowledgeable about the curriculum, after-school activities, and faculty and staff issues and about children who are having learning difficulties (and the helping plans for such children). Hancock (1982) points out that principals are public figures without job tenure who are vulnerable to pressures from various factions in the community and whose position may subject them to intense scrutiny and even litigation. Skilled principals are described as able to facilitate and manage change, disperse power, promote schoolwide commitment to learning, encourage experimentation, strongly support teachers while expecting all teachers to participate in the work of the school, and distribute rewards (Allen-Meares et al., 2014). They also influence the climate in their schools through their administrative and disciplinary styles.

Because of the expectations placed on principals, their interest in and need to know about the activities of school social workers and other school employees who interact with parents and agencies in the community is understandable. Of course, every principal functions according to his or her unique personality and history of relations with past "helpers" (both in and out of the school environment). The attitudes in the community about social workers, as well as their appropriate role and function in the school, will also have an impact on the building administrator.

It is incumbent on school social workers to develop harmonious working relationships with their principals. During the initial phase of their contacts, both parties should articulate and discuss their respective expectations regarding the social work role to avoid future ambiguity and confusion. The common goal of wanting to facilitate the educational experience of the children in the school can serve as the foundation for a solid social worker–principal relationship, which will promote the best interests of the children in the school.

CHILDREN WITH SPECIAL NEEDS

As noted earlier, IDEA 2004 (Public Law 108-446) protects the right of children with disabilities to a free appropriate public education (FAPE) in the least restrictive environment (LRE) and Section 504 of the Rehabilitation Act of

1973 (Public Law 93-112). Before describing the process of identifying such children, we must first review the variety of general terms used currently and in the past to refer to children with special needs. Historically, these children have been referred to as "handicapped," "exceptional," "disabled," "defective," "impaired," and as "children with individual learning differences." When children have more than one special-needs condition, they are referred to as students with multiple disabilities.

However, the legislation refers to "children with disabilities," and its classification system uses terms such as "emotional disturbance," "hearing impairment," and "learning disability" for various categories. Such terms emphasize the *losses* or disruptions created by different physical, emotional, and cognitive conditions. It has been said that these views of disability tend to minimize the humanity of the affected persons (Lavin, 2002).

In view of the pejorative connotations of most of these labels, the terminology of educators seems appropriately sensitive to children's feelings of being "different" from other children. Thus being in "special education" classes or leaving a "regular," or general education, classroom to go to the "resource room" does not in itself imply inferiority (although the children themselves and their classmates often attach their own negative connotations to these terms).

A child may be born with a disabling condition or may become disabled through an accident or injury. Attitudes toward children with disabilities have gradually become more accepting, with emphasis on what the children *can* do rather than on his or her limitations. Those who prefer to focus on strengths rather than on limitations argue for use of the term "children with special needs."

Parents of Special-Needs Children

Despite efforts to destigmatize children with special needs, the parents of such a child suffer greatly upon learning definitively about their child's specific condition. All parents want their children to be well and to possess the necessary innate abilities to deal effectively with life. When parents are told (either at birth or later by a pediatrician or other specialist) that there is something wrong with their child, this information stirs up a barrage of feelings, including anger, denial, guilt, and tremendous sadness. Olshansky (1962) coined the expression "chronic sorrow" to refer to the grief of parents in response to the diagnosis of their child's disability and to the recurrence (i.e., chronicity) of that grief throughout the child's life, when it becomes repeatedly apparent that the child's condition requires special assistance from a variety of professionals. Social workers who have ongoing contact with parents of classified children tend to support the view that these parents' grief is chronic and requires sensitive response from school personnel (Rothschild, 1986). The social worker's goals in counseling the parents of a special child, according to Rothschild (1986, p. 42), are (1) to increase the parents' acceptance of living with and adjusting to their disabled child and (2) to help the parents develop the tools they need to increase their child's skills through "translating" the processes of the child's education to the parents. Ideally, the social worker can assist the parents of a disabled child to focus on his or her abilities and positive features, rather than on the child's limitations.

Some special education programs offer support groups for parents of special-needs children, including such nationally affiliated groups as special education parent–teacher associations (SEPTAs), the Learning Disabilities Association of America (LDA), Children and Adults with Attention-Deficit/Hyperactivity Disorder (CHADD), and the Autism Society. Such groups give these parents the opportunity to listen to and discuss both positive and negative feelings and to contribute to and benefit from the solutions of other parents who have similar frustrations and pressures. Dillard, Donenberg, and Glickman (1986, p. 50) point out that "just as a child may experience negative affect and feel separated from the mainstream of school life when placed in a special education class or program, parents may experience similar negative feelings." However, some students thrive and are very happy in smaller classroom settings such as those provided by special education. This might be a helpful fact to point out to parents to lessen their tendency to have negative feelings about their child's special needs.

The Three-Tiered Identification Process

Before a child can be referred for evaluation for special education services, school personnel are required to show evidence of implementation of appropriate interventions that have had little or no impact on the child's current educational progress. The term "response to intervention" (RTI) signifies that the student has been identified as being evaluated on one of the following three tiers of intervention. Tier 1 indicates that the student is not progressing satisfactorily. The student then moves through each successive tier (Tiers 2 and 3) until he or she has been successful (Mellard, 2005). If, at the end of Tier 3 intervention implementation, the student is still struggling, he or she will be referred for a formal eligibility evaluation under the requirements of IDEA 2004 (Harader & Fullwood, 2010).

Federal legislation requires that all schools receiving federal funding follow specific procedures in assessing children who have been referred to the IEP team for a comprehensive evaluation. The steps in this evaluation process, according to the New York State Department of Education's (2009) guide for parents, are the following:

- Referral
- Evaluation
- Eligibility
- IEP
- Placement

- Instruction
- Annual review

The guide describes each step, with clear guidelines for parents regarding how to exercise their own and their child's rights to an appropriate educational placement.

Section 504 of the Rehabilitation Act of 1973 requires agencies to provide information regarding federal and state laws on their websites; these can be found through the department of education or education agency for each state, as well as through U.S. Government websites. The information is presented in a user-friendly description of the special education process in order to provide parents with the knowledge they need to ensure that appropriate educational programs are provided for their children with special needs. Involvement of the parents is basic to the various procedures, beginning with the referral, which requires written parental consent before the evaluation can proceed.

Components of a Comprehensive Evaluation

Once a request for an evaluation has been received, the IEP team has met, and the parents have given their written consent, a team of specialists prepares a comprehensive assessment of the child's skills and abilities. IDEA 2004 states that to conduct the full individual evaluation, a local education agency (LEA) must "use a variety of assessment tools and strategies to gather relevant functional, developmental, and academic information, including information provided by the parent" (NICHCY, 2010). It also states that (1) the LEA must "not use any single measure or assessment as the sole criterion for determining whether a child has a disability or for determining an appropriate educational program for the child," and (2) it must "use technically sound instruments that may assess the relative contribution of cognitive and behavioral factors, in addition to physical or developmental factors."

The components of a full individual evaluation are outlined in Table 9.2. The IEP team arranges to obtain the necessary information through a variety of assessment tools and strategies within 60 days of receiving written parental consent for evaluation and to schedule discussion of these findings at an IEP team meeting, in which the district must make every effort to ensure parental participation. The goal of the evaluation is to arrive at a recommendation that summarizes a child's present level of educational performance, establishes educational goals and objectives for each school year, describes program components needed to meet these goals, and lists ways to systematically monitor the child's ongoing progress.

A child may be found ineligible for special education when the IEP team finds that the student cannot be identified as having one of the disabling conditions defined in Table 9.1. Such "ineligible" children may, however, qualify for a variety of educationally related support services (e.g., short-term counseling or speech–language improvement services) through Section 504 of the

TABLE 9.2. Components of a Comprehensive Education

An initial evaluation to determine [a] child's needs must include:

- A physical examination
- A psychological evaluation (if determined appropriate for school-age students, but mandatory for preschool children)
- A social history
- Observation of [the] child in his or her current education setting
- Other tests or assessments that are appropriate for [the] child (such as speech and language assessment or a functional behavioral assessment)
- Vocational assessments (required at age 12)

Note. From New York State Department of Education (2002a, p. 5).

Rehabilitation Act of 1973. Under Section 504, " 'no qualified individual with a disability shall be excluded from, denied the benefits of, or be subjected to discrimination under' any program or activity that either receives Federal financial assistance or is conducted by an Executive agency of the United States Postal Service" (U.S. Department of Justice, 2009, p. 19). FAPE means the provision of general or special education and related aids and services designed to meet the student's individual educational needs as adequately as the needs of nondisabled students are met. According to the U.S. Department of Education, an appropriate education for "a student with a disability under the Section 504 regulations could consist of education in regular classrooms, education in regular classes with supplementary services, and/or special education and related services" (Office for Civil Rights, 2009). These services may be developed and implemented through a "504 plan."

On the other hand, when a child is found to be eligible for special education services, the IEP should detail the specific nature of the recommended educational placements, accommodations, modifications, and related services, following the principle of LRE. For example, if a child's abilities in a specific area (e.g., math) qualify him or her to participate in a "regular," or general education, math class, this placement must be implemented. Special class instruction, when indicated, will specify conditions such as student–teacher ratio, accommodations and modifications required, supplementary aids and services to be included, related services to be provided, and teacher training required, along with the student being grouped according to the similarity of his or her learning needs to those of other children.

The Role of the Social Worker in Special Education

Some school social workers work primarily or exclusively in special education programs, but the job descriptions of most school social workers include working both with children who have been classified as disabled and with children in the general school population. The specific responsibilities of the social worker related to special education include contact with parents; counseling parents through the evaluation period (and afterward, when indicated); obtaining and writing children's social histories; participating in IEP team meetings; advocating for the children; and working with the teachers, special education staff, building administrator, and families to implement the goals of children's IEPs. Sometimes the social worker provides individual counseling with a child and/or parent or family counseling (which may include home visits). In addition, the worker may provide group interventions with children, as well as with parents who have similar needs.

In summary, the role and functions of the social worker in special education programs are similar to those of any school social worker. However, the special education social worker must also have specialized knowledge regarding disability categories and procedures, as well as the skill and sensitivity to implement this knowledge with other professionals and with parents. Some of these functions are illustrated in the following case, which is a composite of typical cases.

THE CASE OF PEDRO, AGE 7

Family Information

Family Members in the Child's Household

Paternal grandmother	Mrs. Lopez, age mid-60s.
Father	Mr. Lopez, age 30; itinerant construction worker.
Child client	Pedro, age 7, first grade (see the following for details of classification and educational placement).

Other Family Members

Mother (deceased)	Anna, died abruptly of complications from a heart attack when Pedro was 4.

This is a South American family. Mr. Lopez immigrated to the United States from Ecuador when he was 22 years old, settling in New York. He met and married Anna 2 years later, and Pedro was born a year after that. There was considerable discord in the marriage, and on several occasions Mrs. Lopez left, taking Pedro with her to live with her parents in Florida. Anna was a native of Peru and was bilingual in Spanish and English, as was Mr. Lopez. The couple spoke to each other and to Pedro in English. Pedro had exposure to Spanish and learned to speak it during his first 3 years, when he visited his maternal grandparents' home.

Shortly after the Lopezes' last reconciliation, Anna died in her sleep from a heart attack. Pedro, then age 4, had been sleeping with her at the time. When Mrs. Lopez's body was discovered late the next morning, Pedro was found lying on the bed in a fetal position, crying. Within a month, Mr. Lopez took Pedro back to Ecuador, where they would both have the support of his family. While there, Pedro began attending the Spanish-speaking local school. Mr. Lopez stayed with Pedro for several months and then returned to the United States to work, leaving his son with his parents. Pedro spent a total of 2 years in Ecuador with his grandparents, and Mr. Lopez visited periodically. Tragically, the area in which they lived was struck by an earthquake, and Pedro witnessed the devastation of his school and community. A month later, Mr. Lopez brought his mother and Pedro back to the United States to live.

Presenting Problem

Soon after returning to the United States with Pedro, Mr. Lopez went to the neighborhood school and asked to speak to someone about his son, whom he had just registered for the new school year. He was referred to the school social worker and the school psychologist. Mr. Lopez was proactive in apprising the school of his son's unusual and traumatic history in anticipation that he would have special needs. Mr. Lopez also reported significant difficulties with Pedro's behavior at home. He described his son as extremely hyperactive, with difficulty sleeping at night, very finicky eating habits, and disturbing oppositional behavior. Pedro became easily frustrated and physically aggressive (throwing himself and/or objects to the floor) when he did not get his way. Furthermore, he rarely spoke or made eye contact.

Summary

Pedro was a 6-year-old child, about to begin school in a new community after being schooled in another country in another language for the previous 2 years. He had just survived the trauma of a devastating earthquake, which may have rekindled the previous trauma of his mother's sudden death. Pedro was also adjusting to living again with his father and being reintroduced to the English language.

Mr. Lopez explained that prior to the latest trauma of the earthquake, there had been serious concerns about Pedro's academic and behavioral functioning in the school he attended in Ecuador. Had they remained there, Pedro would have been retained in first grade. His highly distractible and impulsive behavior had prompted the school there to make a referral to a psychologist, who diagnosed Pedro with ADHD. Mr. Lopez had not yet followed up on the recommendation for a trial of medication when they left Ecuador and returned to the United States.

School Placement

Pedro began school the next day and was placed in a first-grade class, based on his history of difficulties. He presented as a very physically appealing child with dark brown hair and sparkling brown eyes. He was quiet and understandably anxious, and he did not make eye contact. However, he appeared to understand when spoken to. Over the course of the next few weeks, as Pedro became acclimated to his new school environment, patterns of behavior emerged that were of great concern. The boy was very hyperactive, distractible, and impulsive. He disrupted the class by making animal noises, crawling on the floor, spitting at his classmates, licking the furniture, and laughing inappropriately. When he did not get his way, he would sometimes become physically aggressive, attempting to bite, kick, or hit his classmates. Sometimes he would purposely fall off his chair and repeatedly bang his head on the floor. Pedro also showed compulsive behaviors, such as washing his hands and the furniture repeatedly. If allowed to, he would sharpen pencils all day. Although his classmates were taken aback by his behavior, some of them did try to befriend Pedro. But he did not seem interested in social interaction and showed a clear preference for playing alone.

Pedro's academic skills were very limited. He could recognize only a few letters and numbers. At home, Pedro would have violent tantrums when asked to do anything that he did not want to. Mr. Lopez, having recently assumed primary parenting responsibility for Pedro for the first time, was feeling overwhelmed, helpless, and depressed.

Interventions

Pedro was a puzzle. There were so many variables at play in his young life that it was difficult to determine with any certainty what was influencing his behavior. Although there were several diagnostic possibilities, including ADHD, PTSD, depression, anxiety, or just the utter frustration of all the losses, transitions, and upheavals in his life, it was difficult to draw any diagnostic conclusions. From the standpoint of the school, however, certain immediate concerns had to be addressed: (1) Pedro's aggressive behavior, which posed a safety concern for both the boy and his classmates and which would prompt the school to consider RTI Tier 3 interventions; (2) Pedro's disruptive behavior, which affected both his own learning and that of his classmates; (3) Pedro's low academic functioning, which cast doubt on the appropriateness of his placement in a mainstream first-grade class. He clearly needed more individualized and intensive attention, both academically and behaviorally, in order to function in a school setting. Also, Mr. Lopez desperately needed help in managing Pedro's behavior at home. Furthermore, there needed to be consistency between the school and the home in terms of behavior management. In response to these concerns, the school social worker initiated several interventions to address both the school and home issues.

Referral and Consultation with Mental Health Agency

The social worker made an immediate referral to a local mental health agency to arrange a psychiatric evaluation and therapy and to provide Pedro's father with consultation regarding parenting, as well as psychotherapy to address his own depression. With Mr. Lopez's written permission, the social worker served as the liaison between the school and the mental health agency, updating the therapist on Pedro's progress at school and providing feedback regarding the effectiveness of the medication that was prescribed.

The therapist and psychiatrist remained baffled for a time regarding Pedro's diagnosis and treatment. They proceeded with the working diagnostic hypothesis of ADHD complicated by PTSD. After several months of treatment with minimal progress, Mr. Lopez brought Pedro to the county medical center, where he had a pediatric neurodevelopment evaluation. It was there that Pedro was diagnosed with autism. This diagnosis was initially difficult for Mr. Lopez to accept, although it was a relief to arrive at a diagnosis that seemed to explain this boy's behavior. Although Pedro had certainly endured multiple traumas, the key to this diagnosis was a careful review of the boy's early development (notably behavior problems and truncated speech development) prior to his mother's death.

Classroom Behavior

In collaboration with the school psychologist and classroom teacher, a behavior intervention and supports plan (BIP) was designed and implemented in the classroom, whereby Pedro was rewarded for compliant behavior. Given his limited attention span and tolerance for frustration, Pedro initially received reinforcement for very brief intervals of compliance. After 2 weeks of slight behavior improvement, the intervals were gradually lengthened. Pedro was rewarded with either tangibles (a sticker or pretzels) or a favored activity, such as coloring. A time-out procedure was also implemented, minimizing the disruptive impact of Pedro's behavior on the rest of the class. These interventions were followed and monitored for 3 months with an evaluation at the end of each week indicating either some, little, or no progress.

Data Collection

Unfortunately, records from Pedro's previous school in Ecuador were not available. Mr. Lopez did, however, give written permission to obtain psychological and speech records from Florida, where Pedro had been evaluated just prior to his mother's death. These proved to be very telling. When Pedro was about 4 years old, his parents sought the help of a psychologist out of concern about his unmanageable behavior. At that time he would have frequent tantrums and mood swings. Although Pedro's speech and language development was normal when he was a toddler, he suddenly stopped speaking at about 3 years of age and began pointing to what he wanted. Just as Pedro had begun treatment, his mother died, and he moved to Ecuador with his father. This report was helpful in that it revealed that there were significant issues with Pedro even *prior* to his mother's death.

Referral to the IEP Committee

After interventions were implemented and Pedro's progress was reported as minimal, a referral was made to the IEP team. The committee met to determine whether there was sufficient evidence to warrant a full individual evaluation. All IEP team members discussed Pedro's educational, medical, social, and communication problems and decided an evaluation for eligibility for special education services was appropriate. This involved a thorough evaluation of Pedro's cognitive ability, academic skills, communication functioning, social competence, physical and medical needs, and speech–language functioning and a social history.

Once the IEP team met to review evaluation data and determine eligibility, they decided that Pedro would benefit from a one-to-one aide to monitor the BIP (behavior intervention plan), and he began to receive special education instruction that was tailored to his level of academic and social functioning. He also began speech–language therapy. In addition to services for Pedro, it was clear that Mr. Lopez would need a tremendous amount of support and guidance. It was decided to schedule monthly team meetings with Mr. Lopez, the special education teacher, and the social worker so that there could be a mutual exchange of information about Pedro's school and home functioning.

Information and Community Resources

The social worker provided Mr. Lopez with educational materials and information about autism, as well as resources for parent support networks. One of these resources was another parent in the school district who had a child with autism. This parent was a dynamic advocate for her own child within the school system and was very knowledgeable about community resources. She made herself available to other parents who needed information and support. (A helpful reference for parents of autistic children is Ozonoff, Dawson, & McPartland, 2002; a book on the topic for children is *Russell Is Extra Special* [Amenta, 1992].)

Child Care

Mr. Lopez's mother was Pedro's after-school caretaker. She was easily overwhelmed by her grandson's behavior and tended to give in to him rather than establish boundaries and limits. The decision was made for the social worker to arrange after-school child care at a local day care center. The social worker discussed Pedro's special needs with the director of the day care center, thereby helping to pave the way for a child such as Pedro.

Financial Assistance

Mr. Lopez's financial situation was often strained. The social worker apprised him of Pedro's probable eligibility for Social Security Disability Insurance based on his special needs (he was born in the United States, which automatically made him a U.S. citizen). This additional source of revenue was a help to the family. Often school personnel will assist a parent with the completion of these applications, because they are often daunting to parents, especially those who are not fluent in English.

Camp and Respite Services

The social worker researched and provided to Mr. Lopez information regarding recreational and respite programs that catered to children with special needs. These would provide a much-needed occasional break for Mr. Lopez and his mother and provide Pedro with additional opportunities for social stimulation and fun.

Summary

Over the course of 2 years, adjustments were made to Pedro's medication and his IEP, and to his BIP and academic program. Pedro made slow but steady progress academically, socially, and behaviorally. A sustained coordinated effort by the school (and the various school professionals within the school), the home, and outside agencies was necessary to ensure Pedro's growth. The school social worker was instrumental in establishing and sustaining these linkages.

The prevalence of autism has increased in the last decade to a rate as high as 1 in 250 children (Calohan & Peeler, 2007). The Centers for Disease Control and Prevention (2018) in their biennial update reports a prevalence rate for autism spectrum disorder as 1 in 59 children (1 in 37 boys and 1 in 151 girls). This represents an increase in prevalence of 15% from the previous report. Two treatments have been found to be effective: applied behavior analysis and medication (Ballan & Hoban, 2006; Bullock, 2009; Calohan & Peeler, 2007). Pedro benefited from both.

In applied behavioral analysis, skills are broken down into small steps and may include simple tasks such as making eye contact, as well as appropriate forms of social interactions. "Each step is initially taught using a specific range from physical guidance to verbal cues to very discrete gestures" (Ballan & Hoban, 2006, p. 152). Most researchers emphasize that the earlier treatment begins, the better, and that parents and other significant people in the child's life should be trained to follow similar procedures as those implemented by the school and/or mental health specialist. Although this chapter cannot cover all the interesting and complex details about autism and its variations (autism spectrum disorder), because children with this disability are present with increasing frequency in schools, it is incumbent upon school social workers to be familiar with the types of treatments that can be most helpful.

The issue of providing appropriate schooling for immigrant and refugee children has become quite significant, as families and children have fled from dangerous violence in their homelands. Chapter 16 deals with this topic in detail.

Although this chapter has focused on the various challenges of the school social worker in elementary school settings, we must acknowledge that social workers also play an important role in middle school settings and in high schools. Concerns about bullying and the rising rates of suicides in middle schools attest to the compelling need to have knowledgeable social workers available to children and staff who must respond to these alarming situations. Chapter 15 focuses on the topic of bullying and also the related concerns about the impact of social media on the escalation of suicides among middle school children.

CONCLUDING COMMENTS

The complex role of the school social worker demands great versatility, the ability to think on one's feet, and awareness of the reciprocity of multiple interacting systems. Liking children and wanting to advocate for their best interests in the school are only the beginning of the job qualifications of a school social worker. In addition, as illustrated in this chapter, the school social worker must understand and be able to communicate and collaborate with parents, as well as with the various professionals who also participate in and contribute to the child's educational experience.

The whole range of social work knowledge and skills is epitomized in the role of the school social worker, whose regular activities in the course of a week may include such diverse responsibilities as obtaining data and writing a social history, attending and participating in an IEP team meeting, identifying and reporting sexual and/or physical abuse, counseling children on an individual or group basis, conferring with teachers about specific children, working with outside agencies and making referrals, conducting parent group meetings, and consulting with the building administrator about special programs in response to parent concerns about community violence. This demanding role includes the satisfaction of being a child advocate in a manner that seeks to help not only the individual child but also an entire school community of children.

DISCUSSION QUESTIONS

1. Discuss some of the special challenges related to working in a "host" setting, such as a school. How can the social worker maintain a strong sense of professional identity when working with professionals from many different disciplines?
2. What is meant by "the best interests of the child," and how does this apply to the work of school social workers?
3. How can the school social worker create and maintain harmonious and effective relationships with the principal?
4. Consider the various issues that might be raised in an ongoing support group for parents of children with special needs. What is the ideal role for the social worker in such a group?
5. What legislation and terminology related to special education are important for social workers to be well acquainted with to work effectively with various school personnel?

PART IV

HELPING CHILDREN IN SPECIAL CIRCUMSTANCES

CHAPTER 10

Children Living in Kinship and Foster Home Placements

Once upon a time, everyone assumed that children would be raised in a home with their mothers, fathers, brothers, and sisters and that they would remain at home until they married and moved away to start a family of their own. Is this story realistic today, or does it resemble a fairy tale? If it still has some validity, does it apply to *all* children or mainly to children in economically secure families, in which the traditional roles of father as breadwinner and mother as homemaker permit the children to grow up in a tight and secure circle of nuclear family, church, school, and community? Today, many mothers work, even in economically secure families. But how is this view of children in two-parent families currently altered because of never-married and divorced working mothers, who must arrange out-of-home child care for their children? What about children whose own parents cannot care for them and who then are placed in kinship homes or in foster homes? How strongly do we continue to subscribe to the ideal that children *should* be raised, whenever possible, by two biological parents?

This chapter reviews the role of social workers in the child welfare field, emphasizing both the generic and specialized skills that this work requires. After describing some of the responsibilities of child welfare workers, several case examples will be included to illustrate both the challenges and the special rewards of this work.

BELIEFS ABOUT THE BEST INTERESTS OF THE CHILD

Times have changed, but many people still adhere to values inherent in a lifestyle of the past that no longer conform to current reality. However, the portrayal of children as safe in the bosom of the home was more of an ideal, rather than a universal reality. Certainly it was not applicable to many poor and immigrant families at the beginning of the 20th century, when many mothers worked in factories, on farms, or in sweatshops, sometimes bringing their dependent children to work with them. This belief about the importance of raising children within their family and cultural groups also did not prove true for those who ran the "orphan train" programs that removed thousands of immigrant children in New York from their parents between 1854 and 1930 and sent them to the country to offer the children the benefits of fresh air, good food, and a "wholesome" atmosphere—factors supposedly not present in their urban environment (Hall, 1992). Finally, this fairy tale does not apply to the single mother today who relies on limited public assistance to meet the costs of raising her children. The essential question, in the second decade of the 21st century, as in the 1850s, when the child welfare movement began, pertains to the relative importance of parental bonds as compared with other factors in determining the best interests of the child.

Although some parents become overwhelmed and voluntarily place their children out of the home and others relinquish their infants for adoption, the majority of children in foster and residential placements are there because their parents have been found by the courts to be abusive or neglectful (Berrick, Needell, Barth, & Jonson-Reid, 1998; Children's Defense Fund, 2012; Mannes, 2001; Kelly, 2014). "Children who are found to be neglected, abused, or at high risk in their family situations require specialized protective services from the community and its social agencies . . . *neglect and abuse constitute the major reason for placement of children in foster care*" (Brieland, Costin, & Atherton, 1985, p. 240; emphasis added). This continues to be true, with about 81% of children reported to state child protective service agencies being victims of neglect, 10% victims of physical abuse, and 3% victims of sexual abuse (Kelly, 2014). Neglect occurs when a parent or caregiver fails to provide adequate food, shelter, medical care, or supervision for the child (without any physical injury). Exercising the principle of *parens patriae* (which can be roughly translated as "the state as guardian"), the court uses its power to protect a dependent child by removing the child from the home and placing him or her in a foster home or institution.

Approximately half of all children in placement are from minority groups, and many are recipients of social work services. Because of the number of children orphaned by the AIDS epidemic (Michaels & Levine, 1992) and the large number of children essentially abandoned by substance-addicted and incarcerated parents, it seems understandable that the number of U.S. children in foster care increased by 23% during the late 1980s and early 1990s (National Association of Social Workers, 1993) and by 35% between 1990 and 1998 (Children's Defense Fund, 2000). However, these statistics changed in the first decade of the 21st century, with a 20% decline between 2005 and 2012 due to policy and practice improvements (Children's Bureau, 2014). This trend did not continue in 2014, when there was a slight increase in entries into foster care. Parental substance abuse and other problems continue to interfere with the efforts of social workers to keep children in their own homes.

When parents abandon their children because of addiction or are found to have been abusive or neglectful, grandparents may step in and assume child care because of their love for their grandchildren and their sense of shame, guilt, and failure about what has happened in their family (Tonning, 1999; Shapiro, Shapiro, & Paret, 2001b; Children's Bureau, 2016). There has been a dramatic increase in the number of children living with their grandparents during the last few decades. According to 2010 census data, 4.9 million American children were being raised solely by their grandparents. This number is almost double that of the 2000 census (Makin, 2014). In 2016 the number of grandparents raising grandchildren was up 7% from 2009 (Cancino, 2016). This form of child care, sometimes referred to as "kinship care," is most prevalent among children of color. Reasons for the growth in grandparent placement include parental drug abuse, teen pregnancy, divorce, single-parent households, child abuse and neglect, and the incarceration of parents. Kinship care may also be provided by aunts, uncles, and other family members. These arrangements may be either informal, with no court involvement, or those in which the court has granted temporary guardianship or legal custody.

The focus of this chapter is on methods of helping children who are placed in foster care or who are being raised by grandparents and other kin. The value base of family preservation programs includes the belief that the family is the best context in which to rear a child and that the entire family, rather than the individual child or parent, is the client (Hodges, Morgan, & Johnston, 1993; Ronnau, 2001). Protective intervention through social services often comes at a late stage of a family's problems, after heavy stresses have culminated in neglect or abuse (Brieland et al., 1985) and relatives may be unable or unwilling to assume care for the children. When a child has no grandparents or other family members who can provide care, foster care and small-group homes serve as necessary alternatives that do not necessarily have devastating effects on children but that do involve a complete change of residence for children, who are moved without knowing any of the people with whom they will be living.

This chapter presents the challenge of helping children and their families when the children are living with family members or in foster care. Whenever family members are available, they must be included as partners in the helping process; when they cannot be located or when they are unable or unwilling, children will need to be helped to identify and resolve their feelings about their lost or absent home and relatives. A child's sense of identity is connected to his or her family, and the process of helping the child requires that the family be included in work with the child, either in real life or symbolically.

THE IMPACT OF NEGLECT, ABUSE, AND PLACEMENT ON A CHILD

Before proceeding with the discussion of placement alternatives and the various levels of care options for a child who has been neglected and/or abused, it is essential to emphasize the repercussions on a young child of growing up in a family in which his or her needs have been ignored and/or in which he or she may have been physically or sexually abused. As discussed in previous chapters, a growing child needs security, love, dependability, and consistent care—all of which may be missing or greatly deficient in the family situations being described in this chapter. All the components that constitute a secure attachment may be completely absent or insufficient for normal development for children in families in which their parents are addicted and whose primary focus is on seeking and using drugs. The children's basic needs are ignored, and there may be little or no demonstrations of affection or other meaningful interactions between the parents and the children. In some families, the children are physically or sexually abused, thereby causing the children to lose trust in their parents and to experience elevated stress hormone levels due to fear and anxiety about their safety. The person who is supposed to love them hurts them. Studies have shown that parental abuse interferes with children's normal development and their ability to relate to others (Siegel, 2012).

When a child is moved from his or her parental home to a different location, he or she suffers multiple losses, and it is essential for the child welfare worker to be sensitive to these. A home where violence and abuse may have occurred frequently at least has a sense of familiarity lacking in a completely new environment. Placement with grandparents or other kin usually is more comfortable for children than a foster or group home with unknown adults. When placed out of their homes, children of school age often have to adjust to a new school environment with unknown teachers and peers, and this adds considerably to the child's stress. Understandably, the child is removed from his or her parental home because it is considered unsafe, but it is important to acknowledge that there inevitably will be *new stresses* in the new environment, and this adjustment may take some time for the child to adapt to. The goal of making placement decisions "in the child's best interest" can be very complicated and challenging.

DETERMINING THE NEED FOR PLACEMENT

What is the impact of relocating a child to another family for foster placement compared with arranging for the child to move in with a grandparent or other relative? With tongue in cheek, Mishne (1983) points out that many wealthy parents voluntarily send their children to boarding school, with no expectation that the young people will be harmed by the experience of separation from home. Obviously, it is not primarily the *separation* that threatens a child but the circumstances that precipitated the separation in the first place. If, as previously indicated, the main reason for involuntary placement is parental abuse or neglect, a separation can be viewed as the culmination of *many* past experiences of emotional and/or physical distress because of the adults' behavior. The separation is frequently the outcome of a long, sad history, which often leads the child to mistrust adults. These life experiences of abuse or neglect also contribute to the child's poor ego development and reduced ability to deal with even the everyday difficulties of life, let alone situations of extreme stress. Because every placement decision is different, the interacting influence of many factors must be weighed in determining the specific meaning of the placement to each individual child and family and in outlining a realistic treatment plan.

Evaluating Placement as Crisis: The Use of Tripartite Assessment

In several previous publications (Webb, 1991, 1993, 1999, 2001, 2007, 2010), I have presented the use of tripartite assessment as a method of evaluating the impact of a specific crisis or traumatic experience on a child. As noted also in Chapter 4 of this book, tripartite assessment looks at the interaction of three groups of factors: those related to (1) the individual, (2) the situation, and (3) the support system of family and community. When used by child welfare practitioners, tripartite assessment will assist in evaluating the need for the placement and in weighing the prospects for returning the child to his or her family. It is essential that child welfare workers become aware of the neurological effects on the child's brain of early trauma such as abuse or erratic parenting behavior. These experiences can compromise the child's later ability to trust adults and to cope with stress (Perry, 2006; Webb, 2006b).

A "crisis" is defined by Gilliland and James (2001, p. 3) as "a perception of an event or situation as an intolerable difficulty that exceeds the resources and coping mechanisms of the person." The out-of-home involuntary placement of a child provokes many feelings in the child and the family, including varying degrees of shame, guilt, and anger. The parents have been publicly exposed as unfit to care for their own child, with the result that the family may experience a loss of face and accompanying loss of self-respect. The child, in turn, may feel guilty about his or her perceived role in precipitating the placement. This form of loss generates a state of "disenfranchised grief" (Doka, 1989, 2002), because the stigma associated with the child's placement can be neither openly acknowledged nor mourned. These suppressed, complicated feelings must be recognized and understood by child welfare professionals who work with the child and family. The use of tripartite assessment facilitates this understanding, especially of the complex factors that precipitated the placement decision. Workers who recognize the importance of the multiple factors that culminate in the child's placement will be better able to help the child and the family acknowledge the loss experience that the placement represents as the basis for planning realistically for the future. Figure 10.1 diagrams the various factors that apply to the out-of-home placement of a child.

FIGURE 10.1. Interactive components of a tripartite assessment when a child is placed out of the home.

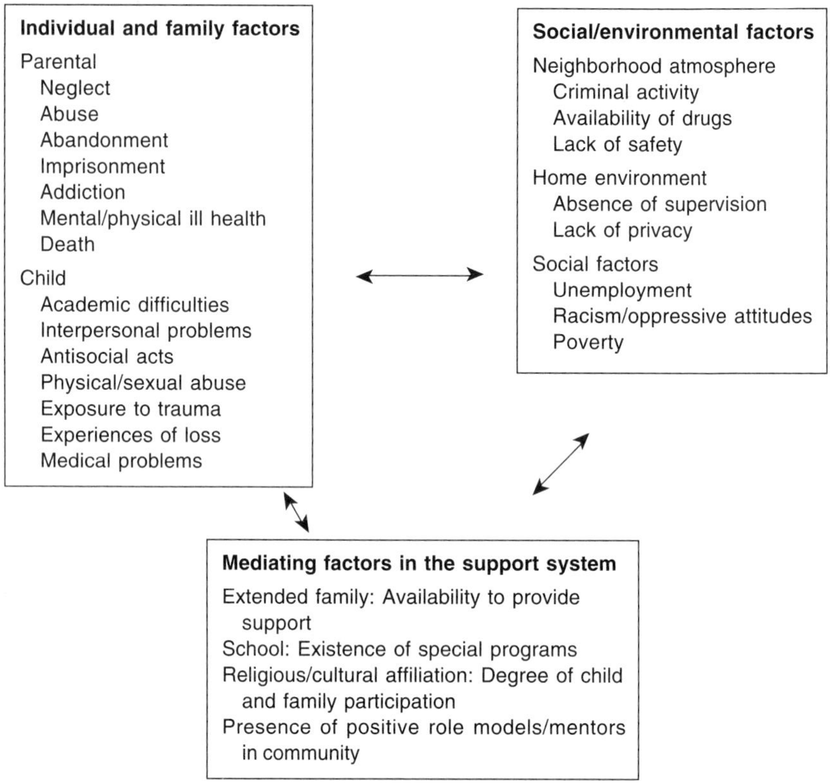

Determining the Factors Precipitating Placement

The decision to move a child from his or her own home to another setting merits the utmost deliberation and review of all relevant facts. As previously mentioned, the majority of children in foster care enter the child welfare system because of family problems related to abuse and neglect. In many instances, this has been chronic. The form in Figure 10.2 allows the child welfare practitioner to record in detail the key factors contributing to the placement, based on the tripartite conceptualization.

Factors related to the family itself and to its ability to nurture the child are often critical in precipitating placement. Some children (e.g., those with autism or ADHD) make excessive demands on their families because of their special needs and the difficulty they have in controlling their emotions and behavior. Other children may have the misfortune to be born at a difficult time in their parents' relationship or when the added demands of child care may prove too much for immature or overwhelmed parents who themselves

FIGURE 10.2. Factors precipitating placement decision.

1. Parental behaviors (list all that apply, identify relevant individual, and give dates):

Abuse (describe) ____

____

Neglect (describe) ____

____

____

Abandonment (describe) ____

____

____

Imprisonment (reason) ____

____

Addiction (describe) ____

____

Physical/mental ill health (describe) ____

____

____

Death (give date and cause of death, including child's involvement) ____________________

____

2. Child behaviors (describe in detail) ____

____

____

Frequency ____

Responses of adults ____

____

____

Child's reactions to adult interventions ____

____

3. Environmental/social conditions (describe the environment in which the child lived prior to placement) ____

____

____

(continued)

From *Social Work Practice with Children, Fourth Edition,* by Nancy Boyd Webb. Copyright © 2019 The Guilford Press. Permission to photocopy this figure is granted to purchasers of this book for personal use or use with clients (see copyright page for details). Purchasers can download enlarged versions of this material (see the box at the end of the table of contents).

FIGURE 10.2. *(continued)*

Presence of after-school activities/sports/recreational programs ____________________

____

____

Neighborhood atmosphere (check applicable items):

Safe _____ Unsafe _____

Presence of drugs: Yes _____ No _____ Not sure _____

Influence of peers: Positive _____ Negative _____

Presence of positive role models: Yes _____ No _____ Not sure _____

4. Traumatizing experiences in child's history (list all that apply):

Physical abuse (specify perpetrator, frequency, and form) ____________________

____

____

____

Sexual abuse (specify perpetrator, frequency, and form) ____________________

____

____

____

Other traumatic experiences, either witnessed or experienced ____________________

____

____

____

feel needy and unfulfilled and who may take out their frustrations on their dependent children. For example, a father who has recently lost his job and whose wife has been diagnosed with cancer may vent his fury on his innocent 9-year-old son, who reminds the father of everything he hoped for in his own life that he now believes has been taken away from him. When the boy asks for money to buy a baseball mitt, the father tells him scornfully that money doesn't grow on trees and that he'd better begin to think about ways to obtain his own money for the things he wants.

One isolated episode like this is not likely to propel a boy into a life of crime. However, when it and others like it are combined with pressure from older neighborhood youngsters who serve as drug runners and decoys for drug dealers, it is comprehensible how the boy could become involved in a life of petty crime—one that later could result in placement in a foster home or a residential treatment facility.

Evaluation of significant influences in child placement often hinges on an understanding of interacting individual and family factors. Figure 10.3 is a form for recording these specific influences on the placement decision.

FIGURE 10.3. Individual and family factors related to placement.

Relevant information from genogram

Position of child in family ______

Extended family (location and degree of involvement) ______

______

Status of parents (current, and at the time of child's birth)

Ages: Mother ______ Father ______

Quality of parental relationship ______

______

______

Employment: Mother ______

Father ______

Medical: Mother ______

Father ______

History of addictions:

Mother ______

Father ______

History of court involvement:

Mother ______

Father ______

Religious/cultural affiliation:

Mother ______

Father ______

Achievements/ego strengths:

Mother ______

Father ______

Status of child

Age and date of birth ______

School grade and adjustment ______

______

______

Educational testing results ______

______

Psychological testing summary ______

______

(continued)

From *Social Work Practice with Children, Fourth Edition*, by Nancy Boyd Webb. Copyright © 2019 The Guilford Press. Permission to photocopy this figure is granted to purchasers of this book for personal use or use with clients (see copyright page for details). Purchasers can download enlarged versions of this material (see the box at the end of the table of contents).

FIGURE 10.3. *(continued)*

Peer involvement (describe in detail) ____________________

____

Names of and relationships with siblings ____________________

____

Medical history ____________________

History of physical/sexual abuse (describe in detail) ____________________

____

____

____

History of exposure to trauma ____________________

____

____

Separation history (including moves and previous placements) ____________________

____

____

Past coping/strengths/typical defenses ____________________

____

____

Home environment

Physical conditions (describe in detail, especially regarding child's sleeping arrangements)

____

____

Persons living in the home (give names and relationships to the child, if any) ____________________

____

____

____

Length of time in current residence ____________________

Previous residences:

Length of time ____________________

Reasons for moving ____________________

DIFFERENT LEVELS OF CARE

Although it is beyond the scope of this chapter to analyze the wide range of child welfare programs for children, it is important to recognize that there is a continuum of services for children who are dependent and/or who have emotional or behavioral difficulties. These include foster care, residential treatment centers, group homes, day treatment programs, shelters, family and psychiatric clinics, and crisis/respite services. Because of space limitations, I focus here primarily on grandparent and foster placement, with case vignettes to demonstrate the varied circumstances that can lead to child placement. Selected methods for helping children in placement to cope with their feelings about their life situations are presented later in the chapter.

Foster Care

Foster care consists of a *temporary* arrangement for child care in a substitute home when the parents cannot take care of their own child because of some serious difficulty. The expectation is that the child will return to the parents' home when the conditions precipitating the foster placement have been corrected.

The intent of the Adoption Assistance and Child Welfare Reform Act (Public Law 96-272, 1980) is to provide permanent homes for children who are in the foster care system, either by returning them to their biological parents or by placing them with relatives. The third best alternative is a legally permanent adoptive family, and the fourth best placement is a reasonably permanent foster family (University of Kentucky College of Social Work, 1989; Whittaker, 1987). It is important to note that this law requires that "a variety of placement prevention services . . . ensure that 'reasonable efforts' have been made to preserve the family before a child [is] placed in substitute care" (Pecora, Reed-Ashcraft, & Kirk, 2001, p. 15). Therefore, we can speculate that children who are placed with nonrelatives probably come from families with fewer supports and resources.

In 2015 there were approximately 408,000 children in foster care, with a median age of 7.8 years (Child Welfare Information Gateway, 2017). Although foster care is supposed to be temporary (limited to 18 months), it is often much longer. Frequently, children have difficulty adjusting in the new home, where they may not be able to trust the foster parent or conform to a new routine and expectations. Unable to adapt, many children act out; then they are moved from one foster placement to another, with increasingly negative effects on their sense of security and self-esteem. The length of a child's stay in foster care varies greatly, from a few days to a few years. The average length is approximately 2 years. Whenever possible, siblings are kept together. The longer a child stays in foster care, the smaller the child's chances are of obtaining a permanent home, according to Brieland et al. (1985).

Kinship Foster Care

The fastest growing form of out-of-home placement in the United States is kinship foster care. In 2016, more than 2.7 million grandparents in the United States were raising their own grandchildren because the children's own parents were unavailable or unable to care for them (Annie E. Casey Foundation, 2017). About one-fifth of these grandparents live below the poverty line; many are over 60 years old, and about a quarter of these have a disability. Therefore, this arrangement can come with its own problems.

Grandparents provide at least half of the kinship care in this country, and estimates suggest that the great majority of these arrangements are made informally between family members in response to emergencies or other situations of need. Other times, grandparents or other relatives are *recruited* to take care of children of their relatives, and they may enter the formal child welfare system with reimbursement as approved foster parents. Although kinship care is viewed as preferable to placement in a home of nonrelatives because it preserves the family, children in kinship foster care are less likely to return to their biological parents and are less likely to be adopted than are children in placements with nonrelated foster parents (Barth, Courtney, Berrick, & Albert, 1994).

There is a long tradition of kinship care in African American and Hispanic families, in which family and kin networks are utilized when child care is needed (Bean, McAllister, & Hudgins, 2001; Patterson & Marsiglia, 2000). However, the tremendous growth of grandparent-headed households between 1990 and 1997 was not just an African American or Hispanic phenomenon, as might be believed. The growth of European American grandparent-headed households was the most dramatic during this period (Bean et al., 2001). As reported by AARP, based on a Metropolitan Life Report and the U.S. Census of 2010, 2.7 million grandparents were raising their grandchildren at that time.

Even when the care of children by grandparents is culturally supported and frequent, they may find it burdensome because of health and economic worries of their own. According to Casper and Bryson (1998; quoted in Shapiro et al., 2001b, p. 126), "children who live in grandparent-maintained households, with or without a parent, are more likely to be without health insurance, living in families below the poverty line, and receiving public assistance."

Other stresses in these families can include ongoing family conflicts regarding the custody of the child, especially when the child's mother has a substance abuse problem and the grandparent doubts that her rehabilitation will last. This was the situation in the case of Ricky, discussed later in the chapter. Other difficulties can occur when the child still longs for the mother and wants to return to her despite the grandparent's love and good care. This

---

Note. I acknowledge the contribution of Nadine Bean, PhD, in the preparation of this section and in the Kayla case.

situation creates a loyalty conflict for the child similar to that felt by many children in divorcing families who feel torn between their parents (Tonning, 1999; Edelstein, Burge, & Waterman, 2002).

Group and Institutional Care

Some children are too conflicted to function well in a foster home, either with grandparents or with unrelated foster parents. Their complex behavioral/psychological problems require specialized services that are more likely to be available in residential treatment settings with intensive programs and a multidisciplinary staff. This type of placement should be considered when children demonstrate the following:

- Poorly developed impulse control
- Low self-image
- Poorly developed modulation of emotion
- Deficiencies in forming relationships
- Special learning disabilities
- Limited play skills

Of course, some of these characteristics are found in many children in foster care, as well as in the population at large. All too often, when the child has multiple difficulties, the foster parents cannot manage, and the child is moved to a new home. Repeated placements with repeated failure to adjust create an overlay of additional problems for the child, who often is blamed for the placement failure. A deeper understanding of the child's psychological state suggests that the abusive and/or erratic parenting he or she received in infancy and early childhood caused him or her to develop an insecure attachment as a baby and toddler (Davies, 2011). Not knowing from moment to moment whether he or she will receive a hug or a hit, the child remains wary and mistrustful (Doyle & Stoop, 1999). This condition can be treated, but foster parents will need both education and support to relate to such a child with patience and continued consistency.

TYPICAL ISSUES FOR CHILDREN IN PLACEMENT

The families of children who require placement have histories of living in homes characterized by substance abuse, homelessness, domestic violence, AIDS, emotional disturbance, poverty, and incarceration (Children's Defense Fund, 2000). Children born and growing up in families struggling with these problems suffer consequences in the form of attachment, trust, identity, and loss difficulties. Often their development has been compromised because of environmental factors that have left their parent(s) overwhelmed, helpless, and hopeless. Growing awareness of the importance of helping the family has resulted in programs that are family centered and focused on family preservation. Many practitioners now believe that it is artificial and faulty to separate children's issues from family issues (Walton et al., 2001). I have repeatedly maintained in this book my own belief that helping the family is essential to helping the child. However, I want to emphasize that a family focus may not be sufficient to help a child whose development has been seriously compromised. Many of these children need individual professional help to overcome the aftermath of their traumatic histories of neglect and abuse.

Social workers and other practitioners must be sensitive to the impact of a child's history on his or her development and be knowledgeable about some specific child-focused methods for helping. In my opinion, working *only* with the family without devoting additional special attention to the child's individual needs cannot repair the damage and attachment issues caused by years of neglect and/or abuse. Many children in foster care and in other forms of out-of-home placement require interventions specifically aimed at assisting them with their grief work, with traumatic memories, and with issues related to their identities. In turn, foster parents who assume the care of children with multiple losses need assistance in understanding the children's extensive needs to respond to them sympathetically and realistically. The past cannot be erased, and developing trust in adults may take some time. The range of intervention methods to meet these diverse needs includes family, group, and individual helping approaches.

INTERVENTIONS WITH THE CHILDREN

Most (if not all) children in foster care and in residential treatment have experienced losses, ranging from multiple moves to parental separation, death, or abandonment. Many of these experiences qualify as traumatic, and the children's behavior may be partly explained as derived from PTSD. The fact that these experiences are frequent does not make them easier for the child. A child who must enter new schools several times during his or her elementary school years is required to make repeated efforts to make friends and establish "credibility" among children who have already formed peer relationships and who may not enthusiastically welcome newcomers, especially when they are different because they are not residing with their own parents. Some schools routinely have time-limited groups in the fall of each year to help integrate new students into the school and also to provide them with a ready-made group of peers with whom to establish friendships. These groups would be helpful to foster children who have been placed in a new school district. Unfortunately, however, the transfers do not always occur at the beginning of the year, and therefore the groups may not be available when most needed. In any case, the school social worker should be notified when a foster child enters a new school so that this professional can try to provide appropriate services to the child.

The Case of Dave Pelzer: A Foster Child with a History of Abuse

In three autobiographical accounts (1995, 1997, 2000), Dave Pelzer describes the repeated physical and psychological abuse he suffered at the hands of his mother. Eventually he was removed from his home after school personnel on several occasions noticed his serious bruises. He had difficulty adjusting to a series of different foster homes in which he was placed between the ages of 9 and 12. Pelzer describes how he had feared his mother's wrath if he revealed "the secret" about his abuse to anyone. After his placement, he kept asking himself whether his mother had ever loved him and why she had treated him the way she did. He was admittedly confused and felt that somehow he must have deserved the abuse.

Pelzer refers to experiences that are common among foster children, namely, his difficulty making friends in school and his discomfort about having to admit to his peers that he didn't live with his parents. He also reports his willingness to steal to gain acceptance from other children. Fortunately, one of his foster mothers had a great deal of experience and the ability to deal effectively with children who had very troubled backgrounds. Her approach emphasized the children's strengths. She acknowledged Pelzer's potential and warned him that he could end up in residential treatment if he continued to get into trouble. Pelzer's three memoirs present an insider's view about foster care that includes his gratitude toward the foster care system, which he credits with saving him.

The Case of Maria: An HIV-Positive Foster Child

In the previous editions of this book, I wrote about the case of Maria, age 10, who was in foster care because her mother had died of AIDS and because she had no known relatives who could care for her. She and her 13-year-old brother, Mario, were placed in a foster home. The foster parents, who had three of their own children, wanted to adopt Maria, but she felt conflicted because the foster parents did not intend to adopt Mario, who had acted out against them and was subsequently placed in a residential treatment center.

Part of my work with Maria consisted of helping her understand and connect with her past, so that she could grieve her serious losses. This was accomplished by having her create a lifebook and write a letter to her deceased mother and by taking Maria and Mario to visit their mother's grave. These interventions, which can be adapted for use with other children in placement, are discussed next.

Specific Methods for Helping Children with Grief Work

The following interventions can be used with children in foster placements to help them mourn their losses. They may be used in individual sessions, in tandem meetings with siblings, or with a group of bereaved children. See Webb (1993, 2001, 2010) for detailed case illustrations demonstrating the use of these methods.

Lifebooks

A "lifebook" is a document in which an individual records his or her unique life story (Aust, 1981; Backhaus, 1984). When created for the benefit of children in placement, it contains stories and/or factual accounts dictated or written by the child about his or her memories; it also contains the child's own drawings and may include photographs, if available. The use of a "time line" in the lifebook helps the child depict the significant events of each year of his or her life, clarifying various moves and the significant people at each location (Doyle & Stoop, 1991). The purpose of making the lifebook is to help the child understand his or her own history and simultaneously to provide the opportunity for validation and release of feelings connected to the powerful memories. Since the first publications in the 1980s describing the use of lifebooks with children, there has been a flood of materials on the market to guide practitioners in helping foster and adoptive parents to assist their children with the process of recording and reclaiming their own past histories. See various publications listed on the Internet under "lifebooks" to uncover booklets and manuals such as *My Foster Care Journey* (O'Malley, 2006) and *The Child's Own Story: Life Story Work with Traumatized Children* (Rose & Philpot, 2005).

Letters to Absent or Deceased Family Members and Others

An essential part of grief work involves the expression of feelings related to the unexpected death or departure of a family member. Often when a death or other loss, such as abandonment, occurs, the family members are left wanting to see the person again so that they can ask or tell them something important. This "unfinished business" sometimes consists of expressing anger or sadness at being left. Writing letters to the missing or dead person and reading these aloud in an appropriate setting can relieve the person of some of the burden of sadness, guilt, or anger. This may be relevant for foster children who feel unfairly treated or who have been abused, as well as for children (and adults) who have suffered a loss through death. (See Figure 10.4 for a form letter to a person who died.) The healing dynamic in writing such a letter relates to the individual's taking action in a situation in which he or she previously felt powerless. It is not necessary for the letter to be delivered for it to have a positive

FIGURE 10.4. Form letter to a person who died.

On this page, write a letter to the person who died. Tell this person all the things you wanted to say but never had the chance. Tell him or her all that is in your heart. Tell the person what you miss about him or her, and what you don't miss, too.

Dear ______________________________,

____

____

____

____

____

____

____

____

____

____

____

____

____

____

____

From *Social Work Practice with Children, Fourth Edition,* by Nancy Boyd Webb. Copyright © 2019 The Guilford Press. Permission to photocopy this figure is granted to purchasers of this book for personal use or use with clients (see copyright page for details). Purchasers can download enlarged versions of this material (see the box at the end of the table of contents).

effect. However, I do recommend the creation of a ritual or ceremony in which the person can read the letter in front of a picture of the absent person and/or at a meaningful place or time.

The content of such a letter, whether to a deceased or absent parent, might include reporting something important about the child's life and expressing whatever feelings he or she has when thinking about the absent person in the present. Letters can even be written to unknown parents. Children who never knew a parent often have many fantasies and questions about that parent, including questions about the nature of his or her relationship with the other parent. Although letters to an unknown parent will not be answered, they help the child by putting their questions in writing. The young child should be told in as sensitive a manner as possible that because the parent is dead he or she cannot write a response. When the child shares the letter with the social worker, this provides the opportunity to validate (and sometimes to clarify) his or her feelings and concerns.

Visiting a Parent's Grave and/or the Child's Birthplace

Sometimes it is possible to arrange a visit to a parent's grave, whether or not the child has been there previously, if he or she wants to do this. This was a very powerful and significant experience for Maria and Mario, who had each written letters to their dead mother prior to the visit. They read these silently to her as they stood by her grave.

Documentation of the Child's History

When a child in placement lacks knowledge about a parent's death or about the circumstances of his or her own birth, it can be helpful to try to obtain death and/or birth certificates and even, where feasible, to visit the hospital where the child was born or the home in which his or her early childhood years were spent. In most families parents keep photo albums and tell children stories about their early lives. However, the child who was placed at an early age may not have such stories in his or her memory. These children lack a family narrative that helps create a sense of a family identity and contributes to the child's development of a coherent sense of self (Shapiro et al., 2001b). The creation of a lifebook and the other activities described here can help serve this purpose in the absence of parental input.

The Case of Ricky: A Child Living with a Grandparent

Tonning (1999) presented the case of Ricky, age 3, who was removed from his mother's home for chronic abuse and neglect after she left him home alone with his 6-year-old brother for 3 days when he was 18 months old. The mother, who was addicted to crack cocaine, was subsequently incarcerated for a year, and Ricky was placed with his paternal grandmother, who was also caring for the 2½-year-old daughter of another son at that time. The grandmother was concerned about Ricky because he seemed angry, unhappy, and oppositional.

In this African American family, Ricky had quite a bit of contact with his extended family, including weekend visits with his father, who would sometimes leave him with his mother, despite her background of having abused Ricky previously. The boy also would occasionally visit his half-brother, who had been diagnosed with ADHD and was living with his paternal grandparents. According to the grandmother, Ricky would return from these visits to his father greatly regressed. She knew that the visits were hard on him, but she nonetheless was unable to set limits and implement a less stressful (shorter) visiting plan, even when she learned after one extended stay that his mother had beaten him. The parents were seeking to regain custody of their son, and the grandmother apparently felt that she should not stand between a father and his son. She probably also feared that if she did so she would jeopardize her relationship with her own son. The family abruptly withdrew from counseling in the middle of the custody dispute, and the social worker commented that "the intergenerational conflict over where Ricky belonged and who was his rightful caregiver proved impossible to resolve" (Tonning, 1999, p. 221). Clearly, this child was caught in the middle, and his disturbed behavior could be understood as reactive to the chaos around him. The case also demonstrates the frustration of the caseworker and the limitations on her ability to help. Unfortunately, these cases do not always have happy endings.

The Case of Kayla: A Child Living with Her Grandmother

This case involved a German Jewish grandmother who had custody of her severely emotionally disabled 2-year-old granddaughter (Bean et al., 2001). Kayla had been placed with her grandmother after having been removed from her mother's care three times due to neglect. Both parents were addicted to heroin. Kayla's father (the grandmother's son) was incarcerated for drug trafficking, and her mother had a history of numerous arrests for prostitution. There was the suspicion that Kayla had been sexually abused by various caretakers.

Nadine Bean, with several colleagues, interviewed grandparents and great-grandparents raising grandchildren from various cultures in the United States. This research study looked for recurrent themes in the experiences of the kinship parents. Kayla's grandmother was particularly eloquent in expressing her anguish at seeing her granddaughter so terribly afraid of men and so clingy and fearful. The pain of the grandmother's empathy nearly caused her to end her role as a kinship foster parent, but she changed her mind in view of the child's great needs and the presence of guidance from a supportive social worker. I mention this case to emphasize the great importance of ongoing counseling and support for all foster parents.

INTERVENTIONS WITH THE FOSTER PARENTS

Most foster parents experience considerable stress in carrying out their parenting responsibilities. Whether the child is related by blood or not, the likelihood is that he or she comes into the placement experience with multiple problems that often include difficulties trusting others, aggressive behavior, sleep and eating difficulties, and possible antisocial behavior, such as stealing. The foster parents must be firm and patient and realize that it will take time before the child develops some sense of trust. They also need help understanding that the child's behavior is often based on his or her *past negative experiences with adults*, and that it is not in response to the current life situation in the foster home. In other words, the foster parents could be doing a very good job, and yet the child in placement continues to act out against them. The role of the social worker is to provide consistent support to prevent the foster parents from giving up their efforts.

All foster parents would benefit from either individual or group counseling. A parenting support group consisting of other foster parents can provide an outlet and a resource for them. Visitation with the child's biological parents often stirs up feelings of resentment, competition, and conflicts about custody. It is important for the foster parents to have a safe place to discuss their feelings. If and when the child is reunited with his or her biological family, the reunion should be accomplished gradually and with sensitivity to the feelings of all. Obviously, this did not happen in the case of Ricky, despite the social worker's best efforts. Every change of placement is a loss experience for all involved. It is important to find a way to help everyone grieve their losses so that they can accept new relationships.

THE ROLE OF THE SOCIAL WORKER IN CHILD WELFARE

Social workers in child welfare settings have a multifaceted role—one that includes direct work with culturally diverse children and families, work with the family court and the department of social services, and the necessity of functioning on an interdisciplinary team. A social worker often serves as a case manager, coordinating the progress reports of a child's residential staff, educational and psychological reports, and all matters related to setting goals and evaluating the child's progress.

It is important for social workers in this field of practice to have a solid knowledge base in child assessment, including diagnostic classifications, family systems assessment, substance abuse assessment, and evaluation of the impact of trauma on children (especially that resulting from physical and sexual abuse). An administrator of a large residential treatment center identified the issues of substance abuse, HIV/AIDS, neglect, and physical abuse as typical of about 80% of the center's population (Webb, 1995). Because many children in foster care and residential treatment have experienced multigenerational losses from AIDS, it is imperative for social workers attempting to help these children to understand the impact of disenfranchised grief (Doka, 2002) and to be knowledgeable about methods for assisting with mourning. Because of HIV/AIDS, it is increasingly common for multiple siblings in a family to enter care simultaneously. It may become the social worker's responsibility to coordinate the work with these siblings, which will be greatly facilitated when the children's care is managed by the same agency rather than by several agencies. Social workers need skills in conducting sibling sessions to maintain and enhance the children's family ties.

Special Challenges

Some of the special challenges to the social worker in child welfare settings relate to the need to work with very resistant and overwhelmed families in a political climate in which funding is decreasing. Sometimes the worker's own feelings of discouragement can be an obstacle, especially when the worker assumes too much responsibility for a child or family and in the process fails to respect appropriate professional boundaries. The worker who shares *all* the pain of his or her clients will soon suffer burnout and become ineffective. The last chapter of this book discusses the topic of vicarious traumatization, which is a great risk for child welfare workers. It is essential for practitioners to understand the personal dangers of their work and to learn to establish appropriate boundaries to avoid becoming overwhelmed and ineffective. Regular supervision and self-care practices can help workers retain their personal balance and enthusiasm for their work.

Special Rewards

The child welfare worker does experience moments of great satisfaction in his or her work, despite the difficulty and heart-wrenching circumstances of so many cases. One positive response to my survey question about satisfaction in this work (Webb, 1995) mentioned "seeing children go from depression and hopelessness to trust and belief in the possibility of a happy future." Another respondent referred to "clinical moments" at which children are able to verbalize important understandings about their lives, as in the case of a child who finally developed enough trust in his caseworker to tell her how ashamed he felt because no one in his family wanted him! These significant moments help the child welfare worker appreciate the importance of his or her role and (let us hope) will lead to retention of competent workers in the system. There are probably few settings that make as many demands on social workers or in which dedicated workers are more desperately needed. Our profession must acknowledge more fully the vital importance of this work.

CONCLUDING COMMENTS

Children in foster care, through no fault of their own, grow up without the security of a stable family. When extended family members are not available to assume their care, they are thrust into the child welfare system. Unresolved mourning is a vital issue for these children. Children who are moved from one family to another and who may lose contact with their biological parents through either death or abandonment, need assistance to put their experience into perspective and to realize that they were not to blame. This is a great challenge to the profession, and one that can reap substantial rewards.

DISCUSSION QUESTIONS AND ROLE-PLAY EXERCISE

1. Discuss the pros and cons of kinship foster care and foster care by nonrelatives. What safeguards could the social worker implement to avoid custody battles in the family? Role-play a family session with the mother, father, and grandmother in the case of Ricky, in which the custody issue is the focus.
2. Consider the matter of a family secret involving a foster child whose parent has a history of substance abuse and physical abuse of the child when drinking and drugging. What kind of help does the child require prior to resuming visitation with this parent? What kind of help should the parent receive?
3. What are some of the key personal issues for the social worker who is employed in a child welfare agency? Describe some ways to avoid burnout.
4. Discuss the implications of the position that clinical issues and larger societal issues overlap in child welfare.

CHAPTER 11

Children in Single-Parent, Divorcing, and Blended Families

Children in the 21st century come from many different types of families. No longer can teachers or others working with children assume that a child lives in a family with his or her biological father and mother and the siblings from that marriage, although this family form still remains the most common structure. In 2016, about 69% of children were living with both parents, 23% lived with a single mother, and 4% lived with only their father (U.S. Bureau of the Census, 2016). Of the 50.7 million children living with two parents, 47.7 million lived with two *married* parents, and 3 million lived with two *unmarried* parents (U.S. Census, 2016). About 16% of all children lived in blended families that included a stepparent, half siblings, or stepsiblings (U.S. Bureau of the Census, 2011). Eleven percent of children were living with a never-married single parent; the father was the absent parent in 86% of single-parent situations. Thus, although all children begin life as the result of the biological union of a man and a woman, many of them do not grow up with these two individuals, and a few never even know the identity of one or both of their biological parents. A study in 2014 (Pew Research, 2015) found that fewer than half of U.S. children live in a "traditional family," meaning that having a stepparent and living in a blended family is as "normal" for many children as it would be for them to live in a "traditional" two-parent home.

Because of the prevalence of divorce and the upheaval in children's lives that often accompanies the separation of their parents, this chapter focuses on helping children in divorcing families and in the new families that are formed when a parent establishes a new household with a new partner. The chapter also addresses issues that may occur for children in single-parent families. In my own clinical practice, I have had contact with children from numerous divorced families in which each parent developed relationships with new partners who also had children. Sometimes these new unions produced new children who were half siblings of the child from the divorced family. The world of these children, therefore, consisted not only of their mother, father, and brothers and sisters but also of a stepmother and her children as well as a stepfather and his children, and frequently new half siblings. Often the child changed residences on weekends and vacations because of custody agreements, and the change of residence might mean that the child would have to share a previously private sleeping space with the new stepsiblings. Other times he or she would be the one to move in on a stepsibling, who might or might not welcome him or her. Furthermore, the child often had to develop relationships with the extended family of his or her stepsiblings who might be visiting at the same time, including grandparents, aunts, uncles, and cousins. I purposely list these extended family members to emphasize the *numerous* new family contacts that children in blended families may be expected to establish and sustain.

The term "blended family," sometimes called a "reconstituted family," refers to a family in which one or both partners have been married before and in which they are combining two families into one. Over 50% of U.S. families are remarried or recoupled, meaning that blended families are as common as "traditional" formats. A helpful workbook for children living in blended families allows the child to document different relationships (Evans, 1986).

Despite society's growing tolerance of divorce, remarriage, and single parenthood by choice, children living in these and in various other family arrangements often suffer multiple stresses that are not usually experienced by children in intact, "traditional" nuclear families. These stresses include the following:

- Lower socioeconomic status.
- Custody battles.
- Divided loyalties.
- Changes in school and home environments.
- Reduced or absent communication with the noncustodial parent.
- Adjustment to stepparents, stepsiblings, and other new relatives.
- Divergent rules and lifestyles in different homes.
- Uncertainty about information that they are permitted to share with others.
- Confused feelings about where they belong.
- Prejudice or disapproval related to their family's lifestyle.

Of course, every family is unique, but I believe that children in divorcing and blended families have some important issues in common and that we need to consider these issues in our efforts to help them. The most important issues relate to experiences of loss and multiple stressors.

ISSUES OF LOSS AND MULTIPLE STRESSORS

Loss

In popular books and on television, the traditional nuclear family is most typically portrayed as consisting of mother, father, and children. Preschoolers learn before they begin kindergarten that everyone has a mommy and a daddy. When there is no father in the home, a child will usually ask about him, and, depending on what the child is told, he or she may either accept the explanation or continue to mull it over and wonder when Daddy is going to appear. If a never-married mother speaks disparagingly to her child about the man who impregnated her and then disappeared, the child picks up the underlying message that his or her father was "bad." This perception may have an ongoing influence on the child's feelings about men and relationships, as well as on his or her own sense of identity.

Another example of an absent father involves a single, never-married lesbian mother in a gay relationship who wants a child and arranges to become impregnated with the help of an anonymous sperm donor. This mother must find a way to explain to her child the fact that he or she has two mothers but no father who is part of their family.

On the other hand, the preschool child in a blended family who has a stepfather and also has ongoing contact with his or her biological father may accept the mother's statement that the child is lucky to have *two* daddies. However, as this same child grows to school age, he or she may intuit differences in the way the stepfather treats him or her compared with his biological children; the child may then begin to want more time with his or her "real" father, beyond the usual once-a-week visitation. This child may question both parents about why they don't get married or live together anymore.

Absent ("lost") parents remain significant presences for children in divorced, single, remarried, and homosexual families. Similarly, the "ghosts" of missing parents also continue as important influences among adopted children who do not have information about their biological parents (LeVine & Sallee, 1992). My own experience with children confirms that absent parents play important symbolic roles in these children's lives and that the children grieve for the lost parents on significant holidays (e.g., Mother's Day or Father's Day, the child's own birthday, Thanksgiving, and other major holidays when rituals emphasize family togetherness). In psychodynamic terms, such a child has suffered an "object loss," namely the loss of a major attachment figure. Feelings of longing and anger about this loss may persist indefinitely. Sometimes the imagined presence of a "lost" parent serves an important comforting role for a child, similar to the manner in which a child may retain and benefit from the memory of a deceased parent (Silverman & Worden, 1992). An unfortunate aspect of the child's loss in a family with a missing parent, however, is the child's inability to speak openly about it because the adults with whom the child currently lives usually prefer to deny or minimize the child's feelings of longing for or positive connection with this person. The custodial parent's anger toward the spouse may prevent any sympathy or acknowledgment of the child's feelings. The child is unsupported in his or her grief, which cannot be openly acknowledged or worked out. As noted in Chapter 10, Doka (2002) refers to this type of mourning as "disenfranchised grief."

Other losses experienced by many children in divorcing and blended families relate to the reduced economic status and possible changes in schools and living arrangements that often accompany divorce, remarriage, or a period of single parenthood. Furthermore, when a parent's marital status changes, relationships with the kinship network also usually alter; in fact, a child may lose contact with an entire group of grandparents, uncles, and aunts because the custodial parent no longer feels comfortable in their presence. This is an example of the adult's needs eclipsing those of the child.

In the single-parent home following a divorce, a parent may work long hours and want to devote some time to adult relationships without the child (or children). This can cause a child to feel resentful, rejected, and lonely. A child in a single-parent household may also be expected to share in performing chores and/or to accompany the parent to the supermarket or laundromat. Sometimes the single parent unwisely begins to confide in the child, almost as if the child were an adult. In these situations the child may take on the role parental caretaker. This blurring of parent–child boundaries causes the child to worry about adult concerns prematurely, and this may interfere with the freedom to focus on his or her own developmental tasks (Siegel, 2007). When this happens, the child is losing his or her very childhood.

Multiple Stressors

Children do not like to be different; as early as elementary school, many want to dress in a certain way to resemble their peers and to participate in after-school activities with their friends. A parent's reduced income and/or lack of time to go shopping with the child or attend a school event may mean that the child dresses differently from peers and misses out on activities with them. This may contribute to a feeling of alienation or "difference" from friends whose parents are able to spend more time, money, and attention on their children.

Furthermore, a child's worry about finances may preclude his or her even asking to participate in certain after-school activities (e.g., baseball or cheerleading, which would involve expenses for a uniform). In times of financial prosperity, many schools have scholarship funds to accommodate the needs of children who cannot, without assistance, afford to participate in sports and other after-school activities. Unfortunately, in times of fiscal constraint, these special funds are not available in many school districts, and children are expected to pay for even basic school supplies. The impact of tighter economic conditions at home and in the community means that children whose family incomes are limited are deprived of certain "extras" that might enrich their lives. It would be understandable if this deprivation, together with the other stresses and losses, resulted in reduced self-esteem and increased anger and alienation. In fact, according to Allen-Meares et al. (2000), children in single-parent families are at greater risk of educational difficulties than children living with two parents: "They score lower on standardized tests, get lower grades in school, and are twice as likely to drop out of high school before graduation" (p. 63). Another source of stress for children in divorced families occurs when they are "put in the middle" (Garrity & Baris, 1994) and asked by one parent to convey messages to or keep secrets from the other. This behavior creates disturbing feelings of divided loyalties in the children. According to Wallerstein and Kelly (1980, p. 49),

> school age children particularly appeared to conceptualize the divorce as a struggle in which each participant demanded one's primary loyalty, and this conception greatly increased the conflict and unhappiness of [such a] child. For, by its logic, a step in the direction of one parent was experienced by the child . . . as a betrayal of the other, a move likely to evoke anger and further rejection.

The case example later in this chapter illustrates a loyalty conflict such as this for a child whose parents were in a custody battle.

Other stresses that may preoccupy children in single, divorced, and blended families relate to worries about their parents' happiness and their own uncertain futures. Rather than assuming that their lives will continue on a certain course, children in these families know that conflict can lead to ruptured relationships and major life changes. Custodial parents may be angry or depressed and thus may lack energy to focus on their children. The children may worry about both the parent with whom they live and the absent parent, in addition to their own futures. These children have personally experienced the fragility and the complexity of life; this experience, although strengthening the coping capacities of some, may also lead to premature suffering and strong feelings of personal vulnerability.

Even children in stable single-parent households and in single-parent, divorced, or blended families that are not suffering economic hardship may experience stress related to the curiosity, prejudice, and disapproval expressed by some adults and peers about their families. This could happen, for example, when a divorced mother moves with her children into her boyfriend's home without any plans for marriage. Her children may like the boyfriend and his children and feel comfortable within their new home environment; however, they may find it difficult to explain to their teacher and friends that the man in their new home is neither their father nor their stepfather, but their mother's friend. Children may feel stigmatized when their families differ from society's norm. Support groups such as Banana Splits (see Chapter 8) for children in divorced and blended families can help significantly in lessening children's feelings of isolation and difference.

ASSESSMENT OF THE IMPACT OF FAMILY CIRCUMSTANCES ON THE CHILD

Many distinctive factors interact to affect any given child's reaction to a parent's unmarried status, divorce, or remarriage. It is not the parent's status itself that causes stress for the child but rather the many circumstances associated with it that may affect the child adversely. Because children are self-centered, the overriding issue for them is how much their lives are affected. Certainly, not all children in single-parent, divorcing, or blended families develop problems. A child's temperament, a family's overall functioning, and the presence of an effective support system can all balance the negative effects of stress on the child.

As discussed in Chapter 10 regarding the interactive components of child placement, a tripartite conceptualization (Webb, 1999, 2001, 2007) can help us understand the reactions of an individual to a specific situation, based on analysis of three groups of factors that interact and determine the outcome of a specific crisis state: (1) the nature of the crisis situation, (2) the characteristics of the individual, and (3) the strengths and weaknesses of the support system. Originally developed for crisis situations and later adapted to bereavement, this tripartite model can be further adapted to make it specifically relevant to children living in single, divorcing, or blended families. In Figure 11.1, I have diagrammed the factors to be considered in the tripartite assessment of children in single-parent, divorcing, or blending families. This diagram may help the practitioner understand why one child has difficulties adjusting to a divorce and changed family situation, whereas another does not.

Figure 11.2 presents a form to facilitate the practitioner's use of tripartite assessment to organize, summarize, and understand the unique circumstances pertaining to a child living in a single-parent, divorcing, or blended family. The practitioner fills out this form based on information available in the family's record and interviews with various family members. Use of the form, together with information from the child's developmental history, will help identify sources of possible stress for the child (and, therefore, areas for possible intervention).

GOALS FOR HELPING CHILDREN IN DIVORCING OR BLENDED FAMILIES

Depending on the circumstances of each case, individual, family, or group methods can help children in single-parent, divorcing, or blended families express and resolve some of their feelings of loss and stress. Regardless of the method, the work must emphasize that the *adults* are responsible for creating and resolving the family difficulties. Children must be reminded repeatedly that they did not cause the situation and that, because they are children, they cannot remedy it. The adults involved must free the children to proceed with their lives and to leave adult concerns to adults. This is generally easier said

FIGURE 11.1. Interactive components for a tripartite assessment of a child in a single-parent, divorcing, or blended family.

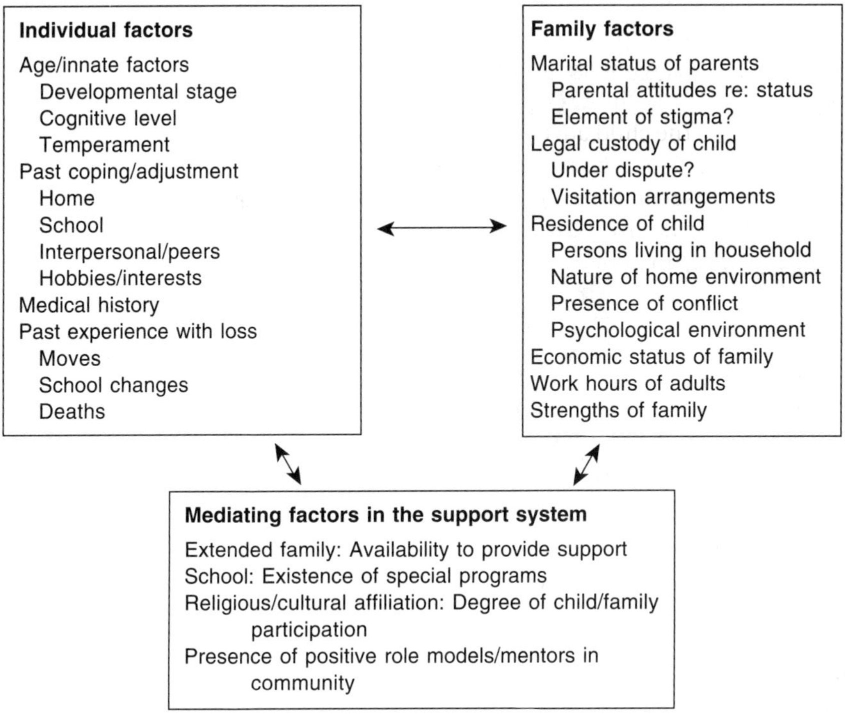

than done, both for the adults and for the children, who become accustomed to sharing adult conflicts and worries.

Wallerstein (1983) and Wallerstein and Blakeslee (1989) describe six "psychological tasks" that children of divorce must successfully resolve. I propose that these same tasks, with minor adaptations, also apply to children of single (never-married) parents and to children in remarried (blended) families. The tasks are as follows:

1. *Acknowledging the reality* (of the marital rupture, of a parent's remarriage, or of a parent's single status). Children may deny the reality or fantasize about a status or outcome they would prefer. The adults can help the children by providing them with information in terms that they can comprehend, including the reason for the current living situation. This should be done with consideration for the children's feelings and for their limited ability to understand complex adult motivations.

2. *Disengaging from parental conflicts and distress and resuming their own customary, age-appropriate pursuits.* As mentioned earlier, it is

FIGURE 11.2. Tripartite assessment of family circumstances.

Marital status of parents

Mother: Never married ____ Divorced ____ (date) ____ Remarried ____ (date) __________

Father: Never married ____ Divorced ____ (date) ____ Remarried ____ (date) __________

Parental attitudes re: status

Mother: Accepting ____ Angry ____ Ashamed ____

Father: Accepting ____ Angry ____ Ashamed ____

Family composition

With whom is child currently living? (check all that apply)

Mother ____ Father ____ Stepmother ____ Stepfather ____ Mother's boyfriend ____

Mother's lesbian partner ____ Father's girlfriend ____ Father's gay partner ____

Grandparent(s) (specify) __________

Siblings: No ____ Yes ____ Ages ____

Stepsiblings: No ____ Yes ____ Ages ____

Half-siblings: No ____ Yes ____ Ages ____

Others living in family with the child __________

With whom does noncustodial parent live? __________

Are there children from this relationship? No ____ Yes ____ Ages __________

Child's contacts with parent(s)

Does child have contact with mother?

Yes ____ How frequently? __________

No ____ Why not? __________

Does child have contact with father?

Yes ____ How frequently? __________

No ____ Why not? __________

What child has been told about whereabouts of absent parent(s)

Does child know where parent is? Yes ____ No ____

If no, has child asked about the absent parent? No ____ Yes ____

If yes, at what age? ____ What was child told? __________

____

Contacts with extended family

Does child have contact with members of the extended family?

No ____ Yes ____

If yes, with whom? __________ How frequently? __________

Changes in child's life over past year

Has there been a change in the family's economic status during the last year?

No ____ Yes ____ If yes, explain __________

____

(continued)

From *Social Work Practice with Children, Fourth Edition*, by Nancy Boyd Webb. Copyright © 2019 The Guilford Press. Permission to photocopy this figure is granted to purchasers of this book for personal use or use with clients (see copyright page for details). Purchasers can download enlarged versions of this material (see the box at the end of the table of contents).

Has there been a change in the custodial parent's work hours? No ____ Yes ____

If yes, give details ____

If yes, does this affect the child's schedule? No ____ Yes ____

If yes, give details ____

Child's housing history

How long has child lived in current residence? ______________________

Where did child live previously? ______________________________

How long lived there? __________ Why moved? ______________________

Does child share a bedroom? No ____ Yes ____ If yes, with whom? __________

Did child share a bedroom in previous residence? No ____ Yes ____

If yes, with whom? ____

Child's school history

Current grade ______________ Appropriate grade for child's age? Yes ____ No ____

If no, explain ____

Current academic performance: Good ____ Fair ____ Poor ____

How long has child been enrolled in present school? ________________

Was child enrolled in a different school last year? No ____ Yes ____

Child's academic performance in previous school: Good ____ Fair ____ Poor ____

Why has child changed schools? (give details) ______________________

____

Custody issues

Who presently has legal custody of the child?

Mother ____ Father ____ Other (specify) ______________________

Is the child's custody under dispute? No ____ Yes ____ If yes, give details __________

____

Presence of conflict

Are the child's parents in conflict? No ____ Yes ____ If yes, give details __________

____

____

Is there conflict in custodial parent's home? No ____ Yes ____ If yes, give details ______

____

Psychological environment of custodial home

Level of custodial parent's functioning: Good ____ Fair ____ Poor ____

Give details ____

____

Strengths in custodial family (give details) ______________________

____

____

Problems in custodial family (give details) ______________________

____

____

contraindicated for children to spend their time worrying about their parents. This worry takes energy and consumes time and effort that the children otherwise would be able to put into schoolwork or social activities. Parents who may (knowingly or unknowingly) use their children as confidants need to be counseled to find peers or a therapist with whom to share their concerns.

3. *Resolving the loss.* This refers to a child's feelings of confusion and rejection about an absent parent. Children should be encouraged to talk about their feelings in group or individual counseling, as well as with their parents in parent–child sessions. Those who have grown up in a single-parent family and have never known the other parent need to acknowledge that they have two parents but that for many complicated reasons their parents decided not to live together. The emphasis should be on the fact that this was an *adult* decision.

4. *Resolving anger and self-blame.* It is very common in situations of divorce for children to feel great anger toward one or both parents. Even when they have witnessed years of painful conflict between their parents, many children still cling to the belief that the divorce was preventable. Some children also blame themselves for causing or contributing to the divorce because their parents argued about them or because they did something that upset the parents. Sometimes a child in a single-parent family feels that he or she is a burden to the parent and possibly the reason for the parent's not remarrying. In a blended family, the child's anger may be projected onto the stepparent, whom the child may view as the cause of the divorce and of all subsequent difficulties.

Resolving children's anger and self-blame takes time. Parents have an important role in this process, and the children may require additional help in the form of group, parent–child, or individual counseling. There are numerous books written for children of various ages to help them realize that other children have struggled with many of the same complicated, disturbing feelings. (See the resources section at the end of this chapter for a list of selected books for children of different ages in divorced and reconstituting families.)

5. *Accepting the relative permanence of the parental status* (divorce, remarriage, or single). This goal encourages children to give up their hope of turning back the clock and magically remaking their families according to their own preferences. Although as adults we know that nothing in life is truly permanent, children who hang on to a fantasy that their parents will reunite or that their father or mother will leave a new relationship are depriving themselves of the opportunity to invest emotionally in the family in which they presently live. If we are always hoping for something different, we lose what we have.

6. *Achieving realistic hope regarding future relationships.* Some of the longitudinal research on children in divorced families (Wallerstein & Blakeslee, 1989; Guidubaldi, 1989; Wallerstein, Lewis, & Blakeslee, 2000) shows that children of divorce struggle with feelings of anxiety about love and commitment in their own intimate relationships. Hetherington and Kelly

(2002), in a study of 1,400 families, found that about 20–25% of children of divorced parents had later difficulties adjusting socially and establishing trusting relationships themselves. Because they had witnessed unsuccessful marriages, they feared that they would have similar marriages themselves and, as a result, had problems with intimacy. However, in an interview with *The New York Times* (Duenwald, 2002), Hetherington emphasized that, although some children of divorce had problems 30 years later, the *majority* were functioning quite well. Another researcher, Elizabeth Marquardt (2006), however, found very different results in a national survey of 1,500 young adults from divorced and intact families. Marquart concluded that children of divorced parents are more likely to struggle in adulthood with feelings of loss, isolation, loneliness, and suffering. These differing opinions may attest to the varying experiences of children in divorcing families and to their own unique abilities to deal with the stress, confusion, and anxiety that a divorce automatically creates. As we know, the same experience can have distinctly different consequences on the various people involved.

CUSTODY DISPUTES: CHILDREN "CAUGHT IN THE MIDDLE"

Approximately 10–15% of divorcing parents take their struggles to court in the form of disputes about visitation, financial support, and custody of the children (Wallerstein et al., 2000; Hetherington & Kelly, 2002). In such cases the parents are usually angry and embittered toward each other, and each turns to the court in an adversary proceeding designed to win a judgment that will force certain concessions from the former partner. These proceedings are totally contrary to the recommendations discussed herein for assisting children in adjusting to this major change in their lives. Frequently, according to Wallerstein and Kelly (1980), one or both parents will deliberately attempt to sway a child to their side; each does this by denigrating the other parent and questioning that parent's interest in and love for the child (Bing, Nelson, & Wesolowski, 2009).

Under these circumstances, it is no surprise that children often become upset and anxious. They are encouraged to take sides, which then interferes with their own attempts to disengage from the parents' hostility. One child graphically referred to the experience as similar to "being cut down the middle with a hatchet." Another said, poignantly, "My mother doesn't realize that when she shoots arrows at my father they have to go through my body before they reach him!" (Wallerstein & Kelly, 1980, p. 71). A drawing by a 10-year-old in the middle of a custody battle shows a child with tears coming down her cheeks and with her nerves exposed along the entire exterior of her body (see Figure 11.3). The words printed on the drawing say, "Oh my God, I cant believe this" and "I am so scared and upset," and also "What do I do?" This poignant drawing clearly pictures a child's sense of agony and upset over her parents' ongoing custody battle.

FIGURE 11.3. 10-year-old girl's Draw-A-Person.

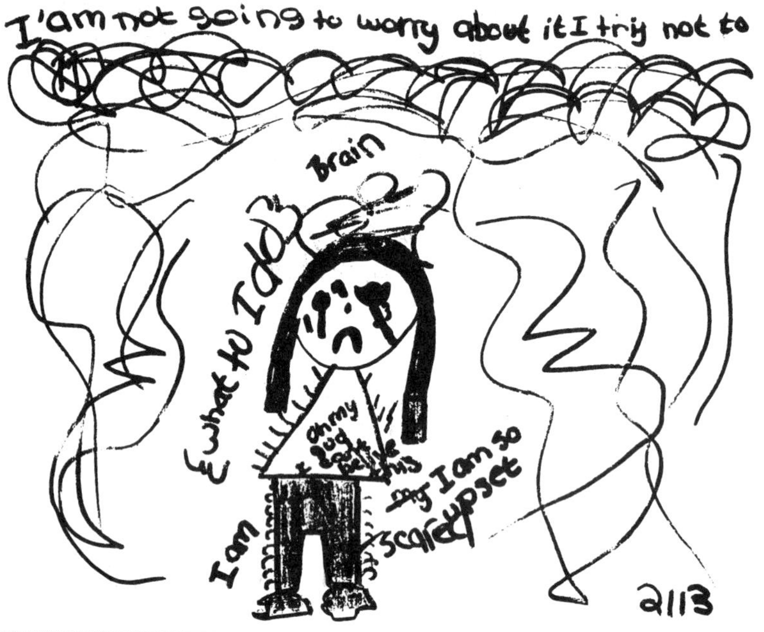

Effects on Children

It is not surprising that, in these sad situations, many children develop such problems as deteriorating schoolwork, aggression toward siblings and peers, sleep disturbances, and somatic complaints. Regression is common but is not always present, because mediating influences may exist in the extended family, the child's school, and the community. Figure 11.2 can help practitioners identify children who are at risk because of intense family hostility and lack of compensatory supports. These children often come to the attention of social workers and other practitioners through the recommendation of the court when it becomes evident that the children are reacting to an embattled family situation and the family court judge orders that the children receive counseling. In some cases, the judge may also appoint a guardian *ad litem* to represent a child's best interests. The case of Charlie, described in the next section, provides an illustration of these circumstances.

The Court-Appointed Guardian

Sometimes referred to as a "mediator" (Rice & Rice, 1986) and in many states as a "guardian *ad litem*" (literally, "guardian at law"), an individual may be hired by the court to represent the best interests of the child and to advocate for the child's welfare. The guardian, often a lawyer, may interview both parents and the child preparatory to making recommendations to the judge. In addition, the guardian may recommend psychological and psychiatric exams for the child and the parents, in addition to counseling for the child.

At best, the guardian remains neutral and objective and helps a child feel protected from the warring parents. At worst, a child may be intimidated by the perceived power of this person to decide monumental issues in his or her life, such as which parent he or she will live with.

According to Koocher and Keith-Spiegel (1990), most states subscribe to the concept of "the best interests of the child" in making legal decisions in court custody cases. The following factors are considered in making such a determination:

- The nature of the child's relationship with each parent.
- The capacity and willingness of each parent to care for the child.
- The presence of a stable environment and the length of time the child has spent in that environment.
- The likelihood that the home will serve as a family unit.
- The nature of the child's adjustment at school and in the community.
- The moral fitness of each parent.
- The physical and mental fitness of each parent.
- The child's own preference.

The next section describes how the guardian *ad litem* and the social worker attempted to weigh these factors in the case of an 11-year-old boy whose parents were in a custody battle.

THE CASE OF CHARLIE, AGE 11

(This case is a composite based on the case of Malcolm in the second edition of this book and on my extensive clinical experience with similar cases under dispute. Any similarity to real individuals is purely coincidental.)

Family Information

Mother	Brenda, age 30, cashier at a big box store; history of depression, on medication.
Father	Ray, discharged from Army; abandoned mother and Charlie, when boy was age 2.
Child client	Charlie, age 11, fifth grade.

This was an African American family with an absent father. Charlie's parents had divorced when he was a preschooler, and his father enlisted in the army soon after. The boy had only sporadic telephone contact with his father in the intervening years, and he knew that his father had remarried.

Presenting Problem

Charlie's father had recently received a medical discharge from the army after stepping on a mine in Afghanistan and losing one leg in the explosion. He contacted the family for the purpose of obtaining custody of his son. The father had remarried, and he wanted Charlie to live with him and his new wife and her 14-year-old daughter. The father hired a lawyer to represent him in the custody dispute, and the mother had a court-appointed lawyer. Because of the hostility between the parents, a guardian *ad litem* was appointed to represent Charlie's best interests. A referral to a family agency was made to help Charlie deal with these stressful circumstances.

Background

Soon after Charlie's parents married, his mother became pregnant. Their relationship was always stormy, and Ray abandoned his wife and young son when Charlie was about 2 years old. Brenda then decided to move in with her mother, who had cancer that was in remission and who worked several nights a week as a waitress. It was a busy household, but it functioned fairly well because the women shared the housekeeping responsibilities and child care. Brenda relied a great deal on her mother to take care of Charlie after school when she was working.

Charlie's mother stated to the social worker that her work was quite demanding, and she often felt overwhelmed and exhausted. She had been on medication for several years to help with her depressed feelings after a relationship with a boyfriend was broken off. She had been in the habit of spending several nights a week at her boyfriend's apartment, because she felt that she needed "a break," and her mother would care for Charlie at these times. She became pregnant but had a miscarriage and then became quite depressed for several months. During the time when she was preoccupied with her pregnancy and her boyfriend, Brenda sometimes would forget to take Charlie for his routine dentist and doctor's appointments. Charlie's father later used this information against Brenda in the custody dispute.

When his father reappeared and wanted to have Charlie in his life again, the boy was initially pleased, and weekend visits were arranged. Charlie was nervous about his father's amputation but was relieved to later find out that his father had a prosthesis and that he could walk without assistance. Charlie reported that his dad's wife and her daughter were "nice" but that he was often bored there. He didn't like it when, during the drive back home to his mother, the father would say very negative things about his mother and her family and imply that the mother had prevented him from visiting all those years. Charlie was afraid to ask his father directly why he didn't come and visit him, stating that he thought his father might hit him if he asked (although there was no reported history of abuse).

It soon became evident that Ray's goal was to try to obtain full custody of his son. Neither Charlie nor his mother wanted this; nor could Brenda and Ray agree on a visitation schedule. Realizing that the family was at an impasse, the family judge appointed a guardian *ad litem* to represent the child's best interests. The judge also ordered psychological evaluations of each parent and of Charlie and recommended that Charlie receive counseling services. A referral was made to the local family service agency.

Assessment and Plan for Intervention

The plan was for the social worker to see Charlie for weekly play therapy sessions, to maintain contact with each parent on a monthly basis, and to communicate regularly by telephone with the court-appointed guardian. The social worker realized that both father and mother would probably try to present themselves as the preferred custodial parent and that Charlie himself was probably in turmoil over the dilemma of having both parents pulling him in separate directions. It would be the guardian's responsibility to make a recommendation to the judge, based on the reports of the psychologist and the child's therapist.

First Session

In the initial meeting, Charlie was guarded at first but warmed up quickly when some drawing activities were introduced. The predictions about his anxiety proved quite accurate when Charlie, asked to draw a person, drew a figure he called "little boy Frankenstein." The face had a very sad expression, and when the social worker asked Charlie to tell her about the picture, he replied that Frankenstein was lonely and different from everyone else. He felt both sad and mad. The worker asked Charlie if he ever felt that way, and Charlie agreed that he had some of the same feelings and, in addition, that he was worried because he didn't know where he would be living.

Second Session

In the next session, the worker introduced a version of the therapeutic drawing exercise called the "Squiggle Story Drawing" (Winnicott, 1971b; Webb, 1999). She presented the exercise to Charlie as a "fun art game." This drawing exercise consists of the child and therapist making alternating "scribbles" on a piece of paper, then trying to convert these into drawings of real or imaginary figures.

SOCIAL WORKER: Tell me about your picture.

CHARLIE: It's a boy and he's thinking about getting on a small boat and sailing to a special island made of money.

SOCIAL WORKER: And when he gets there?

CHARLIE: He's going to take as much of it back with him as he can.

SOCIAL WORKER: To use for?

CHARLIE: Clothes and candy and toys and toys and toys!

SOCIAL WORKER: Oh, has he been needing that stuff?

CHARLIE: Not really. But he wants MORE!!

SOCIAL WORKER: (*laughing*) Does he go on the trip with anyone?

CHARLIE: Oh no, he goes by himself and comes back to surprise everyone. That way they suddenly find out they don't have to fight about money anymore.

SOCIAL WORKER: Who are "they"?

CHARLIE: His mom and dad.

SOCIAL WORKER: Do yours fight about that?

CHARLIE: Maybe. But they won't miss me on this trip because it's a magic trip; it's a long way off but I'll get there in just seconds, and then back again. So, we don't have to miss each other that way.

SOCIAL WORKER: Who would miss who?

CHARLIE: I'd miss my family.

SOCIAL WORKER: Can you tell me who in particular?

CHARLIE: My mom and sister and father and grandmother.

SOCIAL WORKER: So, it sounds like you want to magically solve things so that no one has to miss anyone. You can spend all the time you need to spend with everyone.

CHARLIE: That's right.

SOCIAL WORKER: If only things were that simple! Life's not that easy, is it? You can't live with both Mom and Dad at the same time.

CHARLIE: Why can't they just let me do what I want? Live with Mom and see Dad whenever I can?

The social worker then tried to explain how both his parents wanted him in their life and that the judge would be the person who decided what was best for him.

Third Session

Charlie asked if he could play the drawing game again, and this time he called the resulting picture a "big storm" and said that he was in the middle of it. He described how he was falling and that he was afraid because he didn't know where he was going to land. He also referred to other things blowing around and said that he was afraid of being hit.

The social worker identified the scared feelings connected to this situation, and Charlie added that he couldn't control what was happening because of the strong winds.

Because the connection between Charlie's own life and his story was so clear, the social worker asked him if he had some of the same feelings about his life. Charlie then openly discussed his frustration at the long time the legal proceedings were taking, and he said he wanted to write a letter to the judge. The social worker supported this idea and offered to help him with it.

Summary of the Next 6 Months

A psychologist met with both parents and submitted a report to the guardian recommending that Charlie should live with his mother but spend 2 months in the summer with his father, plus 3 weekends a month during the school year. Charlie was not at all happy about this plan and asked his father about the arrangements for regular contact with his mother over the summer. The father did not give Charlie any assurance that he would, in fact, be able to see his mother, stating that it "would be up to her." The father planned to enroll Charlie in a summer camp program, but Charlie did not want to leave his home, his neighborhood, friends, and family. Also, he really didn't want to go to camp because he didn't know how to swim. He did not want to move in with his father for an extended visit of this kind. He told his father that he wanted to be with him for only 1 month and that he didn't want to go to camp. He wrote a letter to the judge expressing his feelings. The judge then reconsidered and permitted Charlie to remain with his mother over the summer, with weekend visits with his father. The father evidently could not accept this plan, and he subsequently informed Charlie that he would see him in the fall, again disappearing from the boy's life.

Discussion

The events of this case prevented the child from having an ongoing, nonconflictual relationship with both parents. How could Charlie disengage from the conflict when it had such ongoing repercussions for his life? How could this child participate in age-appropriate pursuits when he was being pulled in two directions and remained uncertain about where he would live?

This case illustrates many of the issues typical for children in divorced and blended families: multiple losses and stressors, custody battles, loyalty conflicts, reduced or absent communication with the noncustodial parent, and adjustment to a stepparent and stepsiblings. It also demonstrates the unfortunate reality that help for a child may not be obtained until after years of family instability and stress.

The balancing factors in predicting Charlie's future adjustment are his own and his mother's strengths, the ability of both to express their feelings appropriately, and their willingness to engage in a helping process to obtain the support they need. The court ordered that Charlie continue in counseling, and he and his mother agreed about this. His mother stated that she did not want him to have similar relationship problems when he grew up. The social worker wanted to give him the opportunity to participate in a support group of peers from divorced and remarried families, and she planned to help identify and involve a male role model to demonstrate the qualities of dependability and caring.

According to Garrity and Baris (1994), children who are pressured to take sides between their divorcing parents often pay the price of "denial of the sense of self" (p. 87). "Lacking the freedom to form their own opinions . . . children grow to doubt their own feelings. Therefore, the most important goal of therapy is to encourage the emergence of the child's separate sense of self" (p. 90). The methods for helping children "in the middle" include the range of play therapy techniques illustrated throughout this book.

ETHICAL ISSUES FOR PRACTITIONERS

Goldman et al. (1983, p. 4) note astutely:

> In working with children, many ethical issues should be expected to arise. Because children are dependent upon others who are legally responsible for them, and because parents are often at legal odds with one another or with juvenile authorities, there are many times when the [practitioner] will be called upon to consider at what point the child is truly served.

Whether or not there is a guardian *ad litem* involved, the practitioner must always support the child's best interests and try to help disentangle him or her from the parents' disputes.

The matter of access to the child's records constitutes a problematic ethical issue. The legal rights of divorced parents are unclear regarding who is entitled to see reports of a child's psychiatric/psychological evaluations and counseling sessions. Often a custodial parent brings a child for an evaluation, hoping to use the resulting information on his or her own behalf in a subsequent divorce proceeding. The noncustodial parent, later learning of this evaluation, may demand to see the record. As discussed in Chapter 2, both parents have the right to see their child's record in some states; in others, only the parent with legal custody of the child is legally entitled to the information. Practitioners should know the status of the law in their state.

I have argued previously against guaranteeing confidentiality between parent and child because of the unfortunate communication barrier this creates. Because it is virtually impossible to promise confidentiality, the practitioner must make process notes with the assumption that these may become open to both parents or to the court at a later date. In situations in which families are involved in litigation, the practitioner must be prepared to have his or her notes subpoenaed. This may present great difficulty, for example, in a situation in which a child has reported instances of verbal abuse and the practitioner wants to explore the matter further before taking action. The practitioner must exercise care in writing detailed notes about matters that may subsequently be used as part of a custody determination. Furthermore, the fact that the record may later be shared with others puts distinct constraints on the relationship, and the practitioner may need to discuss these with the child. According to the 2016 revision of the NASW code of ethics, the worker has an *obligation* to clarify with all individuals the matter of "which individuals will be considered clients and the nature of the social worker's professional obligations to the various individuals who are receiving services" (NASW, 2016, Section 1.06d).

Another matter that may cause an ethical conflict for the practitioner relates to the relationship between the practitioner and the guardian *ad litem*. When a child enters counseling, the guardian may expect the child's practitioner to offer an opinion regarding the child's and parents' mental state and attitudes. This can cause an ethical dilemma for the worker, because these matters often take considerable time and thought and because the outcome is so critical in terms of the child's future. Many social workers are not prepared to offer a firm opinion about which parent a child should live with, believing that the child's optimal adjustment depends on his or her maintaining an ongoing relationship with *both* parents.

These difficult ethical matters deserve more attention in schools of social work to prepare practitioners who work with children for the likelihood that they will be faced with these dilemmas in their future practice.

CONCLUDING COMMENTS

Children who live in single-parent, divorcing, and reconstituted families must cope with numerous stressors and losses. All children are responsive to the conflicts within their families and to the attitudes of others toward their families. When parents divorce, remarry, or decide to remain single, their children must cope not only with their anxieties about their own lives but also with the responses of people in their school and peer networks to the changes and lack of stability in their families.

Individual, family, and group helping methods can assist children with their confused feelings. However, in situations involving divorce and custody disputes, the children have often experienced years of conflict between their parents before they are referred for counseling. There are probably few other situations in which family therapy is more necessary; it is imperative to reduce the ongoing recriminations and hostility between partners, which continue to damage the child's relationship with each parent. Although the marriage may be beyond repair, the parents should nonetheless be enjoined to act in the best interests of their child or children to prevent further pain for them. The court could play an important preventive role in this regard by insisting on a minimum of three sessions of counseling for divorcing parents, to attempt to orient them to and educate them about their children's needs.

Single parents need support of a different kind, to provide them with respite from the fatigue of full-time parenting. Peer groups located in the community at day care centers and schools could help connect single parents with their counterparts; this would enable them to offer both emotional and concrete help to one another.

Regardless of the family structure, we must affirm that such families may be different without being deviant. Because of our mission to respect individual differences, we must do everything possible to ease the stresses on the children in these families and to help them mourn their losses so that they may continue with their age-appropriate development

DISCUSSION QUESTIONS AND ROLE-PLAY EXERCISE

1. How can a practitioner help a single mother tell her preschool child about the child's father, who abandoned her when he learned about the pregnancy? (Imagine that the father is now in jail for crimes committed in connection with drug abuse and that the mother has not seen him since before the child's birth.) Role-play this interaction.
2. Many schools offer Banana Splits groups to help children in divorced families talk about their experiences and offer support to one another. What kinds of supports and/or programs would you suggest for children with never-married parents?
3. Consider ways in which the court might collaborate with a family agency to assist children and families in the midst of divorce proceedings. What guidelines would you propose in providing services to parents and to children? What would be the purposes and goals of such collaboration?
4. How can the practitioner resolve his or her own feelings of disappointment when a parent continues to put the child in the middle, as in the case of Charlie?

RESOURCES FOR CHILDREN IN DIVORCED AND BLENDED FAMILIES

Note. Ages are specified when indicated.

Brown, L. K., & Brown, M. (1986). *Dinosaurs divorce.* New York: Trumpet Club. [Reprinted by Little, Brown, Boston, MA.] (Preschool–early school age)

Ekster, C. G., & Rama, S. (2008). *Where am I sleeping tonight? (A story of divorce).* Weaverville, CA: Boulden. (Ages 9–12)

Evans, M. D. (1986). *This is me and my two families: An awareness scrapbook/journal for children living in stepfamilies.* New York: Magination Press. (Parents and children)

Hazen, B. S. (1978). *Two homes to live in: A child's-eye view of divorce.* New York: Human Sciences Press.

Heegaard, M. (1991). *When Mom and Dad separate: Children can learn to cope with grief from divorce.* Minneapolis, MN: Woodland Press.

Heegaard, M. (1993). *When a parent marries again: Children can learn to cope with family change.* Minneapolis, MN: Woodland Press.

Krementz, J. (1988). *How it feels when parents divorce.* New York: Knopf. (Ages 7–16)

Levin, S. (2006). *Was it the chocolate pudding?: A story for little kids about divorce.* Washington, DC: American Psychological Association. (Ages 4–8)

Masurel, C., & Denton, K. M. (2003). *Two homes.* Somerville, MA: Candlewick. (Preschool)

Moore, K. D. (2008). *They both love you: Two separate houses, one common love.* Bloomington, IN: AuthorHouse.

Prokop, M. S. (1996). *Divorce happens to the nicest kids.* Warren, OH: Alegra House. (Ages 9–12).

Winchester, K., & Beyer, K. (2001). *What in the world do you do when your parents divorce?: A survival guide for kids.* Minneapolis, MN: Free Spirit.

CHAPTER 12

Children in Families Affected by Illness and Death

All children, in the normal course of their development, learn about being sick, and most, by the time they enter school, have at least rudimentary understanding of the word "dead" through the experience of seeing dead insects and animals. However, when a young child lives in a family in which a parent has a recurring illness such as cancer and/or in which an older sibling dies suddenly of a drug overdose, the child's confusion and anxiety about his or her own personal survival and that of the well parent are entirely understandable. In the case outlined here and described throughout this chapter, we see that this was the family context of illness and death in which young Sabrina completed kindergarten and entered first grade.

THE CASE OF SABRINA, AGE 5¾

Family Information

Child client	Sabrina Rossi, age 5¾, completing kindergarten.
Mother	Lida Rossi, age 46, psychologist (currently unemployed).
Father	Dan Rossi, age 40, editor at publishing house.
Half brother	John Sand, age 18, unemployed; former college student.
Paternal grandparents	In 70s, living nearby.
Paternal aunt	Carol, age 44, living nearby.

Cousins	Carol's children, Katie and Greg, ages 10 and 4.
Maternal grandmother	Age 70, living out of state.
Maternal aunt	Ann, age 45, living out of state.
Cousin	Ann's son, Steve, age 6.
Maternal aunt	Jean, age 43, living out of state.

Mrs. Rossi had been married previously; her first husband had died of a heart attack at the age of 45, when John was 14. She stated that her husband had a history of depression and alcoholism and that they had been separated since John was 2½. Neither she nor John had contact with any of her first husband's relatives. In fact, she stated that she did not know their whereabouts.

Mr. and Mrs. Rossi have been married 8 years. They are of different religious backgrounds: The father and his relatives are Catholic and Italian, whereas the mother is Protestant and of northern European descent. However, neither Mr. nor Mrs. Rossi attends church services, and both have been interested in Eastern religions; they have a large statue of the Buddha in their living room.

Presenting Problem

Mrs. Rossi telephoned to request help for her family because she was facing major surgery, and she was concerned about how they would cope with her projected long postoperative period. Lida had a large tumor that required removal, necessitating both a colostomy and a vaginectomy. She stated that there was a lot of tension and conflict between her husband and her son and that she was quite worried about how they would manage without her presence as a buffer. Although the operation was not considered life threatening, Mrs. Rossi said that she wanted to work with a therapist who was experienced with both family and bereavement issues.

Assessment and Plan for Intervention

Because the operation was to occur in 10 days, time was limited. Mrs. Rossi had indicated on the phone her reluctance to include Sabrina in the initial family meeting, so I began by seeing the parents and John to address Mrs. Rossi's specific concerns. It was very evident that Mr. Rossi was angry about John's lack of employment or plans for his future. The boy, who looked more like a 14-year-old than an 18-year-old, had overdosed on cocaine 6 months earlier and since then had dropped out of college. He spent most of his days sleeping and his evenings out with friends, drinking beer and drawing graffiti. There was a great deal of tension between Mr. Rossi and John; nonetheless, Mr. Rossi gave John money every week so he could buy gas to go job hunting. Recently Mrs. Rossi had insisted that John enter therapy, and he had gone for two or three sessions at the time of the first family meeting with me. Mrs. Rossi herself had been engaged in individual therapy for several years.

I sensed that Mrs. Rossi seemed to be trying very hard to "put her house in order" before going into the hospital. She wanted John and her husband to promise to help her when she came home, when she herself would be too weak to go shopping or perform routine housekeeping tasks. During the session, we listed the chores and obtained agreements about who would do what. It was evident that everything related to John was a struggle; he resisted the idea of doing his laundry regularly rather than leaving it piled up, and he seemed equally reluctant to promise to feed his own cats or to meet Sabrina's school bus, because he "might be sleeping." He did agree to do the shopping, and Mr. Rossi agreed to vacuum and cook. I made an appointment to see Mr. Rossi and John together the day after Lida's operation.

I also expressed concern about Sabrina's reaction to the impending separation from her mother, especially after Mrs. Rossi told me that the child's kindergarten teacher had commented recently about Sabrina's "spaciness" and inability to concentrate. I encouraged Mrs. Rossi to bring her for one session to prepare her for her mother's absence.

We agreed that couple, family, and/or parent–child sessions would be planned later, depending on Mrs. Rossi's stamina and the family's needs after her operation.

Mother–Child Session

Sabrina brought a stuffed white toy cat named "Sassy" with her. At the beginning of the session she seemed quite anxious, as expressed in silly, teasing behavior in which she had Sassy crawl all over and tickle her mother.

I explained to Sabrina who I was. I then said that I knew her mother was going into the hospital next week and that I wondered what it would be like for *her* without her mom at home. Sabrina said that she was "mad" because she had to stay at her grandmother's. She had her own room there, but it was dark at night, and she didn't like it. Mrs. Rossi immediately said that they would get a nightlight for that room, just like the one she had at home. Sabrina seemed somewhat placated by this idea.

I asked Sabrina to draw a person. The drawing (see Figure 12.1) appeared to be very primitive and almost frightening. The core body was in black, with parts of the hands, legs, and feet outlined in red. Sabrina also outlined the body and arms in purple. The features of the face were minimal, and the figure had no hair. Sabrina declined my invitation to tell me about this person. I considered that it might reflect the child's fantasy about surgery (the distinctive red color could signify blood). I decided to prepare Sabrina for the experience of seeing her mother hooked up to intravenous (IV) lines. I knew that Mr. Rossi planned to take her to the hospital to visit soon after the operation. Therefore, I made a crude drawing of a person in a hospital bed

FIGURE 12.1. Sabrina's Draw-A-Person before her mother's surgery.

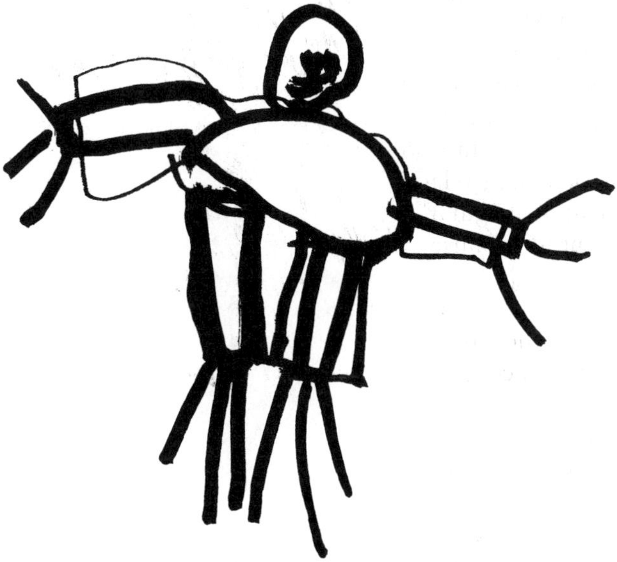

with the IV stand next to it, with connections to the patient (see Figure 12.2). I explained to Sabrina that after an operation people cannot eat as usual and that their food and medicines are given to them in tubes that go into the veins in their hands and noses. Sabrina expressed disgust about the nose tube, but her mother reassured her that it was only for a short time and that it didn't hurt.

I then brought out a doll family and bedroom furniture and suggested that we play out what it would be like to go to visit Mom in the hospital. We set up Sabrina's home in one location, with a toy telephone, and Mom's hospital bed in another, also with a phone. I invited Mrs. Rossi to role-play what it would be like after her operation, suggesting that she tell Sabrina she felt very tired and weak but that she would get stronger later. Mrs. Rossi played this scene with Sabrina very effectively, and at the end Sabrina hugged her mother and said, "I'm glad it's not today!"

Summary of the Next 8 Months

The first several months after Mrs. Rossi's surgery were a period of hope and optimism. Mrs. Rossi had a good recovery from the operation, despite the considerable adjustment in adapting to using the colostomy and urinary bags. No chemotherapy or radiation was prescribed, as Lida had previously undergone a course of radiation in an earlier attempt to shrink the tumor.

FIGURE 12.2. Therapist's drawing of a person in a hospital bed with IV stand and tubes.

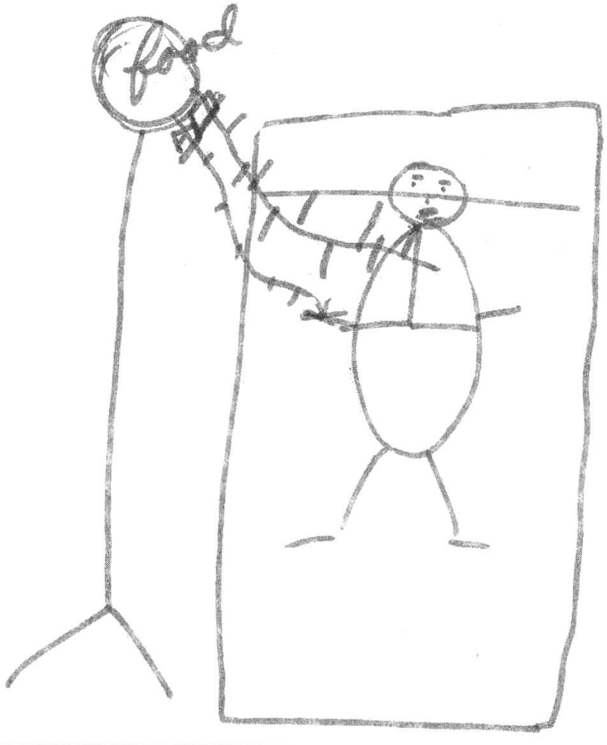

Mr. Rossi was very supportive of his wife and hopeful that they could resume some form of sexual activity, adapted to his wife's limitations. Mr. and Mrs. Rossi and Sabrina went on a vacation together, and Lida was making plans to resume her professional career. John had obtained employment, with the intention of getting his own apartment and returning to school the next semester.

Sabrina was doing well in her first-grade class; she drew a picture of a "princess" (see Figure 12.3) 2 months after she had drawn the primitive, insect-like drawing prior to her mother's hospitalization. Comparing the two drawings now, I believe that the earlier figure reflected the child's fears and regression caused by her anxiety about her mother's upcoming operation and the anticipated separation.

During this period I saw various members of the family at 2-week intervals in different combinations, including the parents together, Sabrina alone, Mr. Rossi and John together, and Mr. Rossi alone. John was continuing sporadically in individual therapy with another therapist. The family mood was positive, despite the ongoing concern about John. Because Sabrina was doing so well in school and at home, it was not necessary to see her weekly.

Eight months after Mrs. Rossi's operation, this period of optimism and hope for the future came to an abrupt and tragic end when John was found dead of a heroin overdose in a friend's apartment. My initial thought upon hearing the news was that it was a suicide, but both Mr. and Mrs. Rossi stressed that John had recently found a job and was in good spirits, talking about getting his own apartment and returning to school. They regarded the death as an accident and believed that John had not used heroin previously. They also criticized the friend who had given it to him because he ignored John when he passed out in a drugged state. Members of both Mr. and Mrs. Rossi's extended families attended the funeral, as did many of John's friends; Sabrina sat in the front row between her parents.

I refer to the Rossi family at the time of John's death to illustrate some typical bereavement reactions throughout the chapter.

FIGURE 12.3. Sabrina's Draw-A-Person (a princess), 2 months after her mother's surgery.

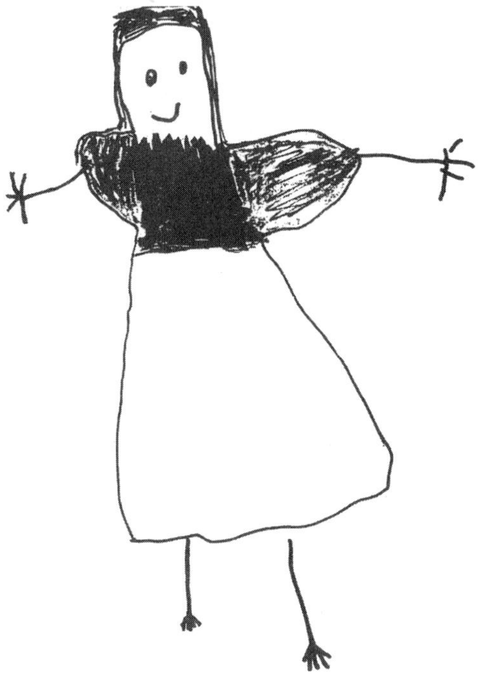

DEVELOPMENTAL INFLUENCES ON CHILDREN'S UNDERSTANDING OF DEATH

The poet who described childhood as "the kingdom where nobody dies" (Millay, 1934/1969, p. 203) presented an idealized picture that certainly is not true in this age of television, war, gun violence, and growing awareness among teachers and parents that children should be included in death-related discussions and experiences. Kastenbaum (2001, p. 283) states that "from direct observation, clinical experience, and systematic research there is ample evidence that children do think of death." The child, however, does not begin with the realization that death is inevitable, universal, and final but rather understands it as an experience of separation and loss.

In previous publications (Webb, 2002a, 2002b, 2010), I presented a review of the child's gradual, progressive understanding of death as related to his or her cognitive development. Using Piaget's work as a guide (Piaget, 1955, 1968, 1972; Piaget & Inhelder, 1969), I connected children's developing ideas about death to the three major phases of cognitive development, as summarized in Table 12.1. The age references in the table should not be taken too literally, as development is an individual process and variations occur depending on a child's unique life experiences. Chronological age is only a very general guideline, indicating the typical gradual progression in children's understanding about death.

Let us now apply the concepts in Table 12.1 to the case of Sabrina. Because of Sabrina's young age (6½) when her brother died, her understanding was still at the preoperational stage. She may have thought that something she did or

TABLE 12.1. Children's Cognitive Development and Understanding of Death

Age of child	Piaget's stage	Understanding of death
The young child (ages 2–7)	Preoperational • Magical thinking • Egocentricity	Temporary, reversible, caused by own wishes/deeds
The latency-age child (ages 7–10)	Concrete operational • Reduced egocentricity • Improved reasoning • Awareness of time	Irreversible, final, inevitable (but in future, for "old," not selves); distinction between body and "spirit"[a]
The prepubertal child (ages 11–12)	Formal operational • Logical thinking • Abstract thinking • Tolerance of contradictions and ambiguity	Mature understanding: final, inevitable/universal, irreversible

Note. Adapted from the discussion in Webb (2002a, pp. 4–7). Copyright © 2002 The Guilford Press. Adapted by permission.

[a]Most experts believe that children acquire a realistic perception of the finality and irreversibility of death at the *end* of this period, by age 9 or 10. This understanding is a *gradual* process.

said led her brother to take drugs or alcohol. She may also have thought that he would return, especially because her parents' religious perspective included the concept of reincarnation. This could have been confusing for Sabrina, because children her age are very literal; she could have become angry if she believed John would come back and he did not do so.

THE TRIPARTITE ASSESSMENT OF THE BEREAVED CHILD

Although the child's age and developmental stage should always be considered in assessing the impact of a death experience, these are only a few of the many factors that must be evaluated. In all three editions of my book *Helping Bereaved Children* (Webb, 1993, 2002a, 2010), I present the tripartite assessment of the bereaved child as a method for understanding the specific meaning of a specific death to a specific child. The discussion that follows is a further elaboration of the concepts I originally presented there.

As I have indicated in earlier chapters of the present book, a tripartite assessment weighs the interaction of three groups of factors in considering the reactions of a child following a death. These three groups of factors are as follows:

1. Individual factors.
2. Factors related to the death.
3. Factors in the support system (family, social, religious/cultural factors).

In some situations, individual factors, such as the child's past history of death and loss, may have a compelling impact on his or her response. In other cases, the element of trauma related to the death may exert an overriding influence on the child and family. Finally, regardless of the nature of factors related to the individual and to the death itself, the responses of family, religious/cultural, and social networks must always be considered as balancing factors that either support the grieving individual or do not do so. Figure 12.4 illustrates the specific components and interactions among the three sets of variables.

I have developed four different forms to assist the practitioner in highlighting significant factors in the tripartite assessment of the bereaved child. Blank versions of these forms are provided in the Appendices; in the following discussion, I use filled-in versions to demonstrate their application to Sabrina and her family at the time of John's death.

The first form (Figure 12.5) facilitates the recording of information about the child's life and general level of adjustment prior to the death. A second form (Figure 12.6) records information about the death itself and about the child's degree of involvement in ritual observances connected to the death. A third form (Figure 12.7) permits the recording of information about the

FIGURE 12.4. Interactive components of a tripartite assessment of the bereaved child. Adapted from Webb (2002a, p. 30). Copyright © 2002 The Guilford Press. Adapted by permission.

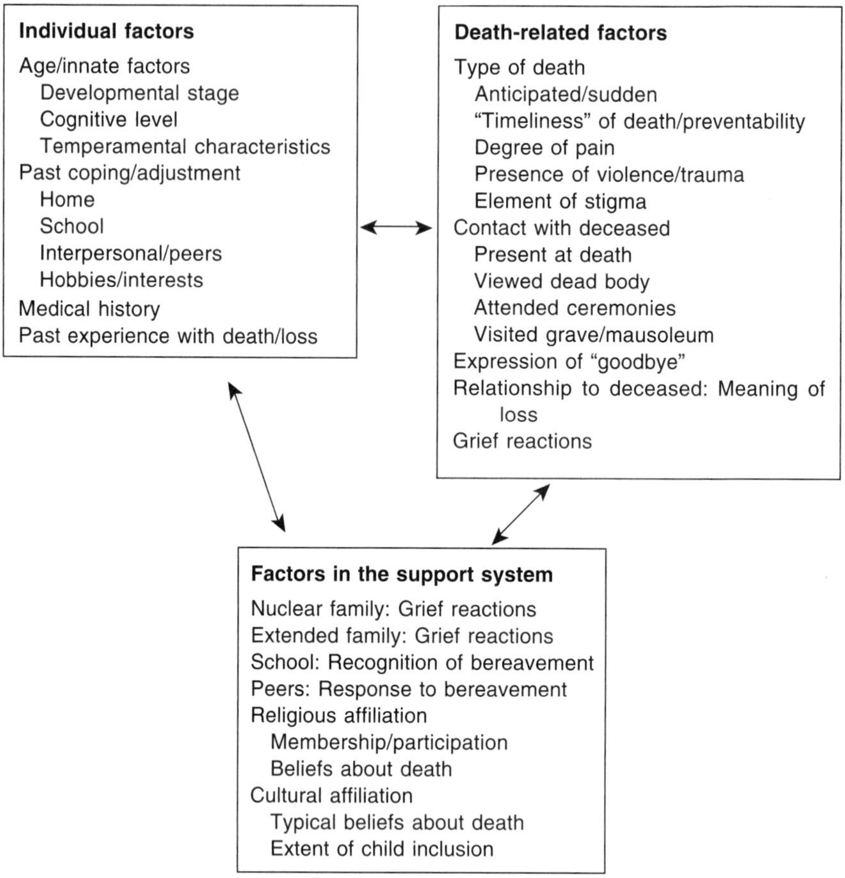

extended family, about the child's school and peer contacts, and about possible religious and cultural influences on the child following the death. A form for recording the nature of the child's grief reactions (Figure 12.8) can be filled out with the assistance of the parent(s) or others who were present following the death. This form probes for specific information related to the nature of the relationship between the child and the person who died.

It appears from Figure 12.5 that this child was developing well, without apparent behavioral or emotional difficulties. The mother's only concern about her was her seeming lack of assertiveness with friends; Mrs. Rossi had noticed that Sabrina was usually a follower, not a leader.

Figure 12.6, which records information related to the death, shows that this family was in shock following John's death. They also felt shame because of John's drug use. Nonetheless, the parents were concerned about Sabrina's reaction and tried to include her as much as possible in the family rituals. The presence of West Coast relatives and cousins who came for the funeral helped Sabrina engage with children her own age during this intensely stressful time.

For the most part, the members of this family were expressing their grief openly and fully, as Figure 12.7 shows.

Sabrina's grief reactions are described in Figure 12.8. Sabrina's teacher said that she was continuing to do well in school (she was now in first grade). However, Mrs. Rossi reported that Sabrina told her she sometimes went into the bathroom at school and cried. Sabrina was also waking up in the night and sometimes sleeping on the couch. She denied that she had bad dreams or that she was thinking about John. These behaviors could be viewed as normal grief reactions in a 6-year-old child.

FIGURE 12.5. Individual factors in childhood bereavement. *Note.* This form is one part of the three-part assessment of the bereaved child, which also includes an assessment of death-related factors (Figure 12.6) and family/social/religious/cultural factors (Figure 12.7). The form itself (not the responses) is from Webb (2002a, p. 31). Copyright © 2002 The Guilford Press. Reprinted by permission.

1. Age _6_ years _6_ months — Date of birth ______ Date of assessment ______

   a. Developmental stage:

   Freud _Late Oedipal/early latency_

   Erikson _Industry vs. inferiority_

   b. Cognitive level:

   Piaget _Preoperational_

   c. Temperamental characteristics:

   Thomas and Chess _Easy_

2. Past coping/adjustment

   a. Home (as reported by parents): Good _X_ Fair ___ Poor ___

   b. School (as reported by parents and teachers): Good _X_ Fair ___ Poor ___

   c. Interpersonal/peers: Good ___ Fair _X_ Poor ___

   d. Hobbies/interests (list) _Brownies, ballet_

3. Medical history (as reported by parents and pediatrician)—describe serious illnesses, operations, and injuries since birth, with dates and outcome _Some earaches and difficult hearing because of allergies; neither problem is severe, according to parents. Otherwise, health is good._

4. Past experience with death/loss—give details with dates and outcome *or* complete Wolfelt's Loss Inventory

   No known experience. Maternal grandfather died before she was born. She may be aware that John's father died 5 years ago; however, Sabrina would have been only a toddler of 18 months at the time

FIGURE 12.6. Death-related factors in childhood bereavement. *Note*. This form is one part of the three-part assessment of the bereaved child, which also includes an assessment of individual factors (Figure 12.5) and family/social/religious/cultural factors (Figure 12.7). The form itself (not the responses) is from Webb (2002a, p. 35). Copyright © 2002 The Guilford Press. Reprinted by permission.

1. Type of death

   Anticipated: Yes ____ No _X_ If yes, how long? __________ or sudden X

   "Timeliness" of death: Age of the deceased 19

   Perception of preventability:

   Definitely preventable _X_ Maybe ____ Not ____

   Degree of pain associated with death:

   None _X_ Some ____ Much ____

   Presence of violence/trauma: Yes ____ No _X_

   If yes, describe, indicating whether the child witnessed, heard about, or was present and experienced the trauma personally. ______________________

   Element of stigma: Yes _X_ No ____

   If yes, describe, indicating nature of death, and degree of openness of family in discussing. Since the death was caused by a drug overdose, the family felt ashamed. Sabrina's grandparents never discussed the death with Lida and Dan, although they did attend the funeral.

2. Contact with deceased

   Present at moment of death? Yes ____ No _X_

   If yes, describe circumstances, including who else was present and whether the deceased said anything specifically to the child. ______________________

   Did the child view the dead body? Yes ____ No _X_

   If yes, describe circumstances, including reactions of the child and others who were present. ______________________

   Did the child attend funeral/memorial service/graveside service?

   Yes _X_ No ____ Which? ______________________

   Child's reactions Child cried at funeral; there was no graveside service, since the body was cremated and the ashes were stored in an urn.

   Has the child visited grave/mausoleum since the death? Yes ____ No _X_

   If yes, describe circumstances. ______________________

3. Did the child make any expression of "goodbye" to the deceased, either spontaneous or suggested? Yes _X_ No ____

   If yes, describe. Sabrina assisted in writing messages on the exterior of John's casket. The message said, "Goodbye, John, we love you." She also drew hearts and flowers next to the words.

FIGURE 12.7. Family/social/religious/cultural factors in childhood bereavement. *Note*. This form is one part of the three-part assessment of the bereaved child, which also includes an assessment of individual factors (Figure 12.5) and death-related factors (Figure 12.6). The form itself (not the responses) is from Webb (2002a, p. 39). Copyright © 2002 The Guilford Press. Reprinted by permission.

1. Family influences

Nuclear family: How responding to death? Describe in terms of relative degree of openness of response.

Very expressive _X_ Moderately expressive ____ Very guarded ____

To what extent is child included in family discussions/rituals related to the deceased?

Some ____ A great deal _X_ Not at all ____

Extended family: How responding to death? Describe, as above, in terms of relative degree of openness of response.

Very expressive _X (Mother's)_ Moderately expressive ____ Very guarded _X (Father's)_

To what extent do the views of the extended family differ or agree with those of the nuclear family with regard to the planning of rituals and inclusion of child?

Very different _Father's_ Very similar _Mother's_

If different, describe the nature of the disagreement _Father's family is Catholic; the service was conducted by a lay reader and held in a funeral home. Since John was not their biological grandchild, this did not prove to be a major issue._

2. School/peer influences

Child's grade in school _First_

Did any of the child's friends/peers attend the funeral/memorial services?

Yes ____ No _X_ (However, cousins her age were present)

Was teacher informed of death? Yes _X_ No ____

Did child receive condolence messages from friends/peers? Yes _X_ No ____

Does child know anyone his/her age who has been bereaved? Yes ____ No ____

Not sure _X_

If yes, has child spoken to this person since the death? Yes ____ No ____

Does child express feelings about wanting or not wanting peers/friends to know about the death? Yes ____ No ____ Not sure _X_

If yes, what has the child said? ________________

3. Religious/cultural influences

What is the child's religion? _Father has recently been taking her to Catholic church with his niece and nephew._

Has he/she been observant? Yes ____ No ____ Only recently

What are the beliefs of the child's religion regarding death? ________________

What about life after death? _The Catholic religion believes in life after death. Furthermore, the Eastern religious beliefs that are part of the parents' views consider death as a journey, and include the possibility of reincarnation. These latter views were expressed in John's funeral service._

Has child expressed any thoughts/feelings about this? _No_

FIGURE 12.8. Recording form for childhood grief reactions. *Note*. This form is an extension of "Death-Related Factors in Childhood Bereavement" (Figure 12.6), focusing specifically on the nature of the child's grief. The form itself (not the responses) is from Webb (2002a, p. 38). Copyright © 2002 The Guilford Press. Reprinted by permission.

Age of child 6 ____ years 6 ____ months   Date of birth ____________

Date of assessment ____________

See the form "Individual Factors in Childhood Bereavement" [Figure 12.5] for recording of personal history factors.

Date of death ____________________

Relationship to deceased Half brother

Favorite activities shared with deceased Playing with his cats

What the child will miss the most His jokes; his music

If the child could see the deceased again for 1 hour, what would he/she like to do or say?

"Why did you have to take that drug?"

Nature of grief reactions (describe) Cried when mother told her that John had died. Now every night when says her prayers, asks God to take good care of John. Mother listens to her prayers and tucks her in and they cry together.

Signs of the following feelings? Y = Yes; N = No

Sadness Y Anger N Confusion N Guilt N Relief N

Other N

Source of information on which this form has been based

X Parent X Observation ____ Other

ISSUES IN SIBLING DEATH

The death of *any* family member constitutes a crisis (Goldberg, 1973). However, when the death is untimely (Bank & Kahn, 1982; McGoldrick & Walsh, 1991) or the circumstances of the death (e.g., a death from suicide, AIDS, or a drug overdose) cannot be openly recognized or socially supported (Doka, 1989, 2002), the impact on the family can be devastating. McGoldrick and Walsh (1991) point out that an untimely death in young adulthood may generate in the surviving family members "a sense of cruel injustice in the ending of a life before its prime" (p. 33); it deprives the deceased of the opportunity to fulfill his or her life plans and causes the family members "pain and survivor guilt [that] may block [them] from continuing their own pursuits" (p. 33).

The responses of siblings to the death of a brother or a sister reflect not only their own unique reactions based on their personal relationship with the deceased sibling but also the responses of other nuclear and extended family members and of the community in which they live. A systems perspective views the reactions of individual family members as reflective of both those of the family and those of their surrounding social network. Therefore, a great outpouring of support from extended family and friends, expressed through attendance at the funeral and messages of condolence, can help reduce some of the feelings of loneliness that accompany mourning.

The professional literature on bereavement in childhood tends to focus on the impact of a death of a parent (Bowlby, 1969, 1979, 1980; Furman, 1974; Gardner, 1983; Grollman, 1967) or on helping a dying child. A volume titled *The Child and Death* (Schowalter et al., 1983) does not contain a single chapter (among 29) devoted to the topic of sibling bereavement. Exceptions to this unfortunate neglect can be found in the work of Bank and Kahn (1982), McGoldrick and Walsh (1991), Raphael (1983), Rosen (1986, 1991), Davies (1988, 1995, 1999), Kaplan and Joslin (1993), and Davies and Limbo (2010). Some of the main points emphasized by these writers include the following:

1. The death of a sibling creates a sense of vulnerability in the surviving siblings, who may begin to fear that they also may die (Rosen, 1991). However, the loss of a sibling does not present a child with the *intense* survival issues posed by the loss of a parent (Rosen, 1986).

2. Grieving parents have reduced energy and time to carry out their usual parental functions with respect to the surviving siblings. Therefore, a child in a bereaved family loses not only a brother or a sister but also parents who are emotionally available. "The fatality of the sibling casts a shadow across the parents' wounded forms, and thence upon the children" (Bank & Kahn, 1982, p. 273).

3. The child's reaction to the loss depends on how successfully the parents can continue to maintain their parental functions while they mourn (Rosen, 1991). It also may depend on the amount of shared "life space" between the child and the deceased sibling. The greater the shared activities and feelings, the greater the potential for intense stress and disruption during bereavement (Davies, 1988).

4. The child's developmental level has an important effect on his or her bereavement response. The existence of ambivalent and/or hostile feelings toward the deceased sibling may seriously compromise the mourning of survivors. A young, egocentric child may believe that some of his or her earlier hostile thoughts toward the sibling caused the death (Kaplan & Joslin, 1993).

5. The death of any family member requires role realignments and reorganization:

> After a loss, families must be restructured without the dead person, whose roles and functions must be taken over by others. The more important the

> deceased was to the ongoing emotional or practical functioning of the family, the more difficult it is for those remaining to adjust. When a child dies, family restructuring requires finding another focus for the love and care that previously went to that child. (McGoldrick & Walsh, 1991, p. 51)

In the case of the Rossi family, John's death had a different significance for Mr. and Mrs. Rossi and for Sabrina. As a mother, Lida experienced a very strong reaction of anger and terrible sadness; Mr. Rossi was also angry; and Sabrina was very sad. John's death must be understood in terms of the family history and John's role in this remarried family.

Lida and John had lived alone together for about 10 years before Dan entered their lives, and they had gone through some difficult times together. Soon after Lida and Dan married, John was preparing to move in with his own father; unfortunately, however, his father died before that happened. John never accepted Dan's role as stepfather, and their relationship was always stormy. More recently, with John old enough to be on his own, Lida shared Dan's hope that he would find a job or a field of study that interested him. However, this emancipation process did not proceed smoothly. John's involvement with peers who drank and engaged in antisocial behavior worried Lida, especially after the cocaine overdose, which precipitated a short hospitalization followed by months of daytime sleeping and nighttime alcohol use. Lida was concerned that John would become an alcoholic like his father, and she warned him repeatedly about the dangers of alcohol addiction. However, John continued on his own path; he responded with cursing and rude, self-deprecating remarks whenever either his mother or his stepfather tried to engage him in planning for his future.

In short, John had assumed the role of "black sheep" in this family, and Dan had given up on him. They would go for long periods without speaking to each other, and Lida would finally serve as intermediary. Dan kept telling Lida to "cut the cord," and in several counseling sessions I urged both parents to set age-appropriate, reasonable limits and follow through on them. I was also concerned about John's possible depression and urged Lida to speak with John's therapist about his father's history. She did so and informed me that John's therapist did not believe John was depressed.

Once John became employed, Lida gave him an ultimatum to move out by a certain date. John's therapist was supporting the plan, and an apartment was located and the deposit paid. Lida had hopes that "the therapy was working" and that John would finally achieve success in his life. Dan was planning to redecorate John's room for Sabrina, who up to this time had been sharing a bedroom with her parents.

John's death ended the universal dream and hope that Lida shared with all parents—the dream of seeing their children happy and successful. Lida had tried very hard to be a good mother, and now her only son's death of a heroin overdose seemed to point to her failure. Certainly, John's death represented the end of a very difficult chapter in her life, wiping away all traces of her unhappy first marriage. As Raphael (1983) states, "a child is many things: a part of the self, and of the loved partner; a representation of the generations past; the genes of the forebears; the hope of the future; a source of love, pleasure, even narcissistic delight; a tie or a burden; and sometimes a symbol of the worst parts of the self and others" (p. 229).

Lida's rage was widespread; it was directed most intensely toward John's friends, but it also encompassed Dan, John's therapist, her own therapist, and myself. Sabrina was spared, as evidenced in Lida's statement to me that the only people who *really* cared about John were herself and Sabrina. I understood and accepted Lida's anger as a necessary aspect of her bereavement, especially as related to her displaced rage because John had failed to validate all the years of their special relationship. In fact, the nature of his death shamed her and refuted her consistent belief and hope that he could succeed.

An adolescent like John struggles with issues of identity, sexuality, and separation, which can become very complicated in a remarried family: "To the question of 'Who am I?' is added, 'Who am I in this new family?' " (Rosenberg, 1988, p. 225). It seemed clear to me that John did not want to be in this family and that his life had taken a negative trajectory since the death of his father interrupted his own plans to remain with his father in the familiar neighborhood and school environment of his past. My view of John's situation was that his life had come to a standstill at that time and that the boy's incomplete mourning for his own father contributed to his inability to complete the tasks of adolescence without assuming a "negative identity" (Erikson, 1968). John always impressed me, in both his physical appearance and his manner, as a very *young adolescent.* I think he was "stuck" in the persona of a 14-year-old without a father and unwilling to bond to the stepfather who was willing and waiting to take on that role.

Mr. Rossi's reactions of anger over John's death were related to the youth's failure to take advantage of the numerous opportunities he had been given. In addition, Mr. Rossi partially identified with John, because he too had found it difficult to break away from his own family of origin. Undoubtedly these feelings contributed to Mr. Rossi's difficulties in being firmer with John.

Another aspect of Dan's anger was related to the impact of John's behavior on the family. For example, Dan was completely intolerant of John's habit of returning home in the middle of the night and proceeding to cook hamburgers and other food, when the accompanying odors and noise woke other family members in their small apartment. This behavior continued even during Lida's postoperative period and became the "straw that broke the camel's back," totally alienating Mr. Rossi from his stepson. Nonetheless, Dan felt some affection and admiration for the young man, as expressed in his spontaneous funeral tribute that focused on John's charm and potential, together with his unpredictability and self-centeredness.

For Sabrina, her brother's death converted her into the only child in the family. She told her mother that she was jealous of her cousin Katie, who had a brother. However, because of the big age difference between Sabrina and John, their lives had never overlapped very much. Even on the weekends, when both were home, John usually slept until 2 or 3 in the afternoon, when Sabrina typically would be out of the house playing with friends or engaged in other activities. John rarely ate dinner or other meals with the family, so Sabrina's contacts with her brother were few and possibly weighed toward overhearing arguments between him and her parents. Their shared life space was quite limited.

Raphael (1983) comments that "in losing a sibling the child loses a playmate, a companion, someone who is a buffer against the parents, someone who may love and comfort him, someone with whom he identifies and who he admires. In short, he loses someone dearly loved as well as perhaps envied and rivalrously hated" (p. 114). This may not be true in Sabrina's situation, however, because of the great age and gender difference between her and John. It is probable that this sibling bond was not especially strong and that because Sabrina had strong bonds with other family members, she might be able to tolerate this loss without undue developmental interference (Rosen, 1986). This actually proved true in Sabrina's case, as is discussed later.

SELECTED HELPING INTERVENTIONS FOR BEREAVED CHILDREN

The goal in helping bereaved children and their families is to facilitate the mourning process and to assist when needed with the necessary realignment of roles. Because the process of children's grief is different from that of adults (Rando, 1991; Webb, 2002a, 2010; Wolfenstein, 1966), the worker may need to help family members understand these differences, so that they do not misinterpret a child's interest in playing and participating in fun activities in the middle of the mourning period. Actually, it is *helpful* for the child to return to his or her routine as soon as possible, as children have a "short sadness span" (Wolfenstein, 1966) and cannot tolerate the pain of grief for sustained periods of time. Kliman (1989, p. 61) comments that "during latency, mourning is apt to be particularly silent and slow." This may be related to the fact that latency-age children consider crying to be babyish (Furman, 1974), so they try to act "grown up," which for them means being in control of their feelings.

Play Approaches

The rationale for employing play therapy with a young bereaved child relates to children's reluctance to talk about their feelings, possibly because of the fear of being overwhelmed and then breaking down in tears. Through directed play with a worker/counselor, however, the child can express feelings in a displaced way, using dolls, drawing, games, and other techniques. The method of directed or structured play allows the worker/counselor to deliberately select and offer play materials that will encourage the child to project his or her worries onto the materials and thus to experience cathartic relief, clarification of misunderstandings, and a corrective emotional experience (Enzer, 1988).

Play Materials

Many of the same play materials that should be available in any office in which children are seen for counseling can be employed in work with bereaved children. I have found that plain white and colored paper, markers, clay, family dolls, and some card and board games are very effective in helping children express their concerns in a displaced manner. Clay is particularly useful in encouraging the release of pent-up feelings of tension and anger; in addition, it permits the child the mastery experience of creating something and then obliterating it (possibly reflecting the child's feelings about having a loved person "disappear" through death).

Depending on the age of the child and the specific circumstances of the death, it may be useful to offer toys that will encourage reenactment of the circumstances of the illness and death. Toys in this category include toy ambulances, a doctor kit, and the board game Operation (available from Milton Bradley, Springfield, Massachusetts). A therapeutic board game, Gardner's Storytelling Card Game (available from Creative Therapeutics, Cresskill, New Jersey), contains a cemetery picture that requires the player to make up a story about that background scene. In a previous publication (Webb, 2002a), I discussed the productive use of this game with a 9-year-old boy whose grandmother had died.

In recent years, several workbooks have been published that are designed to help children draw pictures and fill in their thoughts and feelings associated with death. These workbooks can guide counselors who lack experience in and confidence about using drawing and play methods with bereaved children, but they should be used *at a very slow pace* that permits a child to reveal and cope with the feelings that will be generated. My advice to students and the workers I supervise is that "less is more," especially when working with the bereaved. Under *no* circumstances should the workbooks be used by the lay public or given to children to fill in without supervision, as the content might overwhelm young children.

Two excellent exercises from the workbook *When Something Terrible Happens: Children Can Learn to Cope with Grief* (Heegaard, 1991) are (1) Feelings Faces and (2) the Body Map of Feelings. In the Feelings Faces exercise, the child is asked to draw faces showing different expressions on five circles, with a different emotion named under each circle: "angry," "sad," "afraid," "worried," and "happy." When I use this exercise, I reduce the number of emotions to three at most; often I ask a child to draw only the primary emotion that matches his or her feelings when he or she thinks about the person who died. I believe that it is counterproductive to expect a bereaved child to draw five different emotions at one time.

The Body Map of Feelings exercise also can be adapted to conform to a child's developmental and emotional capacity. The body map is an outline of a body, on which the child is asked to use seven different colors to indicate the places where seven different emotions are felt: "sad," "afraid," "guilty," "angry," "jealous," "nervous," and "happy." When I use this, I ask the child to choose which of three feelings he or she would like to draw, and generally this task proves to be sufficient for one time. It is also possible to go very slowly and request only one emotion each session. Because the practitioner and the child use the drawing as an opportunity to talk about a time when the child felt this emotion, it is not desirable to rush the experience. In fact, it may be more helpful to expand on the child's recollection by inviting him or her to draw a picture of that experience.

Individual, Family, and Group Approaches

Grief is a family experience, and the helping person must attend to the needs of the family unit, as well as those of the individual members. In Chapter 6 I recommended an integrated child and family model, which is very appropriate for a bereaved family. Typically, I offer to make a home visit when I learn about a death that pertains to a child client. Depending on the circumstances, I may attend the funeral. It is *always* relevant to see the entire family together soon after the death, to offer condolences and to assess the group and individual needs. Following the death of a child, the parents may benefit from some marital counseling, and it also may be useful to see individual family members alone (when this is practical). This latter approach permits the expression of frustration or anger toward other family members without exposing the targets of these strong feelings to the added stress of being blamed when they are already in the throes of grieving. Often it is helpful to see the child with each parent to observe differences in the child's reactions with different parents and to determine each parent's ability to comfort and support the grieving child.

Whenever I see a parent with a child or the family as a unit, I always invite the parent to participate in whatever play activity I make available to the child. Most parents comprehend that their children are communicating symbolically through play, even though they may have difficulty in knowing how to respond. There are examples of parent–child play in the discussion about Sabrina's family that follows.

Referrals to grief support groups should always be considered, depending on the willingness of the family members to involve themselves in this type of counseling. Many schools offer bereavement groups for children, which can help a child realize that he or she is not the only one who has suffered a loss. This type of intervention is especially appropriate following a teacher's death (Doster & McElroy, 1993). Hospice offers ongoing groups for children of different ages. Examples of bereavement groups for children, with detailed process notes illustrating specific interventions and the children's responses, are described in Tait and Depta (1993), Hickey (1993), Dane (2002), Schuurman (2008), and Ruffin and Zimmerman (2010). Chapter 8 deals with some general considerations in setting up and conducting groups for children.

Interventions with Sabrina and Her Parents after John's Death

Initial Interventions

In the month after John's death, I met with Mr. and Mrs. Rossi once, and Mrs. Rossi brought Sabrina for a conjoint session. The meeting with Mr. and Mrs. Rossi was very intense, because Mrs. Rossi was in the throes of grieving and needed to express her anger about John's death. She stated that she did not wish to involve herself with marital counseling because she planned to continue in individual therapy and had also joined a bereavement group. Although I knew that she was angry with me because I had been unable to mend the relationship between John and Dan, Lida did want me to continue to see Sabrina and agreed to bring her alternately with Mr. Rossi.

Dan was very concerned about his wife's pain over John's death. However, he did not feel the same need as his wife did to process the events surrounding the death or to examine how it personally affected him. He declined my offer to meet with him individually, stating that he "might look for a men's group." Perhaps taking his cues from Lida, Mr. Rossi agreed to bring Sabrina for individual play sessions, according to my recommendations.

In the first session with Sabrina after her brother's death, I asked her to draw a picture of John. Sabrina drew a colorful figure, appearing to float in air, with arms outstretched (see Figure 12.9). She declined my invitation to tell me about the drawing, but she did agree to think about some happy memories of John, mentioning sitting on a wall in a favorite park with John and some of his friends.

Individual Session with Sabrina

In a session a month later, Sabrina told me directly that she didn't want to talk about John or "anything else." I then produced a "new" game, Operation; this totally captured Sabrina's interest, insofar as it permitted her to assume a controlling role in "operating" on a helpless patient. The game also permitted me to make connections to her mother's operation. For example, at one point during the play I asked Sabrina whether any of these operations were like those her mother had. Sabrina said, "No, that was *very* different!" I indicated that I knew about the operation and asked Sabrina whether she was worried about her mother now. She said, "Sometimes," but she could not tell me more.

FIGURE 12.9. Sabrina's drawing of John.

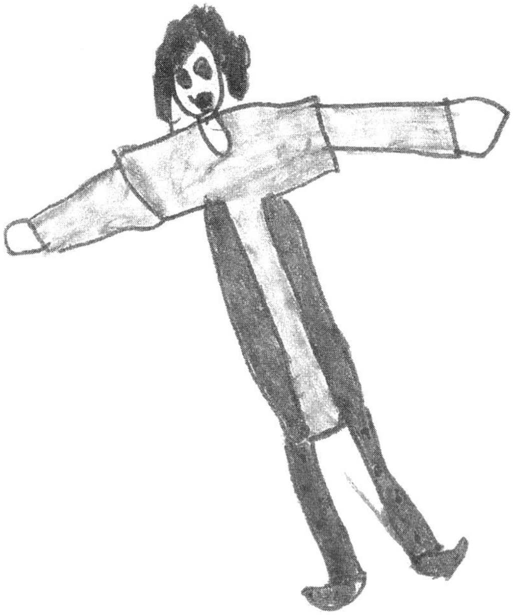

Several times during the play, Sabrina went into the waiting room to say something to her mother. At the end of the session, Sabrina wanted to show her mother the game; she also gave her reward for winning (a wildlife sticker) to her mother.

Session with Sabrina and Her Father

During the first session with Sabrina and her father following the death, I asked how it seemed in the house without John. Sabrina said that she couldn't say, so I suggested that she draw a picture of a face (showing her the Feelings Faces exercise). Sabrina said it was sad and drew a very sad face (see Figure 12.10). The original drawing had one line to denote the mouth, which appeared to convey distress. I responded, "What do we need to help that sad face feel better?" (expecting to lead into a verbal discussion). Sabrina took the marker and drew a full mouth around the straight line she had previously created. I said, "Sometimes we put on a smile when we feel sad inside." Sabrina nodded and then looked toward the doll family and doll furniture she had played with previously. She then proceeded to reenact a scene with the mother doll in the hospital, because "she had to have an operation." The family, around the breakfast table, read the newspaper, and Sabrina announced, "They wrote about Mom in the newspaper." She turned to me (in play) and asked, "What does it say?" I responded, "Mrs. Jones is in the hospital," and

FIGURE 12.10. Sabrina's drawing of a sad face.

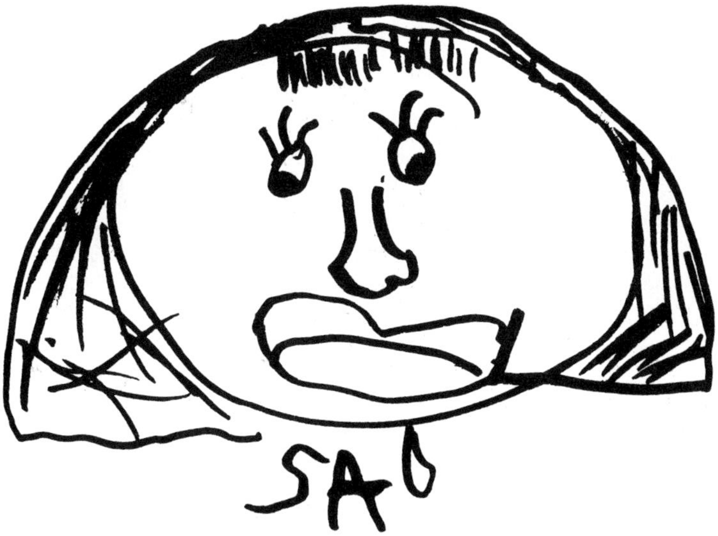

Sabrina interjected, "for a very serious operation." I continued, "She has a very good doctor, and we expect her to recover."

Sabrina then asked to go to the bathroom. During this interval, Mr. Rossi, who was in the room observing this play interaction, stated: "I don't know why she does this; she must associate coming here with Lida's operation." When Sabrina returned, she asked to play Operation.

Session with Sabrina and Her Mother 4 Months after John's Death

Prior to the next session with Sabrina and her mother, I had received a telephone message from Lida stating that one of John's two cats had died.

At the beginning of the session, I noticed how attractive both Lida and Sabrina looked. Lida had lipstick on (for the first time in months), and Sabrina was specially dressed for a birthday party immediately after this session.

Sabrina began by telling me that she forgot to bring the picture she had drawn for me last night in bed. I asked her to describe it, and she said it had "a sun, a house, and grass." She then said, handing me two quarters, that she wanted to give me some money "because you invite me to come here." I was very touched and impressed by the apparent meaning of the sessions to Sabrina. I told her that her father already paid me (through insurance), but she insisted, saying, "I *want* to give it to you!" I thanked her very much, continuing to puzzle about the meaning of this behavior.

Telling Sabrina that I knew about the cat's death and that I was sorry, I asked her whether she was surprised that he died. Sabrina said that she was not sure why he died, and Lida reminded Sabrina that the cat's X-rays had shown an enlarged heart. At this point, Sabrina could not tolerate any more words, and she began crawling around the floor acting out how the cat had wanted to sleep and stay by himself. I asked about how the other cat was responding since the death of her friend, and Sabrina again acted this out by crawling on the floor and making cat sounds.

I introduced the Body Map of Feelings (Heegaard, 1991) and suggested that Sabrina draw on the body in blue where she felt sad. First, she thought this would be in her eyes, but then she said it was in her stomach. She drew a very large blue circle in the center of the body (see Figure 12.11). When I asked Sabrina if she could indicate where in the body she felt afraid, she put a black circle within the blue nucleus of the stomach. She drew orange (nervous) in the neck, and green (jealous) in the head. She said that she couldn't do angry and that happy would be on the face, but she didn't want to mix it with the green color already there.

When we later played Gardner's Storytelling Card Game, one of Sabrina's stories had the theme of feeding a dog, then later calling the dog and he wasn't there.

FIGURE 12.11. Sabrina's Body Map of Feelings. The form is adapted from Heegaard (1991, p. 13). Copyright © 1991 Woodland Press. Adapted by permission.

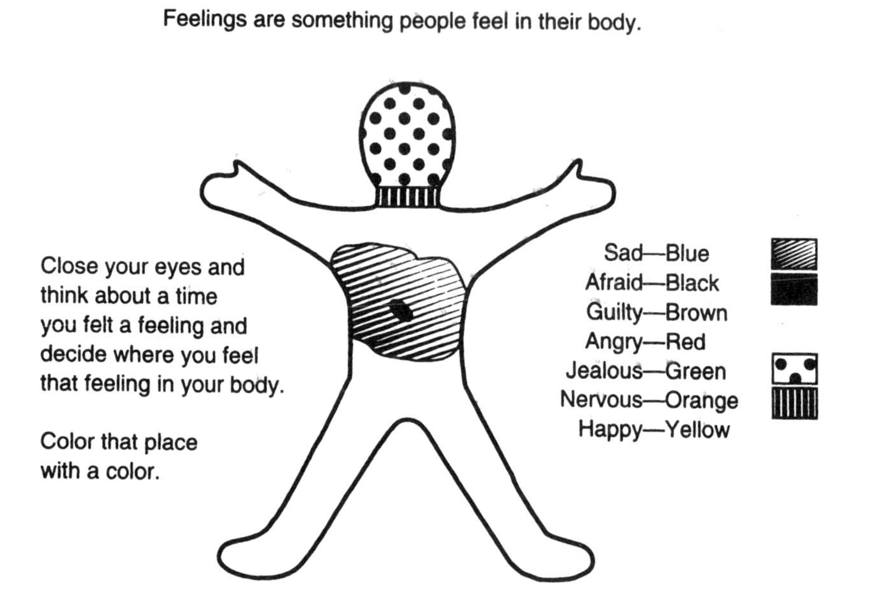

Comment

The accounts of these sessions graphically depict how this latency-age child used a variety of play materials to project her feelings of bereavement and confusion about the two major crises in her life that occurred within an 8-month span, namely, her mother's serious operation and her half-brother's sudden death. Play, in the context of a therapeutic relationship, truly served as an outlet for this child to express her worries about her mother and her sadness about the loss of her brother.

It seems clear from these descriptions that Sabrina continued to be very concerned and protective toward her mother. For example, she presented her mother with her "reward" sticker at the end of a session. In fact, the death of her brother may have assumed major significance to her because it made her mother so very sad. Sabrina continued to be very concerned about her mother's health, which made Mrs. Rossi's prognosis very significant to this child.

Addendum

Approximately a year after John's death, Sabrina's mother died. Gradually, over a 4-month period, Lida's ability to walk and carry on her usual activities had deteriorated. The local hospice provided the necessary nursing and home health care services, and I was seeing Sabrina weekly, sometimes in my office and sometimes at their home.

Even after she was bedridden, Lida could not accept the reality of her impending death. Because I was concerned about preparing Sabrina, I told Lida that it was essential to tell Sabrina about the fact that she (Lida) was not getting better, despite all her medicines and the best efforts of the doctors. Three days after hearing this from me, Sabrina's mother told her, "God wants me and God may be taking me soon." Lida also told Sabrina, "God will take care of you and Daddy, and I'll be watching over both of you." Eight days later, on her own 47th birthday, Lida died.

Update: 8 Years Later

I continued to see Sabrina weekly, sometimes separately and often with her father, over the course of the school year following her mother's death. Typically, she wanted to play Operation, and I used the game to repeat over and over how hard the doctors try, and yet, despite all the operations, the "patient" may die. Sabrina would name the figure in the game, and I would say comforting and soothing things to him. Mr. Rossi did not really understand the importance of this game to Sabrina, and he would try to use the session to talk about how they were managing and about their plans to move to a house adjacent to his parents. After the first anniversary of Lida's death, Sabrina began to want to play other games. I felt that she had moved beyond her need to play and replay the medical situation. She was doing well in school, had friends, and participated in several after-school activities.

During her second-grade year we began to taper off the sessions—initially to biweekly, and then to monthly. In the ensuing years, I have seen Sabrina and her father at least once a year, when I call to invite them to come in together. I usually plan this meeting either around Mother's Day or around the time of John and Lida's deaths. A repeated issue that came up over the years involved their mutual concern about each other's whereabouts. They each became extremely concerned if the other came home late, for example. I addressed this in the context of being "supersensitive" about the possibility of losing each other, as they had experienced two deaths so close together in time. Stahlman (1996) refers to the "overprotectiveness of surviving siblings toward one another following a death," and I believe that this dynamic was operating in this father–daughter relationship as well. A few years after Lida's death, Dan began dating the divorced mother of Sabrina's best friend. When I asked Sabrina (then age 13 and in eighth grade) how she felt about having her father date, she responded, "It's OK but I want to know where he is, and I stay up until he gets home."

Sabrina has maintained contact with her mother's mother and sister on the West Coast, usually going to visit over the summer vacation. When she was 12, she and her father went to a special mountain location there, where they scattered Lida's ashes. In a follow-up session, in preparation for the update in the second edition of this book, Sabrina denied that she thought it was difficult to have two family members die in 1 year. Perhaps trying to present as a "cool" adolescent, Sabrina was not particularly open or responsive to my questions, although she signed the release form without hesitation. Her father told me that he painted her bedroom for her 13th birthday and that she asked him to hang a picture of her (then a 2-year-old toddler) and her mother walking over stones on a beach, with Lida pointing the way for Sabrina to walk. I thought that this seemed a lovely and symbolic way of documenting the "continuing bonds" and the ongoing influence of her mother on this adolescent girl.

CONCLUDING COMMENTS

Children need the stability and security of knowing that the people who love them will remain constant in their lives. When illness and death take precedence over a child's needs, the child may feel abandoned. Children, in fact, do *need* their parents in order to complete certain developmental tasks, such as integrating a firm sense of identity.

It is possible to help children and parents with "the work of mourning" after the death of a family member. These helping methods should be adapted to the age of the individual and to his or her ability to comprehend the reality of what has happened. When a young child is faced with the death of a sibling or the recurring illness of a parent, play techniques can provide the mechanism through which the child can express, in a displaced manner, the conflicts and anxiety he or she is experiencing internally but trying to suppress. The use of directed or structured play therapy can provide such children with relief and the reassurance that an adult comprehends their confused internal state.

DISCUSSION QUESTIONS AND ROLE-PLAY EXERCISES

1. Discuss the implications of young children's magical thinking and egocentricity on their ability to understand death. How can a worker assist a parent in helping a bereaved child who is under 7 years of age? Count off by 3's, with one person taking the role of the worker, another that of a parent of a child under age 7 whose older brother died of a drug overdose, and the third person an observer. After the role play, the observer should comment on helpful responses and suggest other possible ways to communicate effectively with the parent.
2. What issues in a remarried family are illustrated in the Rossi case? If you had been the worker, how would you have dealt with the long-standing conflict between Mr. Rossi and John? Role-play a session in which you address and attempt to modify their hostility toward each other.
3. Consider the pros and cons of having multiple workers/therapists involved in helping a family such as the Rossis. What recommendations would you make to avoid mixed messages and differing goals among the various counselors?
4. How can the worker effectively assist latency-age children who do not wish to talk about their feelings after a death? What play materials might be useful?
5. Compare and contrast the use of individual, family, and group approaches in situations of bereavement.

CHAPTER 13

Children in Substance-Using Families

Many children growing up at the beginning of the 21st century have been exposed repeatedly to the effects of substance use or addiction in their own families, in their schools, and in their communities. Television commercials and programs routinely portray scenes of a father drinking beer as he watches a football game, and news reports often feature drive-by shootings and other crimes committed by drug addicts and dealers. In some families, children receive their first sip of beer or wine from a parent, and even children whose parents are not substance users know that many teenagers and college students brag about "getting loaded" on weekends and that some get into trouble when they are drunk or "high." In urban settings, children may watch addicts buying drugs or "shooting up" in empty lots or the stairways of their own apartment buildings. Older siblings or neighbors may introduce 9- or 10-year-olds into the drug trade by making them "runners," thereby insinuating them into an antisocial adult world that welcomes them primarily because of their immunity from prosecution.

What is the impact of growing up surrounded by older people who regulate their moods through use of chemicals and whose lives seem totally dominated by this experience? And what are the effects on a child when one or both parents are using or addicted to drugs or alcohol?

CLARIFICATION OF TERMINOLOGY

This section begins with a discussion of the terminology related to the use of drugs and alcohol, according to the latest edition of the *Diagnostic and Statistical Manual of Mental Disorders* (American Psychiatric Association, 2013). DSM-5 specifies the categories of substance use and addictive disorders based on the substance that causes a disorder, which may be either alcohol or one of 9 others listed in the diagnostic manual.

DSM-5 no longer uses the terms "substance dependence" or "substance abuse," but instead now uses a single combined category, "substance-related and addictive disorders," which encompasses the use of 10 separate classes of drugs, among these caffeine and tobacco. The addictions are divided into "substance *use* disorders" and "substance-*induced* disorders," and the diagnosis includes an indication of *mild, moderate,* or *severe,* based the presence of 11 different behaviors/activities in an individual over a 12-month period (see American Psychiatric Association, 2013, for specific criteria).

This chapter refers to "substance-using parents" in recognition that even in its early phases this disorder can present problems for the entire family. According to the National Association for Children of Alcoholics (NACoA, n.d.) one in four children under the age of 18 is affected by parental alcohol and/or drug use (Straussner & Donath, 2015). Straussner (1989, 2004, 2014) and Lowinson, Ruiz, Millman, and Langrod (1997) classify different psychoactive drugs in terms of their distinctive effects on the central nervous system and thus on a person's thinking and behavior. Table 13.1 presents an adaptation of these categorizations.

THE IMPACT OF GROWING UP IN A SUBSTANCE-USING FAMILY/ENVIRONMENT

Multiple Stressors

When parents abuse or depend on depressants, stimulants, narcotics/opiates, or psychedelics/hallucinogens, their ability to focus on and respond to their children is significantly impaired. Straussner (1989, p. 149) states that "clinicians and researchers have only recently recognized that growing up with a drug- or alcohol-using parent is frequently a highly traumatizing experience with long-lasting effects." Parental substance use is one of the main reasons why children enter the child welfare system (Barnard & McKeganey, 2004). Furthermore, the traumas and violence they may have personally suffered and/or witnessed during their early development related to the substance use can result in permanent neurological damage for the children (D'Andrea, Ford, Stolbach, Spinazzola, & van der Kolk, 2012). Researchers point out that children in alcoholic families are four to six times as likely to develop alcohol problems themselves (Russell, 1990), and they are at increased risk for anxiety, depression, and externalizing behavior problems (Ellis, Zucker, & Fitzgerald, 1997; Eiden, Edwards, & Leonard, 2007).

Regardless of the eventual outcome of this experience, children growing up in families affected by substance use disorders face multiple stressors, especially the sad reality that a parent's disorder "is likely to take precedence over their own [a child's] basic needs" (Tracy, 1994, p. 535). Other stressors

TABLE 13.1. Effects of Different Categories of Substances on Individuals

Depressants	
Effects on brain:	Slow down, sedate brain tissues; alter judgment and behavior; cause agitation (hangover) in coming off.
Names of substances:	Alcoholic beverages; barbiturates and sedatives/hypnotics; minor tranquilizers (Librium, Valium); low doses of cannabinoids (marijuana and hashish).
Stimulants	
Effects on brain:	Increase or speed up function of brain; can produce acute delirium and psychosis (symptoms may include hallucinations, paranoia, and hypersexuality); violent behavior may occur with use of potent forms of cocaine ("freebase" or "crack").
Names of substances:	Amphetamines; cocaine; caffeine; nicotine.
Narcotics or opiates	
Effects on brain:	Decrease pain; create a sedative and tranquilizing effect; may cause stuporous inactivity (daydreaming/fantasies); may cause physical agitation upon withdrawal (panic and violent behavior may occur at this time).
Names of substances:	Opium, morphine, heroin, codeine, paregoric, methadone; Demerol, Darvon, Prinadol.
Psychedelics/hallucinogens	
Effects on brain:	Produce gross distortions of thoughts and sensory processes (e.g., visual hallucinations, distorted body image); may produce depersonalization, depression, hostility; may lead to violence because of anxiety and misperceptions of reality.
Names of substances:	LSD; PCP ("angel dust"); DOM; STP; mescaline; psilocybin.

Note. Adapted from Straussner (1989, pp. 151–152). Copyright © 1989 New York University Press. Adapted by permission.

on these children, according to Tracy (1994, citing Feig, 1990, and Gittler & McPherson, 1990), include the following:

- Chaotic and often dangerous neighborhoods.
- Poverty and homelessness or unstable housing.
- Parents who lack an extended family and community support system.
- Parents who may have been victimized themselves as children or adults.
- Parents with poor parenting skills and few or no role models for effective coping.

Because the parents' addiction may cause them to value their drugs more than their children and because the parent's behavior and treatment of the child varies when he or she is "under the influence," children of substance-using parents often are treated inconsistently and given confusing and mixed messages (Markowitz, 2014). Understandably, research has shown that children of alcoholics have a higher rate of various forms of insecure attachment than children from nonalcoholic families (Jaeger, Hahn, & Weinraub, 2000). Consider the behavior and responsibilities of Barbie (Chapters 3–5, this volume) with respect to the following quote: "It is not uncommon to see young children taking care of their substance-using parents, cooking meals, and calling the police when their parents get involved in violent fights. They often resist and resent initial attempts to dislodge them from these parental roles" (Copans, 2006, p. 298). The term "parentified child" (Fitzgerald et al., 2008) refers to a child who functions as a caregiver for parents.

Various forms of child maltreatment often occur in families with substance-using parents. These may include neglect, physical abuse, and/or sexual abuse. The concept of "maltreatment" (according to Gonzales-Ramos & Goldstein, 1989, p. 5) refers to *all* physical abuse or marked neglect of children. Specifically, an abused child has parents or caretakers who inflict or permit injury or protracted impairment of physical or emotional health or, due to neglect, allow the risk of such injury. A neglected child has parents or caretakers who fail to supply basic care, supervision, or guardianship or who abandon him or her.

Numerous studies have found a correlation between child maltreatment and substance use disorders, ranging from 40% nationwide (Daro & McCurdy, 1991) to 80–90% in certain localities (Feig, 1990). The National Center on Addiction and Substance Abuse at Columbia University (now called the Center on Addiction) estimated in a 2005 report that substance abuse was a factor in at least 70% of all reported cases of child maltreatment. In 2016 the Administration for Children and Families found an increase of 3% in child maltreatment over the previous 5 years; 18.2% of victims were physically abused, and 8.5% were sexually abused. Maltreated children of substance-using parents are more likely to have poorer physical, intellectual, social, and emotional outcomes and are at greater risk of developing substance use problems themselves (U.S. Department of Health and Human Services, 2003).

The most common form of child maltreatment by parents with substance use disorders is child neglect, according to Black and Mayer (1980). The nature of this neglect may range from a general lack of supervision to "total inattention to such basic needs of children as food and clothing" (U.S. Department of Health and Human Services, 1978, p. 59). Children of substance-using parents are more likely to experience abuse—physical, sexual, or emotional—than children in nonusing households (Lander, Howsare, & Byrne, 2013). Tracy (1994) cites Besharov (1989) as reporting that in New York State over 73% of neglect-related child fatalities are attributed to parental alcohol and drug abuse. Often parents may leave children alone and unsupervised while they go away to procure drugs (Davies, 2011).

Sexual abuse and incest are also common in families that abuse substances (Copans, 1989; Johnson, 1991; Davies, 2011), possibly because of the diffuse parent–child boundaries in such families, which are characterized by role reversals and inappropriate parental role maintenance. Wertz (1986), reported in Copans (2006), suggests that over 50% of physically and sexually abused children come from substance-disordered families. Straussner (1989, p. 151) points out that "any psychoactive substance that produces a state of intoxication . . . can affect parenting because of alterations in the individual's judgment and behavior." Indeed, parents with substance use disorders are often unable to care for *themselves* adequately; thus it is not surprising that they cannot meet the needs of young children, or, in some cases, that they use the children to fulfill their own needs.

However, despite this disturbing picture, we must emphasize that the relationship between child maltreatment and substance use disorders is considered *correlational,* not causal. Moreover, the incidence of maltreatment varies according to type of substance used and other factors. Child abuse has been found most frequently in families in which there is an alcohol- or opiate-addicted mother; in families in which parental violence is common; and in families with low financial status and poor living conditions (Black & Mayer, 1980). Clearly, many elements in addition to substance use contribute to the constellation of family stress in which a young child becomes victimized (Belsky, 1993). Chapter 14 deals with the crisis of family and community violence, situations in which substance use often plays an important role.

The child born into a family affected by a substance use disorder is at risk for a range of problems in addition to maltreatment. Beginning *in utero,* for example, infants of cocaine-using mothers suffer a decreased growth rate, and their behavior as toddlers tends to be hyperexcitable, fussy, and impulsive (Petitti & Coleman, 1990, as reported in Feinberg, 1995; Copans, 2006). Even more startling than this information is the finding that "children who were exposed to cocaine use in the *home* had more serious behavior problems than those exposed in the womb" (Youngstrom, 1991, as reported in Feinberg, 1995, p. 241; emphasis added). In addition to behavior problems, lower intellectual and educational functioning has been found in children whose mothers use drugs of all types (Feinberg, 1995).

According to the Robert Wood Johnson Foundation (2010), more than 40,000 infants are born every year in the United States with fetal alcohol spectrum disorder, a leading preventable cause of birth defects and developmental disabilities. These effects can include physical, mental, behavioral, and/or learning disabilities with possible lifelong implications. Fetal alcohol syndrome is reported to affect approximately 2–5% of school-age children in the United States (May et al., 2009; Smith, 2011). The numerous publications of this foundation emphasize that alcohol is the number one drug of choice among both adolescents and adults and that, furthermore, it is the most widely available drug. Although there has been some decline in alcohol consumption over the past 20 years, it remains the most commonly used drug among young people, who may engage in periodic binge drinking that, in time, may result in alcohol dependence for many individuals (National Organization on Fetal Alcohol Syndrome, 2010).

Multiple Losses

The numerous problems in substance-disordered families make loss an ever-present reality that threatens children's sense of security and safety. On the most basic level, these children are deprived of a structured, predictable routine because of their parents' inconsistent moods and behavior. The children never know when they may have to take complete care of themselves, in addition to their parents. This uncertainty seriously interferes with the children's ability to become involved with peer activities, as the parents' need may take precedence over the children's wishes for more age-appropriate involvement. Often such a child feels embarrassed, "different," and even ashamed of his or her family circumstances. These feelings can lead to social isolation, loneliness, resentment, and depression. The child's very childhood has been lost.

If a child is maltreated and comes to the attention of CPS, separation of the child and parent may be mandated to protect the child from additional harm. This separation, unfortunately, constitutes an even more wrenching loss for the child, if he or she is placed with a foster family of strangers. In an earlier publication (Webb, 2006b) I listed the necessary adjustments a child must make when placed in a foster home as including new people, new food, and different beds, in addition to different expectations about adult rules for appropriate behavior. Older children, who may be aware that their families have been deficient or even destructive compared with those of other children, may develop a sense of shame and loss of self-esteem. These feelings can qualify as a form of "disenfranchised grief" (Doka, 2002) because the stigma of the placement cannot be openly discussed or mourned. The parent, in turn, may feel that the removal of the child is a punitive response to the addiction rather than a remedial effort to help. Certainly, this major loss to the family is one that may be very difficult to reverse in the future, as children from substance-disordered families have low rates of reunification with their biological parents once they enter placement, despite all efforts toward permanency planning (Tracy, 1994, 1999). Often, relatives who disapprove of the parents' substance use have distanced themselves from the family, so they may not be available or willing to take on caregiving roles of the children.

ETHICAL DILEMMAS AND PRESSURES ON PRACTITIONERS

Numerous ethical dilemmas and pressures confront practitioners who work with substance-disordered families. Because the use of many substances is illegal, and because many people consider drug or even alcohol use or dependence a psychological "weakness" rather than a disease, addicted individuals with substance use disorders tend to deny and hide their problems. In addition, denial is an unconscious defense that permits the individuals to continue their substance use. It is understandable that these persons respond with suspicion and rejection to well-meaning helping efforts, in view of society's tendency to denigrate and stigmatize them. Parents with substance use disorders may be oblivious to the havoc of their lives. However, when their behavior puts their young children at risk, then society flexes the muscles of the legal system, challenges these parents' behavior, and insists on detoxification and change as conditional for their retaining custody of their children. The right to self-determination no longer applies to a parent whose disorder interferes with effective parenting and therefore impinges on his or her children's rights.

In circumstances such as this, many ethical dilemmas arise for social workers, who want to advocate for dependent children, yet do not wish to alienate the children's parents or to rupture, through mandatory placement, the bond between children and parents. Sometimes workers agree with society's negative feelings about a mother who neglects her children, not fully understanding that a substance use disorder can seriously compromise an individual's judgment and behavior. Of course, the absent or neglectful father also shares responsibility for his children, but the gender biases of our society exact a higher standard for women; as a result, mothers are often penalized for neglect, whereas similar behavior in men is ignored (Feinberg, 1995; Goldberg, 1995). In many single-parent families headed by women, the fathers are unknown, leaving the job of parenting entirely up to the mothers.

The "Rescue Fantasy"

In teaching, I have found that master's-level social work students working with substance-disordered families often progress from an initial strong stance of wanting to protect ("rescue") dependent children by filing complaints about neglect or abuse to subsequent observation that the children's situations do not improve appreciably in cases in which placement occurs. Furthermore, the students witness much bitterness and unhappiness connected with these placements. Seasoned workers learn through experience that the concept of "the best interests of the child" must be weighed against that of "the least detrimental alternative"; this requires "a realistic appraisal of existing resources" (Kamen & Gewirtz, 1989, p. 180) as a basis for determining the choice of child care in a specific situation. Sometimes *no* good alternative is available, and a concerted effort to help the family members remain together offers the best prospect for "rescuing" a child.

Weighing Differing Needs of Children and Parents

It may be very stressful for a worker to have to determine the degree of risk to a child in two alternative situations, neither of which appears desirable. As Tracy (1994) states, "although the emotional limbo of being in foster care carries its own set of risks, remaining in a substance-abusing home also carries risks" (p. 535).

The separation of a child from his or her family generates intense feelings for *all* parties involved. This serious move, which is intended to protect the child, allows the laws of the state to intervene in family life and to supersede the rights and authority of parents in situations of suspected child maltreatment. However, the goal of permanency planning, as reflected in the Adoption Assistance and Child Welfare Reform Act (Public Law 96-272, 1980), is to provide intensive preventive services for families at risk to reduce the need for placement and to reunify families in a timely manner when placement has occurred. Thus the role of the social worker frequently consists of offering services to parents with substance use disorders (even when they do not want this help) to prevent the out-of-home placement of their children. Tracy (1994) points to the need for demonstrating "reasonable effort" to provide services that address the family circumstances (such as parental substance use disorders) that put the child at risk of placement. Clearly, the primary effort in these cases is to get parents into treatment. This is demonstrated in the case of Vanessa and Vernon later in the chapter.

The federal policy reflected in the Adoption and Safe Families Act of 1997 (ASFA) aims to limit the time a child can be in placement to 15 months to reinforce the need for children to experience consistent caring parenting. Anderson and Seita (2006) discuss the implications of this legislation for substance-using parents who may not be able to complete a successful course of drug or alcohol treatment within this time frame.

In an ideal world, the removal of children from their parents would never be necessary. If parents were negligent or unable to carry out their child care responsibilities, some form of assistance would be offered to families on a temporary basis to provide respite and ensure the well-being of the children. In essence, this is the purpose of foster care: "not to rescue the child, but to offer respite for the family until life becomes manageable" (Minuchin, 1995, p. 253). However, there is a broad gap between the ideal and the real. Effective treatment for substance use disorders takes time, is costly, and is often characterized by recurrence of the addictive behavior. Social workers and others may doubt parents' ability to complete a detoxification and treatment program and/or to sustain their sobriety after discharge. In truth, although treatment is initially costly, it is highly cost-effective *in the long run*.

Knowledge that a substance use disorder is a "family (i.e., intergenerational) disease" (Straussner, 1989) may perpetuate attitudes of determinism and powerlessness among workers who genuinely want to rescue children and who view removal of the children from their "diseased" families as the preferred method of helping. Of course, a child should be removed only if a parent refuses treatment and if neglect or abuse continues.

The Impact of Mandatory Reporting

Although only about 20% of all reported cases of child maltreatment result in court involvement (Kamen & Gewirtz, 1989), every report must be investigated, and the very presence of child protective services can have a profound impact on families because of its implicit challenge to the family's autonomy. Cases involving female victims are more likely to be filed in criminal court and sexual abuse has the highest likelihood of prosecution. Physical neglect was the most common type of maltreatment to result in court filings. Cases involving male perpetrators, older perpetrators, and multiple victims are more likely to be filed for prosecution (Sedlak, Doueck, & Gragg, 2005). It also has a strong impact on the worker, who realizes that his or her report to child protective services will threaten the helping relationship because of the client's inevitable resentment about being reported. A combination of empathy and authority is necessary in working with nonvoluntary court-referred maltreating parents. (See Chapter 14, this volume, as well as Kamen & Gewirtz, 1989, for further discussion of this topic.)

Issues of Confidentiality

Confidentiality has specific limitations in situations in which the court is involved. This can present a formidable additional obstacle in the worker–client relationship, because the client knows that the worker has a legal obligation to report any incidents that indicate recurrence of maltreatment. In such cases, even when the worker informs the client that a report will be made, the parent often deeply resents the worker's actions. A brief case example illustrates this point.

Mrs. Jones, a 25-year-old pregnant mother of three sons (ages 6½, 5½, and 1), was mandated to receive individual therapy with a focus on parenting skills. Her children had been placed in foster care for 8 months because of neglect when she allegedly left them alone for extended periods of time. A neighbor stated that Mrs. Jones took drugs and hung around with drug dealers, but she denied this allegation; she also denied that she had left her children unattended.

Mrs. Jones seemed distant and angry in counseling sessions. She often refused to engage in discussion, answer questions, or talk about her feelings or behavior or about how she was managing now that the children had returned home. She also refused to discuss her pregnancy, stating that she didn't like to have other people "minding her business."

The worker felt that little progress was made in 3½ months, stating in a case summary that "this mother is unresponsive, distant, critical and punitive toward the children, showing them only occasional displays of warmth."

In supervision, the worker recognized that she and the client were both "trapped" in a relationship neither of them wanted. Although the worker admitted her feelings of anger toward the client, she was unable to move beyond this to recognize with the client how the issue of their *mutual* anger and need for control prevented their working together on meeting the children's needs for effective parenting.

This brief vignette illustrates the intense feelings generated by the removal of children from a mother's custody when her allegedly neglectful behavior puts them at risk of potential harm. The possible or even probable substance involvement of a parent merits close attention, but it is not in itself grounds for evidence of child maltreatment in most states (Tracy, 1994, citing English, 1990).

Work with parents who have been charged with some form of child maltreatment requires great sensitivity and skill. Often such parents distrust "the system," and insofar as they view the worker as part of this system, they will be very difficult to engage. The key to effective helping is to discuss a parent's resistance openly, while also identifying the parent's strengths. Referral to a substance use disorder treatment agency in which the chief mode of treatment is group therapy may reduce the parent's denial and sense of stigma, while also offering the support of group members and the possibility of identification with peers who share similar challenges and experiences.

Another situation that requires sensitivity and skill on the part of the worker is that in which a child reveals ongoing abuse but asks the worker to keep this revelation a secret because of fear of destroying his or her family. The worker does not really have a choice in this case, because reporting of abuse is mandatory. *Confidentiality cannot be maintained when a child's safety is in jeopardy.* The worker must make this clear to the child, in a manner that ensures the child's protection and keeps the child from feeling betrayed by the worker. The revised NASW code of ethics (National Association of Social Workers, 2017, Section 1.01) points out that social workers' responsibility to the larger society and/or their specific legal obligations may supersede the loyalty owed to clients and that clients should be advised accordingly.

COMBINING INDIVIDUAL AND FAMILY HELPING METHODS

Because substance use disorders affect individuals, families, and communities, a broad approach to helping is necessary, using a combination of psychological, educational, behavioral, and environmental interventions. The primary focus in such a case must be on the substance use problem itself, because, as Copans (1989) has stated, "treating a family with [a substance-using] member without acknowledging, confronting, focusing on, and dealing with the [substance use] is generally doomed to failure" (p. 277). Furthermore, after treatment, the best chances for lifetime recovery are afforded by ongoing participation in one of the 12-step self-help groups, such as Alcoholics Anonymous (AA), Narcotics Anonymous (NA), or Cocaine Anonymous (CA). Whereas the use of alcohol or drugs previously dominated the life of a person with a substance use disorder, the focus after detoxification (if needed) and treatment must change to a commitment to remain drug and alcohol free. The disorder is not "cured," but, like diabetes, it can be controlled if the individual initiates and sustains a certain lifestyle. This usually entails finding new friends who share the recovering individual's goal of maintaining sobriety. Contacts with the previous network of substance-using peers must cease. Moving to a new neighborhood, when this is possible, symbolizes leaving the past behind and represents a new beginning.

Helping Substance-Using Parents

Most specialists in the field of substance use disorders agree that few individuals enter treatment voluntarily. Because of the denial that characterizes the substance-disordered population, a family member usually must insist on treatment, or another person such as a social worker must threaten to remove a child from parental custody unless the parent agrees to enroll in a detoxification and rehabilitation program.

Many detoxification programs (which are necessary for alcohol and opioid dependence, for instance) are carried out in an inpatient medical or psychiatric unit. This almost always requires a parent–child separation during a 5-day period. Moreover, detoxification is only the first step in treatment; intensive, ongoing educational and other programs are also needed. Goldberg (1995) points out that few treatment programs provide accommodation for children with their mothers, and she believes that the high costs of such programs may limit their widespread development in the future. Ironically, the cost of such treatment is much less than the cost of foster care.

One model program, in existence for more than 40 years, is Meta House in Milwaukee, Wisconsin (*metahouse.org*). This program treats women and children *together,* with the average length of stay between 9 and 18 months. About 25 women complete the program every year (Feinberg, 1995). Treatment is multifaceted and is successful in 90% of cases, with no recidivism. Components of this model program include educational/vocational counseling and training, assistance with housing, monitoring of physical health, legal assistance, and treatment focused on parenting and improvement of the mother–child relationship. Unfortunately, the high cost per family probably precludes broad duplication of this model program, no matter how successful its outcome.

Less costly treatment approaches to helping parents with substance use disorders on an *outpatient* basis following detoxification include day treatment, intensive patient rehabilitation programs, ego-supportive individual treatment, various self-help groups, and intervention with family members (Goldberg, 1995; Straussner, 1989, 2004). Whatever the modality, attention must be paid to environmental factors, such as housing, employment, and health needs, in addition to counseling focused on building the parents' self-esteem and self-confidence.

Family Approaches

Just as addiction develops over time, the response of a family to a substance-using member may vary over time, according to the changing individual and family life cycle stresses that occur during the onset and course of the addictive process (Krestan & Bepko, 1989). Often "the family, as well as the [substance user], develops a rigid system of denial to avoid acknowledgment of the problem" (Krestan & Bepko, 1989, p. 486). When parents are at midlife (mid-40s to mid-60s), they are most likely to seek help for alcohol use disorders; however, this time may come after the children have left home. In contrast, disorders related to the use of illicit drugs may elicit stronger recognition and response by the family, as the addictive process typically is more rapid with drugs than with alcohol. See Straussner (1993, 2004, 2014) for a discussion of the impact of different substances on the family.

Some general guidelines set forth by Deutsch (1982, pp. 127–128) for the treatment of alcohol problems in the family may, with slight revisions, apply also to the family treatment of other substance use disorders. They are adapted here as follows:

- Make a careful assessment of substance use problems in the two prior generations (i.e., look for evidence of the intergenerational persistence of such problems).
- Insist on sobriety/abstinence as a precondition of treatment. Recommend the attendance *at least six times* of the substance-using person at AA, NA, CA, or (when relevant) Parents Anonymous (PA) and of family members at Al-Anon or Alateen.
- Educate the family about substance use and disorder.
- Encourage open discussion of the problem among family members and other families with similar problems.
- Pay attention to the special needs of the children. If they have assumed a parentified role, they need permission to give up that role in favor of more age-appropriate behavior; it may require ongoing work to accomplish this goal.

Helping the Children of Substance-Using Parents

Hereditary Factors

Children in substance-disordered families are at high risk because chemical dependency is a hereditary disease in the same sense in which heart disease, diabetes, and cancer run in some families. Children with a family history of alcoholism are four times more likely to develop alcoholism or chemical dependency, according to five landmark studies (Goodwin, Schulsinger, Hermansen, Guze, & Winokur, 1973; Schuckit, 1985, 1994; Begleiter, 1988; Vaillant, 1983).

Goodwin and colleagues' 1973 study of adopted children showed that children born of alcoholic parents and raised by nonalcoholic parents had a

Note. I acknowledge the contribution of Madeline Zevon, ACSW, CASAC, MAC, in the preparation of this section and the case of Vanessa and Vernon.

very high rate of alcoholism. In other words, it was not the family in which they grew up but their biological inheritance that determined the higher rate of alcoholism. In 1988 Dr. Henri Begleiter of the State University of New York found similar brain wave patterns in alcoholic fathers and sons. In 1994 Mark Schuckit showed that people with the potential for alcoholism metabolize alcohol differently, thereby pointing to a physiological difference predisposing some young people to develop this disease. Further confirmation of hereditary factors came from George Vaillant's 40-year study of 660 men from adolescence to middle age, which found only one consistent predictor of alcoholism: the presence of an alcoholic parent.

Environmental Factors

Despite this compelling research attesting to hereditary factors, we must also acknowledge the role of the environment in the development of chemical dependency. In our society, there are strong pressures on young people to drink and to experiment with drugs (Robert Wood Johnson Foundation, 2001; Nadel & Straussner, 1997). When these influences combine with familial and intrapsychic dynamics and genetic influences, adolescent experimentation may move progressively into substance use disorder (Nadel & Straussner, 1997, citing Feigelman & Feigelman, 1993).

The combination of hereditary and environmental factors puts children of alcoholics and addicts at very high risk. They should be targeted for prevention by giving them factual information about their vulnerability. The emphasis in such preventive education is the message that the disease cannot develop if susceptible individuals abstain from using alcohol and drugs.

Living with a Substance-Using Parent

The concept that alcoholism or other substance misuse is a *family* disease recognizes the stresses experienced by all members of the family system (Ficaro, 1999). Children can be taught about the roles they may play inside and outside of their families as part of a family's denial that a parent is drinking. Five different roles have been identified by Wegscheider (1981) to illustrate that no one escapes in a chemically dependent family. These include:

- The enabler
- The hero
- The scapegoat
- The lost child
- The mascot

Ficaro (1999) points out that each role offers its own payoffs for both the individual and the family and ultimately exacts its own price. It is helpful for children to become aware of these family patterns through discussions in groups with peers who have similar family backgrounds.

GROUPS FOR CHILDREN OF SUBSTANCE-USING PARENTS

Open-ended outpatient after-school groups for children of alcoholics and addicts can be very helpful to children of different ages and their families (Zevon, 1990). Some of these programs permit children to be served on a long-term basis, depending on their needs and family situation. Children can enroll even if their parents are not receiving simultaneous services, although the goal of the program is to provide recovery groups for each family member in parallel treatment tracks. Often parents are or have been in treatment.

Each after-school group consists of 8–10 male and female children within a 2-year age range between the ages of 5 and 18 years. The groups are structured around activities that facilitate open discussion of the impact of alcohol and drug use on family life. One such activity is called the Feelings-in-the-Bottle or Feelings-in-the-Drug-Syringe drawing exercise. The children are given large sheets of poster paper and instructed to draw a bottle, can, syringe, or vial and then to indicate the "feelings" that come out of this container as the substance enters a person's body. Figures 13.1 to Figure 13.3 show some typical drawings that children using this exercise in a group have produced. After the drawings are completed, the group leaders post them on the wall and encourage each child to talk about what he or she drew. This group experience offers a great sense of validation and support to children in substance-disordered families, who up to this point may have felt very alone and isolated with their feelings.

Figure 13.1, for example, reflects an 8-year-old girl's ambivalent feelings—of sadness about a parent's drinking, yet also her feelings of love for the alcoholic parent. Children younger than 8 years often have trouble reconciling two apparently contradictory feelings, such as being angry at someone they love. This would be an important clarifying point for the group leaders to mention as the child displays her drawing.

Figure 13.2, by a 12-year-old girl, is replete with a variety of feelings. She mentions "sad," "angry," and "ashamed," as well as "stupid" and "dumb." It's not clear whether these last two terms refer to herself or her alcoholic parent; however, this child recognizes the impact of the drinking on self-esteem. Another cause for concern is this child's phrase in the lower left corner of the bottle—"like I'm not a real person." This seems to refer to her awareness that the alcohol causes her parent to ignore her individual needs because the alcohol takes precedence in the parent's mind. This child needs reassurance that her needs *are* important, even when her parent ignores them. This recognition would be very supportive not only to the child but also to others in the group who feel as if they are unimportant to their parents.

Figure 13.3, a 15-year-old girl's drawing of a syringe, contains many typical emotions of a child of an injection drug user, including the word "misfit" on the needle. Other feelings mentioned reflect the unhappiness and disgust associated with drug use. Although this girl's age places her beyond the range covered in this book (which does not include the adolescent years), I have

FIGURE 13.1. Feelings-in-the-Bottle drawing by an 8-year-old girl.

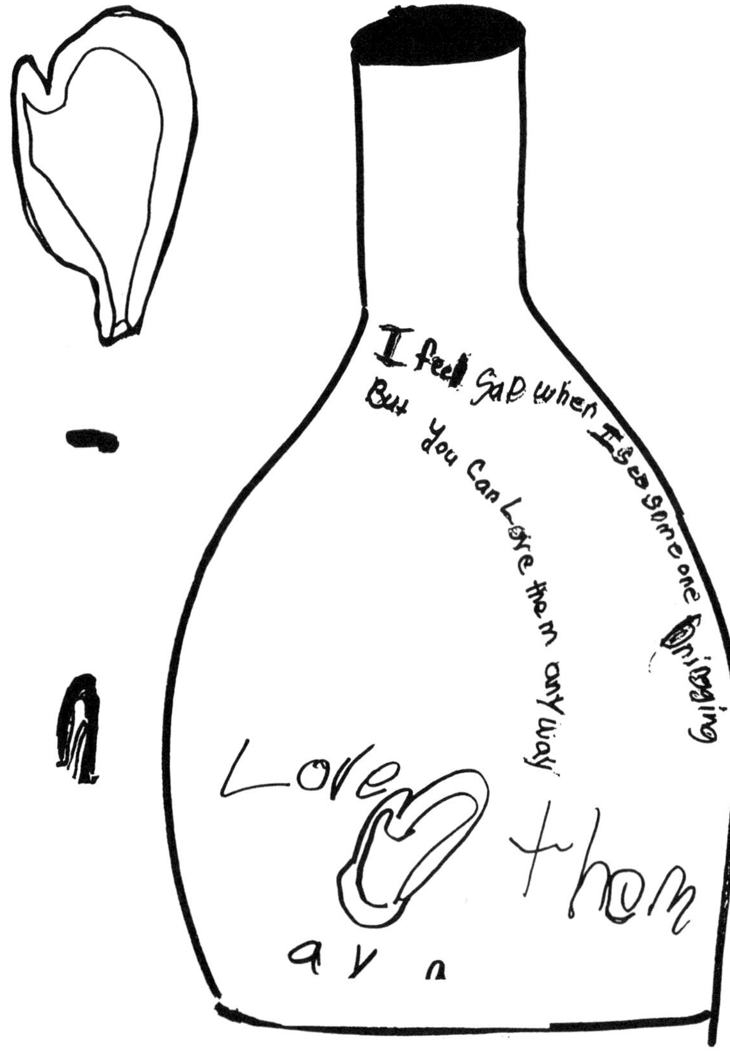

FIGURE 13.2. Feelings-in-the-Bottle drawing by a 12-year-old girl.

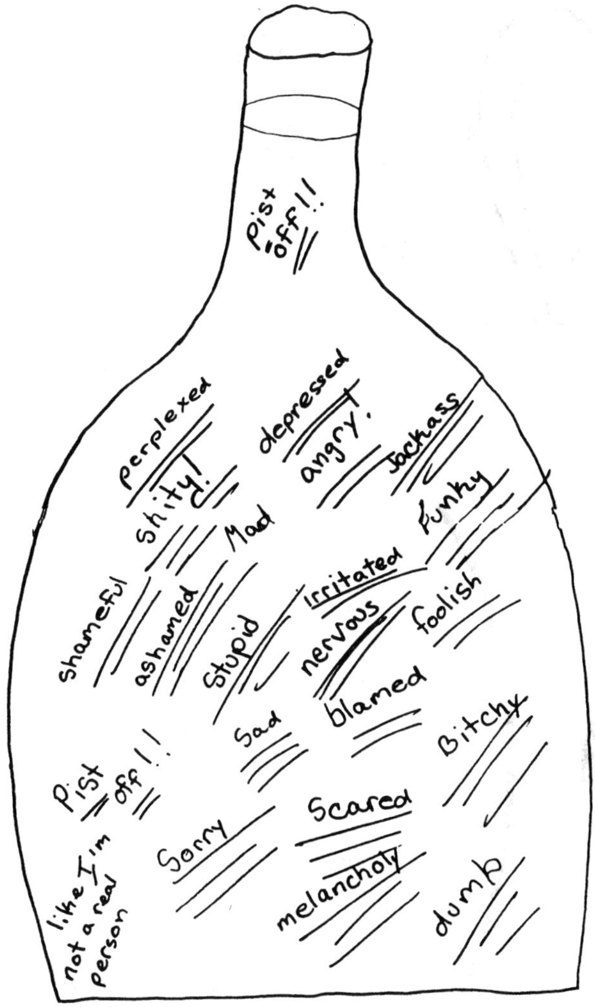

FIGURE 13.3. Feelings-in-the-Drug-Syringe drawing by a 15-year-old girl.

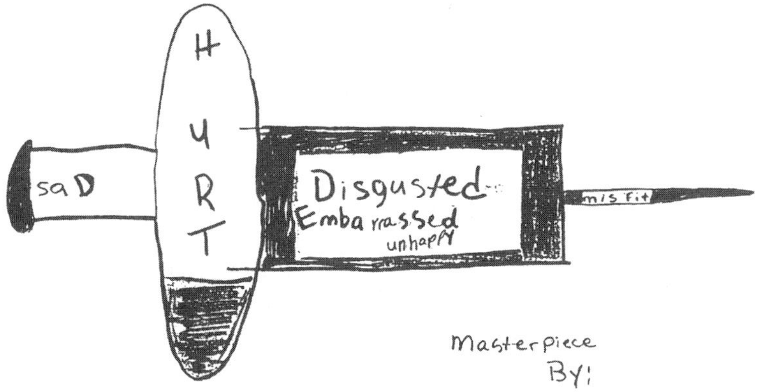

included this drawing here because of the probability that the drawings of teenagers who attend separate groups will be seen by younger children on the walls of the group room and the hallway of the agency. The intention is to have *all* children and their parents exposed to the wide-ranging effects of substance use disorders.

Videotapes/DVDs, Workbooks, and Storybooks for Children

Video and written materials are useful in children's activity and support groups to stimulate discussion and sharing about the experience of growing up in a substance-disordered family. The Resource Materials section at the end of this chapter provides sources of information for obtaining a variety of DVDs, videotapes, workbooks, and children's stories that would be useful to leaders of children's groups.

In using a DVD, workbook, or storybook, the group leader tells the children that other children in other places have also grown up in families with substance use disorders and that the video or book tells about one or more such examples. The leader also mentions that after the planned activity, the children will have the opportunity to talk about their own experience. After trying to elicit from the group some of the universal themes that emerge from the video or book, the leader invites the group members to make comparisons with their own life experiences.

Overview of Group Benefits

The group experience combats the isolation and shame of each child, while making explicit the fact that many other children are going through similar experiences. The challenge to the leaders is to provide support to the children while recognizing each child's need to live in a family in which he or she is important and unique rather than an insignificant family member who must fend for him- or herself.

THE CASE OF VANESSA, AGE 9, AND VERNON, AGE 10

Family Information (at the Time of Assessment)

Mother	Pearl, age 38, African American; active alcoholic.
Father	Josef, age 40, African American; history of crack dependence; in prison for selling drugs.
Child client	Vanessa, age 9, fourth grade; poor school functioning; depressed.
Child client	Vernon, age 10, fifth grade; some acting-out behavior.
Maternal grandmother	Sandra, age 62, resides with daughter and children.

Presenting Problem and Background

Vanessa, age 9, was referred to the outpatient program for children of alcoholics (COA) because her mother had come to school intoxicated on several occasions. This time the crossing guard said the mother had passed out in front of the school when she was with her daughter. Although the CPS agency was contacted, they were unable to effect any change.

Vanessa's grandmother brought her to the program and gave the following history. She described her daughter, Pearl, as a late-stage alcoholic who coughed up blood at times. The father, a drug addict, was currently in jail for drug-related offenses.

Intervention with Different Family Members

The comprehensive outpatient alcohol and drug treatment clinic encourages the whole family to become involved in the recovery process. Therefore, whenever a child enters the program for children of alcoholics or addicts, the other family members are urged to participate in a series of educational sessions. This includes education about the disease of chemical dependency, about the codependency issues of nonalcoholic family members, about children of alcoholics and addicts, and about the recovery process for the entire family.

In this family Vanessa enrolled in a once-a-week after-school group for children of alcoholics and addicts. There were seven other girls in the group between the ages of 9 and 11. Vanessa's mother, Pearl, refused all efforts to become engaged in treatment for herself, as she was in denial about her own alcoholism. However, she allowed her daughter to attend the COA program because of the father's addiction; in fact, she never wanted her daughter to miss a group, and she would call the agency often with complaints when the van to pick up Vanessa was late.

Several months later the father, Josef, was released from jail, and he brought his son, Vernon, age 10, into the COA program. Josef showed much less denial about his addiction than Pearl did about hers, and he enrolled himself in the clinic's day treatment program. Unfortunately, after a few weeks Josef relapsed and was referred to an inpatient rehabilitation program, followed by a long-term residential program.

Pearl telephoned the clinic frequently, usually in a cranky and irritable mood, but she admitted that the children had benefited from the program, and gradually she developed a cordial relationship with the leader of the children's group. One day she came to the agency and asked to go into detox. Her blood alcohol count was 0.342, usually a toxic level. She was rushed to the detox unit of the hospital, where she remained for 5 days. After discharge, she refused to attend the clinic's day treatment program, but she did accept a referral to another site that was more like a private-practice setting. Pearl entered that program and attended it for a year, with very good results.

The Children's Group

The model which served as a guide for the COA groups was Children Are People (Hazelden Foundation, 2002) and Moe (1989, 1993). The topics covered included the following:

- The disease concept of chemical dependency
- Feelings
- Families
- Decision making
- Self-esteem

A variety of toys and techniques were used, including puppets, role plays, therapeutic board games, drawing exercises, and videos. Books were read to initiate discussion of sensitive issues (see the list of resource materials at the end of the chapter). Holidays and birthdays were celebrated.

The drawing exercises proved especially helpful for Vanessa and Vernon. Vernon illustrated his feelings in the outline of a beer can (see Figure 13.4), which suggests that he missed his father and was depressed about his mother's drinking. Vernon was a quiet boy who did well in school and was liked by other children. He was not very verbally expressive, and it seemed unlikely that he would have volunteered these painful feelings without the drawing exercise as a stimulus. In his second drawing (see Figure 13.5), he listed his feelings, and, in showing the drawing to the group, he told why he experienced these feelings. Another drawing exercise on paper plates involved drawing the face you show to the world on one side of the plate (Figure 13.6), and how you feel inside on the other side (Figure 13.7). Vernon's illustrations show that he

FIGURE 13.4. Vernon's drawing of Feelings-in-a-Beer-Can.

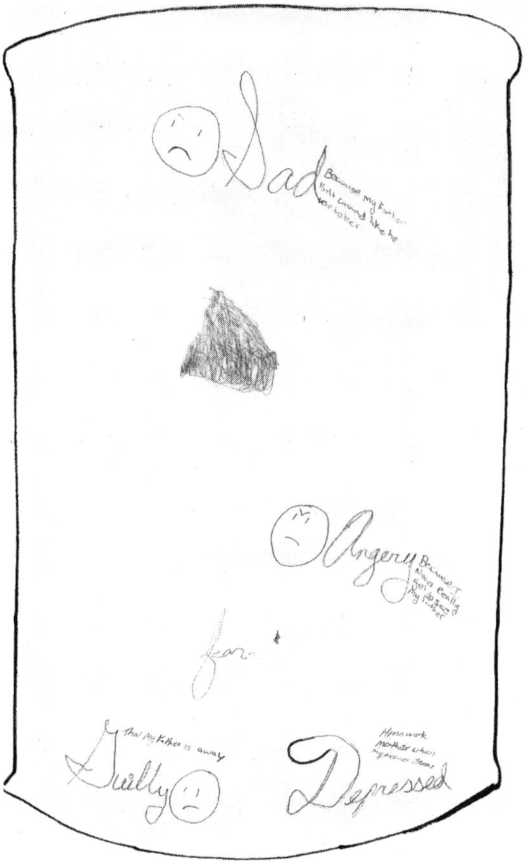

looks happy on the outside but feels disappointed on the inside. This exercise helps children learn about how they defend themselves from anxious feelings.

Vanessa's drawing of her feelings in the bottle showed her mother smoking and the words "My mom is drunk" with a sad face (Figure 13.8). Another drawing (Figure 13.9) indicates that she is worried about her uncle's drinking. There was a strong history of alcoholism and chemical dependency in this family. Vanessa's paper plate (Figure 13.10) shows a happy face on the outside and someone who feels tired and stressed on the inside (Figure 13.11). Vanessa often put her head down and fell asleep in the group. Because her mother reported that she slept well at night, this could be viewed as Vanessa's way of tuning out her unpleasant thoughts. Vanessa was in a special education class in school and appeared to be depressed.

(text resumes on page 307)

FIGURE 13.5. Vernon's list of Feelings-in-a-Beer-Can.

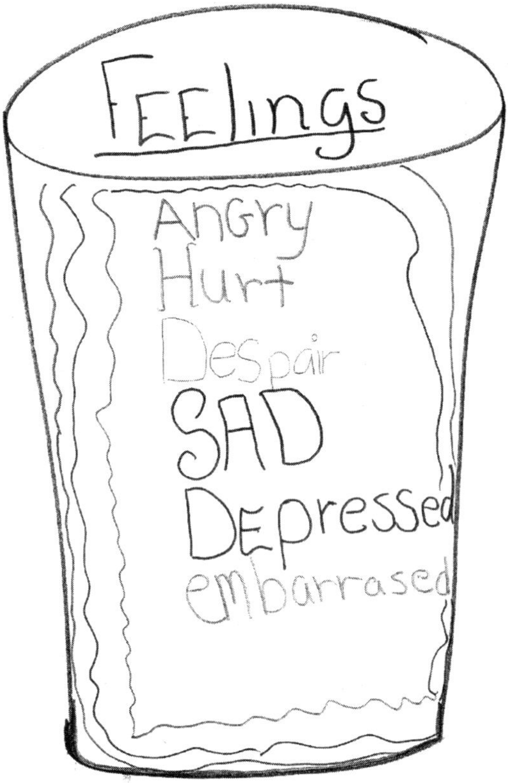

FIGURE 13.6. Vernon's drawing of his happy face (feelings on the outside).

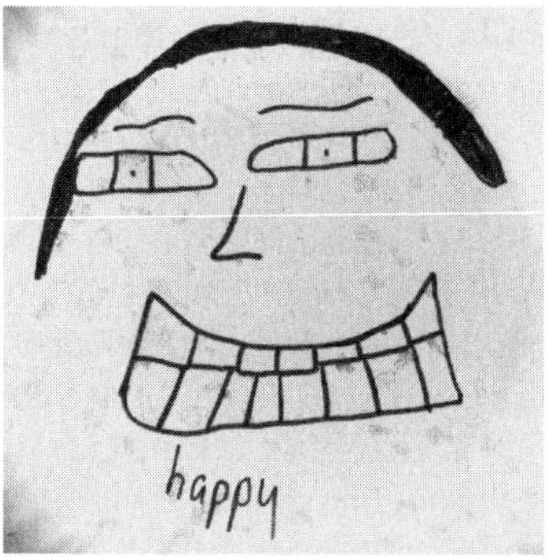

FIGURE 13.7. Vernon's drawing of his disappointed face (feelings on the inside).

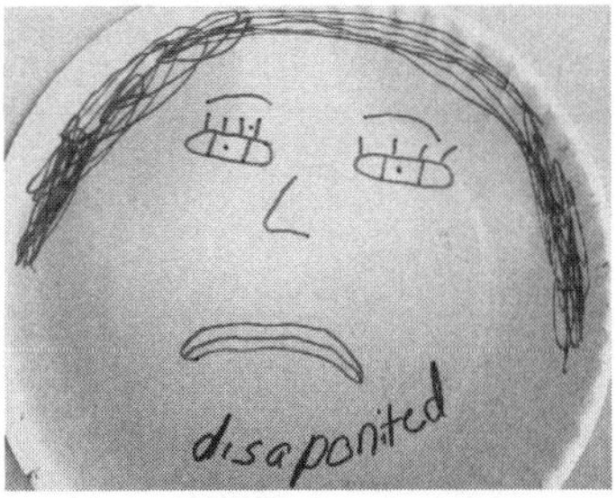

FIGURE 13.8. Vanessa's drawing of Feelings-in-a-Bottle.

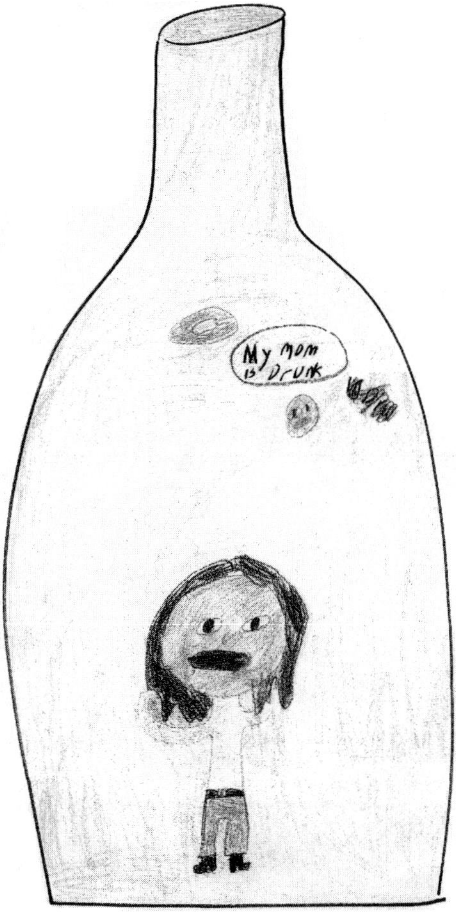

FIGURE 13.9. Vanessa's drawing of her uncle's drinking.

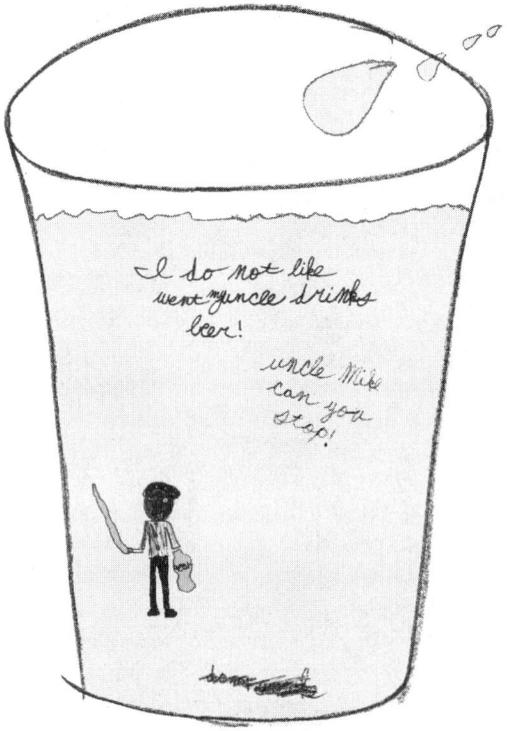

FIGURE 13.10. Vanessa's drawing of her happy face (feelings on the outside).

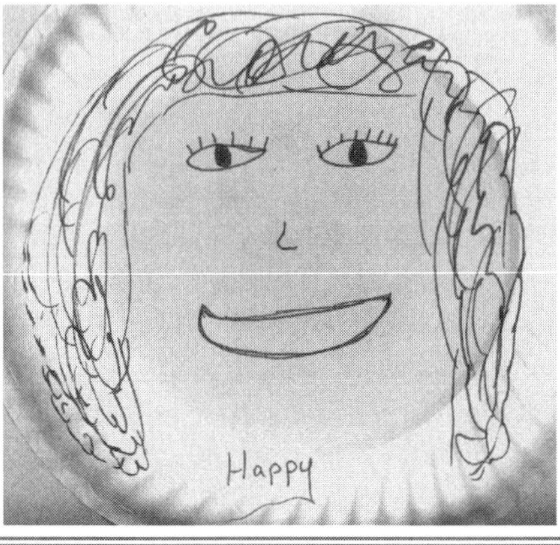

FIGURE 13.11. Vanessa's drawing of her tired, stressed face (feelings on the inside).

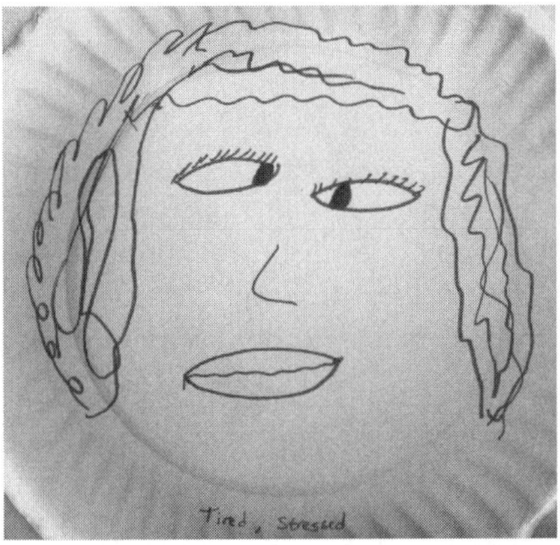

All the children in the group participated in a variety of group activities and developed a good understanding of their parents' addiction. At the end of each group the members formed a circle and recited the serenity prayer: "God grant me the serenity to accept the things I cannot change, courage to change the things I can, and the wisdom to know the difference." The children learn that they cannot change their parents because the parent has an illness and needs treatment. One time, after her mother had been in treatment for a while, Vanessa reported that she still wasn't sure that her mother had stopped drinking; she was so used to her mother's deception that it took Vanessa a while to be trustful.

Outcome and Discussion

Eventually, Pearl got a job and then went back to school. Josef completed the inpatient rehabilitation program, and both parents were reunited and in recovery. Vanessa was in the program for 4 years, and Vernon participated for 3 years. They left the program when they were ages 13 and 14, respectively. This is the age at which experimentation with drugs and alcohol often occurs. However, with their knowledge and awareness of the hereditary aspects of these diseases and the experience of their parents' treatment, it is hoped that the generational cycle of addiction will not be repeated. In terms of Wegscheider's (1981) roles, Vanessa was clearly the lost child and Vernon the family hero.

When working with children of alcoholics or addicts, the worker must involve the parents. In this case, the worker started with the children, and the whole family eventually entered treatment and participated in the recovery process.

CONCLUDING COMMENTS

Unlike many of the topics discussed in this book, substance use disorder is a lifelong problem with repercussions through the generations. Therefore, the first approach to helping must be education about this disorder. Children and adults alike need to understand the implications of having such a disorder, so that they will be able to make rational decisions for themselves and their family members.

Because a substance use disorder affects not only the individual but also all his or her family members and the community in which the individual lives, the approaches to helping must be comprehensive and long term. Interventions must always begin with a commitment to remain substance-free, but that is only the beginning, as extensive life changes and ongoing treatment will be necessary to maintain sobriety. Counseling for the addicted individual and for the family members and special programs for children are necessary to address this problem adequately. Groups help the addicted person and family members realize that they are not alone. The support given and received in groups can help build self-esteem, even as the group constitutes a new friendship network.

Preventive efforts in the schools have been shown to have positive results in reducing substance use disorders. Because of the serious consequences of such disorders, an argument can be made for implementing substance use prevention groups as part of *every* school's curriculum. In addition, every outpatient treatment program for substance use disorders should have a component for children, in order to help them understand the disease and, it is hoped, to prevent its recurrence in the next generation.

DISCUSSION QUESTIONS AND ROLE-PLAY EXERCISES

1. Discuss the implications of the statement that a substance use disorder is a family disease. How does this apply to the question of which family members to see and to setting up short- and long-term goals?
2. Role-play a situation in which a child reveals recurring physical abuse to a social worker but asks the worker "not to tell" because of fear of reprisal. First, demonstrate what you would say to the child; second, show how you would deal with the parent.
3. How can the worker best respond to a parent's anger at "the system" and tendency to view all helpers as critical and threatening?

4. Discuss the tension between "children's rights" and the rights of the parents, as this issue affects appropriate treatment for children in substance-disordered families.
5. Role-play a session in which the worker discusses with a parent the effects of the parent's substance use on his or her children as preparation for the children's beginning treatment.

RESOURCE MATERIALS

National Organizations

National Association for Children of Addiction
10920 Connecticut Avenue, Suite 100
Kensington, MD 20895
888-55-4COAS
https://nacoa.org

Center on Addition and the Family
Locations in California, Florida, Maryland, Massachusetts, Metro DC, New Hampshire, New York, Rhode Island, Texas, Vermont, and Virginia
877-930-0239
www.phoenixhouse.org/family/center-on-addiction-and-the-family

Al-Anon, Alateen Family Group Headquarters
1600 Corporate Landing Parkway
Virginia Beach, VA 23454-5617
757-563-1600
https://al-anon.org

Videotapes/DVDs

Kids Talking to Kids, 17 minutes
You're Not Alone (Elementary), 9 minutesi
Lots of Kids Like Us (Preteen), 28 minutes
My Father's Son (Teen–adult), 33 minutes
End Broken Promises (High school–adult), 24 minutes
The Cat Who Drank and Used Too Much (Elementary–adult), 12 minutes
A Story of Feelings (Grades K–3), 16 minutes
The Dog Who Dared (Elementary), 25 minutes

FMS Productions
P.O. Box 2268
Georgetown, TX 78627
800-421-4609
www.fmsproductions.com

Soft Is the Heart of a Child (Grades 7–12), 35 minutes

Hazelden Publishing
15251 Pleasant Valley Road
P.O. Box 176
Center City, MN 55012-0176
800-328-9000
www.hazelden.org/web/public/publishing.page

Books/Workbooks

Note. Ages are specified when indicated.

Al-Anon Family Groups. (1977). *What's drunk, mama?* New York: Author.
Anth, J. (2007). *Emmy's question.* St. Augustine, FL: Morningside Press.
Black, C. (1979). *My dad loves me, my dad has a disease: A workbook for children of alcoholics.* Newport Beach, CA: Alcoholism, Children, Therapy. Available from Hazelden. (Ages 5–10)
Brooks, C. (1981). *The secret everyone knows.* San Diego, CA: Kroc Foundation. (Older children)
Center for Addiction and Mental Health. (2011). *Wishes and worries: Coping with a parent who drinks too much alcohol.* Toronto, ON, Canada: Tundra Books.
DiGiovanni, K. (1986). *My house is different.* Center City, MN: Hazelden Foundation. (Ages 6 and up)
Duggan, M. H. (1987). *Mommy doesn't live here anymore.* Weaverville, NC: Bonnie Brae Publications. (Ages 5–11)
Hastings, J., & Typpo, M. (1984). *An elephant in the living room.* Minneapolis, MN: Comp Care. (Ages 7–13)
Jones, P. (1983). *The brown bottle: A fable for children of all ages.* Center City, MN: Hazelden Foundation.
Kenney, K., & Krull, H. (1980). *Sometimes my mom drinks too much.* Milwaukee, WI: Raintree Children's Books.
McFarland, R. (1991). *Drugs and your brothers and sisters.* New York: Rosen. (Ages 10 and up)
Melquist, E. (1974). *Pepper.* Frederick, MD: Frederick County Council on Alcoholism. (Ages 5–10)
Operation Cork. (1983). *Winthrop and Munchie talk about alcohol.* La Jolla, CA: Author.
Seixas, J. (1979). *Living with a parent who drinks too much.* New York: Greenwillow Books. (Ages 8–12)
Sheff, D., & Sheff, N. (in press). *Everything you wanted to know about drugs, alcohol, and addiction.* (Tweens and teens)
Smith, T. P., & Brogar, R. J. (2008). *Junior drug awareness: Alcohol.* New York: Facts on File. (Ages 10–12)
Snyder, A. (1975). *First step.* New York: Holt, Rinehart & Winston.
Woods, G., & Woods, H. (1985). *Cocaine.* New York: Watts. (Ages 10–14)

CHAPTER 14

Child Victims and Witnesses of Family and Community Violence

The idea of home as a sanctuary has long and deep roots. Most of us expect to feel safe behind the locked doors of our own homes. The poet May Sarton poignantly refers to "a house where every man may take his ease/May come to shelter from the outer air/A little house where he may find his peace" (1936–1938/1973, p. 43). This romantic view of almost 70 years ago seems like an obsolete ideal at the beginning of the 21st century, when kidnappers snatch children from their beds at night and when many children suffer physical and sexual abuse in their homes at the hands of their parents, relatives, or caretakers.

Similarly, the concept of a safe community neighborhood also is disappearing, especially in large cities where innocent citizens are killed by the shootings of drug dealers and hundreds can die suddenly at the hands of terrorists. Even schools may suffer deaths at the hands of a psychotic or angry killer. Furthermore, the media guarantees that everyone who can see and has a television will be deluged with images of every type of crime, from murder to terrorist bombings. Children are witnessing countless acts of violence in all areas of their lives. Some are themselves victims; others, through constant exposure, will become desensitized and apathetic about the effects of violence on victims (American Psychological Association, 1993; Edleson, 1999). Unfortunately, children who grow up in a context of violence may come to view this as an acceptable way to resolve differences. Thus the attempts of schools and religions to teach that violence is wrong may fall on deaf ears when young people are living in cultures that subscribe to the philosophy that the strongest person is the winner.

This chapter focuses on violence that occurs in the family and in the community and its short- and long-term effects on children. Although some important differences exist between different forms of violence, all can have a major impact on children, and social workers must be familiar with specific treatment strategies to both deal with the existing problem and intervene to prevent the perpetuation of these devastating interactions.

DEFINITION AND SCOPE OF THE PROBLEM

Family Violence

The term "family violence" refers to acts of physical, sexual, or psychological maltreatment, aggression, and violence that occur in a family unit whereby one family member with more power or authority attempts to gain control over another family member (American Psychological Association Ad Hoc Committee, 1996). Victims may be adults or children, and the perpetrators are usually adults but may also be older children.

Gelles (1979), defining violence as "an act carried out with the intention of physically injuring another person," states that people are more likely to be hit, beaten up, physically injured, or even killed in their own homes by another family member than anywhere else or by anyone else in U.S. society. The home, far from being a sanctuary, is a place of danger and fear for many children. Brendler (2006, p. 434) refers to a family's interpersonal walls as an "emotional prison where its members feel alone and disconnected from one another," resulting in their feeling abandoned, controlled, or betrayed. This, obviously, can be a frightening environment for children.

Our patriarchal system traditionally condoned the battering of women, but the topic of domestic violence has attracted growing media attention and increased public awareness and outrage since the mid-1970s. The formation of the National Coalition against Domestic Violence in 1978 raised public consciousness and led to the development of shelters, support groups, and improved legislation to protect battered women. Nonetheless, the problem continues. In the United States, approximately 50% of all murders occur between family members and acquaintances (Corr, Nabe, & Corr, 2000), and one-half of those are spouse killings (Margolin, 1979, as reported in Gilliland & James, 2001). Physical and sexual violence against women committed by current or past partners affects approximately 1.5 million women in the United States annually (Kastenbaum, 2006). In 2005 an average of three women everyday were killed by an intimate partner (O'Hara, 2017).

Many children both witness and personally experience violence in their families. It has been estimated that about 15.5 million children in the U.S. live in families where domestic violence occurred at least once in the previous year (Theresa's Fund, 2018). According to Guterman and Cameron (1997, as reported by Nisivoccia & Lynn, 1999), as many as 80–90% of young children and three out of four elementary and high school students of color in urban areas have witnessed at least one violent act in the home or community (Garbarino, Dubrow, Kostelny, & Pardo, 1992; Lorion & Saltzman, 1993). From 1 to 5% of children may be victims of incest, and several times that number are subjected to serious physical abuse or see their mothers, brothers, and sisters being beaten. In addition, children themselves can become the targets of uncontrolled rage. The National Child Abuse and Neglect Data System (NCANDS) reported an estimated 1,670 child fatalities in 2015 caused by abuse or neglect (Child Welfare Information Gateway, 2017). Three-quarters of these involved children younger than 3 years in 2015, and about half of the fatalities occurred to children younger than 1 year of age (Child Welfare Information Gateway, 2017). Most of these deaths (72%) are the result of caregiver neglect, while about 43% occurred because of physical abuse; some deaths are caused by both (Child Welfare Information Gateway, 2017).

Community Violence

The term "community violence" refers to assaults occurring outside the home, within the neighborhood, city, suburb, or country; these assaults may be committed by known or unknown persons, and they may result in various degrees of injury, from minor damages to fatalities. The violent events may happen to a single individual, as in a beating witnessed on the sidewalk, or to many individuals, as in a bombing or terrorist attack.

Children witness between 10 and 20% of the homicides in the United States, and they either know about or witness approximately 10% of the rapes ("Post-traumatic Stress: Part II," 1991). Reports of children in the cities of New Haven (Marans & Cohen, 1993) and New Orleans (Osofsky, Wewers, Hann, & Fick, 1993) confirm that significant percentages of children are victims of and witnesses to serious acts of violence. It has been estimated that between 3.3 and 10 million children annually witness acts of family violence (Edleson, 1999). Indeed, in 1995, homicide was listed as the third leading cause of death among elementary school children, and all too often many classmates witnessed these tragic deaths (Kochanek & Hudson, 1995). Interpersonal violence among peers, including bullying, is discussed in Chapter 15. Violence in schools is discussed in Chapter 9.

THE IMPACT ON CHILDREN OF EXPOSURE TO VIOLENCE AND IMPLICATIONS FOR TREATMENT

Because children are helpless and terrified in the face of the violent acts of adults, the witnessing and experiencing of this behavior may result in "profound changes in the child's [belief] about the safety and security of future intimate human relationships" (Pynoos & Eth, 1985, p. 27). Unable to trust their parents to serve as protectors, children may be overwhelmed with a sense of fear, betrayal, and loneliness regarding their present and future security (Groves, 2002). Pynoos and Eth (1985) warn that children who witness extreme acts of violence "represent a population at significant risk of developing anxiety, depressive, phobic, conduct, and posttraumatic stress disorders" (p. 19).

The adverse effect on children's behavior caused by exposure to domestic violence has been cited in the literature since the 1980s (Rosenbaum & O'Leary, 1981; Hershorn & Rosenbaum, 1985; Miller, 1989). "A child may be extremely traumatized by violence exerted by an adult against the child's mother, a family pet, or personal property," according to Miller (1989, p. 419). When the child is personally abused, he or she lives with feelings of dread about future possible repetition and may develop defensive reactions, such as distancing, wariness, and avoidance of the frightening parent and/or other adults. The possible impact of abuse on attachment relationships with adults was discussed in Chapter 10 and is reviewed again later in this chapter. Some of the children's responses correspond to the criteria for PTSD, which also is discussed more fully later in this chapter.

> Psychological trauma is especially damaging when it involves a violation of trust and a distortion of family intimacy. For a child who is repeatedly abused physically or sexually, the stress is constant and the threat is always present . . . *the source of terror is also the only source of comfort* . . . abused children understand little of what is happening, since everyone around them is ignoring it or lying about it. They are systematically confused and misled; *incest is disguised as love, beating as discipline* ("Post-traumatic Stress: Part II" 1991, pp. 1–2; emphasis added)

Children who are exposed to abuse and violence in their families may respond with a wide range of behaviors, including somatic complaints, school-related problems, excessive crying and fear, withdrawal, clinging, aggressiveness, tantrums, anxiety, depression, and self-mutilation. Numerous research articles document these findings (Carlson, 1984; Scheeringa & Zeanah, 1995: Groves, 2002; Eiden et al., 2007). Unfortunately, child abuse is significantly more likely to occur in families in which there is domestic violence, with the consequences to the child reported as being pervasive and long-lasting (Anderson & Seita, 2006).

It is often difficult to engage children who have experienced chronic abuse during their formative years. Any person, child or adult, who has been subjected to abuse or trauma begins therapy full of doubts and suspicion about the therapist's motives and ability to help (Herman, 1992). Because of their insecure attachment and inability to form meaningful relationships, it may take from 3 to 11 months for therapists to engage children with attachment disorders, according to Doyle and Bauer (1989).

The process of establishing attachment in older children who have been traumatized may be long and difficult, according to James (1989, 1994, 2009). However, the effort put into this may be "the only hope for [the children] ever forming an intimate bond with another person. . . . Children who have learned not to trust adults and who are intimacy-avoidant may not show signs of relationship development with the therapist for many months" (James, 1994, p. 61). The experience of traumatization, abuse, and lack of parental empathy affects the children's developing ability to value themselves as persons and to identify with the emotional states of others (Jordan, 1991). It is very important for therapists to understand the child's distancing behavior and not terminate treatment prematurely.

Furthermore, when children witness repeated violence between their parents, they learn that violence is a way to settle disagreements. This unfortunate and powerful lesson may affect their own present and future relationships, because these children have no experience of nonviolent methods of resolving controversies and conflicts. In addition, their observation of the failure of adults to restrain themselves may seriously jeopardize the children's confidence in their *own* impulse control (Pynoos & Eth, 1985, p. 26). This may be the operating dynamic when we see a child engaging in uncharacteristic aggressive, reckless, or self-destructive behavior after exposure to adult (especially parental) violence. A literature review and other studies have confirmed that children exposed to violence are more likely to display behavioral and psychological problems than are their nonexposed peers (Shahinfar, Fox, & Leavitt, 2000; Evans, Davies, & DiLillo, 2008).

THE ASSESSMENT OF THE CHILD VICTIM AND/OR WITNESS OF FAMILY VIOLENCE

This section deals with the child as both the victim of and witness to various forms of family violence. The topic encompasses both the physical and sexual abuse of a child by another family member and the witnessing by a child of either form of abuse perpetrated by one family member on another.

After discussing the legal mandate to report suspected abuse, I review the specific signs and symptoms associated with physical and sexual abuse.

The Legal Mandate

The Child Abuse Prevention and Treatment Act (Public Law 93-247, 1974) mandates the reporting of child maltreatment in all states receiving certain federal funds. Social workers interact with children in a variety of settings, and they may become concerned about the possibility of physical or sexual abuse because of certain aspects of a child's behavior or attitude or because of specific physical indications on the child's body.

It is the responsibility of every social worker to know the laws in his or her state about reporting suspected maltreatment, the information that is required in making such a report, and the agency that is responsible for investigating the report. Although reporting to the appropriate agency is *mandatory,* Lukas (1993) cautions about making the decision to report hastily or unilaterally, because of the inevitable complicated repercussions that such a report sets in motion. It is often helpful to a worker to discuss the details of a case with a supervisor or with other experienced workers. Weighing the needs of the child and those of the family may generate ethical dilemmas and pressures on the worker. This is "a powerful responsibility . . . since both a child's safety and the well-being of a family may be at risk" (Lukas, 1993, p. 139). Also, the legal and protective interventions that often follow may be very perplexing and anxiety provoking for the child (Gil, 1994). The worker must convince the child that he or she will do everything possible to ensure the child's safety, even though this may mean that the child will have to live someplace else for a while. This certainly is a very frightening situation for any child.

If it is likely that the child will have to testify in court or to a judge, the worker can help prepare the child for this experience—*not* by rehearsing with the child his or her actual testimony (as this would be considered putting words in the child's mouth) but by briefly and simply explaining the court procedures. It is often helpful to use a workbook for children that shows pictures of a courtroom and describes a child's participation in typical court procedures. (See Schwab, 1986, for a coloring book to prepare children ages 5–12 to go to court.) David Crenshaw (2014) has written about and advocated for the use of "facility" dogs in the courtroom to help allay the anxieties a child may feel when required to testify in court. The NASW has published a guide titled *The Legal Rights of Children* (2010) that contains essential information relevant to the legal status of children and an orientation to the court system and various legal matters that affect children.

Indicators of Physical Abuse

The indicators of physical abuse listed in Figure 14.1 constitute a general guide, rather than positive proof of child abuse, because it is always possible that a child's injuries occurred through play or otherwise accidentally. Obviously, multiple and recurrent injuries and those that do not seem congruent with the description of how they occurred merit further investigation and close monitoring.

THE CASE OF ELISA IZQUIERDO, AGE 6

(All information was reported in *The New York Times* [Bruni, 1995].)

Family Information

Mother	Addicted to crack; history of abuse.
Father	Unknown.
Child client	Elisa, age 6, first grade; in foster care.
Elisa's five siblings	Ages 2–9; two older than Elisa, three younger.

Note. I realize that this is a very old case, and I considered using one from the news accounts of 2018. Unfortunately, the cases I found in the current news reports had details that were distressingly similar to those of Elisa's case. So I decided to keep this one as a reminder that the incidence of parental abuse has not diminished and in the hope that readers will work to find ways to intervene that can help reduce this appallingly persistent problem.

FIGURE 14.1. Physical and behavioral indicators of physical abuse.

Physical indicators	Behavioral indicators
Bruises and welts Marks on face, lips, mouth Marks on torso, back, buttocks, thighs Symmetrical marks on both sides of body (suggesting that the child has been grabbed by two hands; accidental injuries are not symmetrical) Bruises/welts in various stages of healing Clustered bruises indicating repeated contact with an object Patterned bruises that reveal the shape of an object, such as a belt buckle, electric cord, or hairbrush Marks on several different areas Marks regularly appearing after weekends, absences, or vacations *Burns* Cigarette burns, especially on palms, soles, back, or buttocks Immersion burns (matching injuries on both ankles or hands, suggesting that the child was immersed in hot liquid) Patterned burns in the shape of an iron or a curling iron Rope burns on arms, legs, neck, or torso *Fractures* Fractures to skull, nose, face, arms, and legs Fractures in various stages of healing Multiple fractures, with splintering (caused by pulling or twisting) *Lacerations/abrasions/bites* Tears in tissues Tears to mouth, lips, gums, eyes Lacerations to genitalia Bites to buttocks	Wariness of adult contacts Apprehension when other children cry or get hurt Behavioral extremes (aggressiveness or passive withdrawal) Obvious fear of parents Reluctance to go home Reports of injury by parents Frequent weeping in school Self-mutilating behavior

Presenting Problem

The principal of Elisa's school wrote a letter to the family court judge, outlining the school's suspicion that the child had been physically and emotionally abused during her weekend visits with her mother. Among the indicators noticed by school personnel and by neighbors were bruises and welts on the child's body, nightmares, vomiting, withdrawn behavior, fear of using the bathroom, and "walking strangely." Despite these concerns and the letter written to the judge, her mother was granted custody. A year and a half later Elisa was found dead of bleeding caused by a blunt impact wound to her head.

Discussion

A newspaper account of Elisa's death in New York City (Bruni, 1995) illustrates that children who suffer chronic abuse show many physical and behavioral indicators that are noted by their teachers and neighbors. Elisa's case raises the question about whose rights take precedence—those of the child or those of the mother. The newspaper account (Bruni, 1995) portrays Elisa's mother as an abused woman herself, addicted to crack, who took much of her rage out on Elisa because she thought the child was possessed by voodoo. The caseworker should have noticed the different way Elisa's mother treated her compared with the other children in the family. Exploration of the mother's cultural/religious beliefs might possibly have averted this tragedy. Certainly, child safety must always be of paramount concern. Sedlak and Broadhurst (1996) point out that, nationally, approximately 9% of children served by public child welfare agencies are sexually abused and almost 10% are physically abused (reported by Mannes, 2001). Sadly, placement and agency monitoring do not always serve the intended child protective purpose. The U.S. Health and Human Services (2016) predicted that 1 in 4 girls and 1 in 4 boys will be sexually abused before they turn 18 years old.

Elisa was the third of six children, ranging in age from 2 to 9. Although the other children did not show indications of abuse, they certainly were aware that their sister was beaten and that she died at the mother's hands. As witnesses to family violence and homicide, these children were traumatized and will need help for many years.

The *NASW News* of July 2010 featured an article discussing a Capitol Hill briefing that called for greater attention to the rise in child abuse fatalities (Pace, 2010). A report by the Every Child Matters Education Fund (2010) titled *We Can Do Better* outlines the issues and makes suggestions for improvement.

Indicators of Sexual Abuse

Figure 14.2, which lists the physical and behavioral symptoms of sexual abuse, can serve as a general guide for workers who suspect that a child is being sexually abused.

The term "sexual abuse" refers to behaviors in which a child is used for a sexual purpose. This rather simple definition encompasses a broad range of sexual behaviors—from exposing a child to pornographic pictures to touching to various forms of sexual behavior (including oral, anal, or genital intercourse). Lukas (1993) clarifies that the perpetrator may be a man or a woman,

FIGURE 14.2. Physical and behavioral indicators of sexual abuse.

Physical indicators	Behavioral indicators
Pain, bruises, bleeding, or itching in genitals or rectum, or recurrent urinary infections	Sleep disturbances
Venereal disease in mouth, genitals, or rectum	Oversexualized or seductive behavior (including excessive masturbation)
Bedwetting	Preoccupation with own or other children's genitals
Difficulty in walking or sitting	Unwillingness to change for gym or to participate in physical education class
Torn, stained, or bloody underclothing	Poor peer relationships or sudden social withdrawal
Offensive odors	Reports of sexual assault
Preteen or early teen pregnancy	Self-mutilating behavior or suicide attempts
Recurrent vomiting or stomachaches	

that the child involved may be a male or female of any age, and that the abuse may have occurred once or many times. Lukas also reminds us of two important facts about the sexual abuse of children: (1) "Sexual abuse occurs in every race, ethnic group, and economic class in society" (p. 145), and (2) "The perpetrator is most likely to be someone the child knows" (p. 145).

Serious repercussions follow a conviction of sexual abuse, and workers who suspect possible sexual abuse may have to go to court to present the reasons for their concerns. Some guidelines in preparing to document suspicions of sexual abuse include the following:

1. Use open-ended questions in obtaining information from the child (e.g., "Tell me more about that," or "Show me with the dolls what happened," rather than "Did Daddy come into your bed every night?").
2. Record information about what happened in the child's own words, using as many specifics as possible.

The Tripartite Crisis Assessment

Even when multiple physical and behavioral indicators of physical or sexual abuse are apparent, and even when a child has verbally confirmed experiences of abuse, we still do not know the *meaning* of the abusive experience to the child. The child's experience of an event can differ significantly from what adults expect: "An event may or may not be experienced as traumatic by a child, and it may be traumatizing at one stage of a child's development and not at another" (James, 1989, p. 21). A basic tenet of crisis intervention is that it is not the event itself that constitutes the crisis but rather the individual's *perception* of the event. A full assessment of the event, the child, and the surrounding environment therefore permits us to understand more completely the implications of an abuse experience in a child's life.

In previous publications (Webb, 1991, 1993, 1999, 2001, 2003, 2007, 2011), and in several chapters of this book (Chapters 4, 10, 11, and 12), I have utilized variations of tripartite crisis assessment to demonstrate the interactive influences among three groups of factors in evaluating the significance of a specific crisis event or events:

1. Factors related to the individual.
2. Factors related to the crisis situation.
3. Factors in the support system.

FIGURE 14.3. Interactive components of a tripartite crisis assessment. Adapted from Webb (1999, p. 5). Copyright © 1999 The Guilford Press.

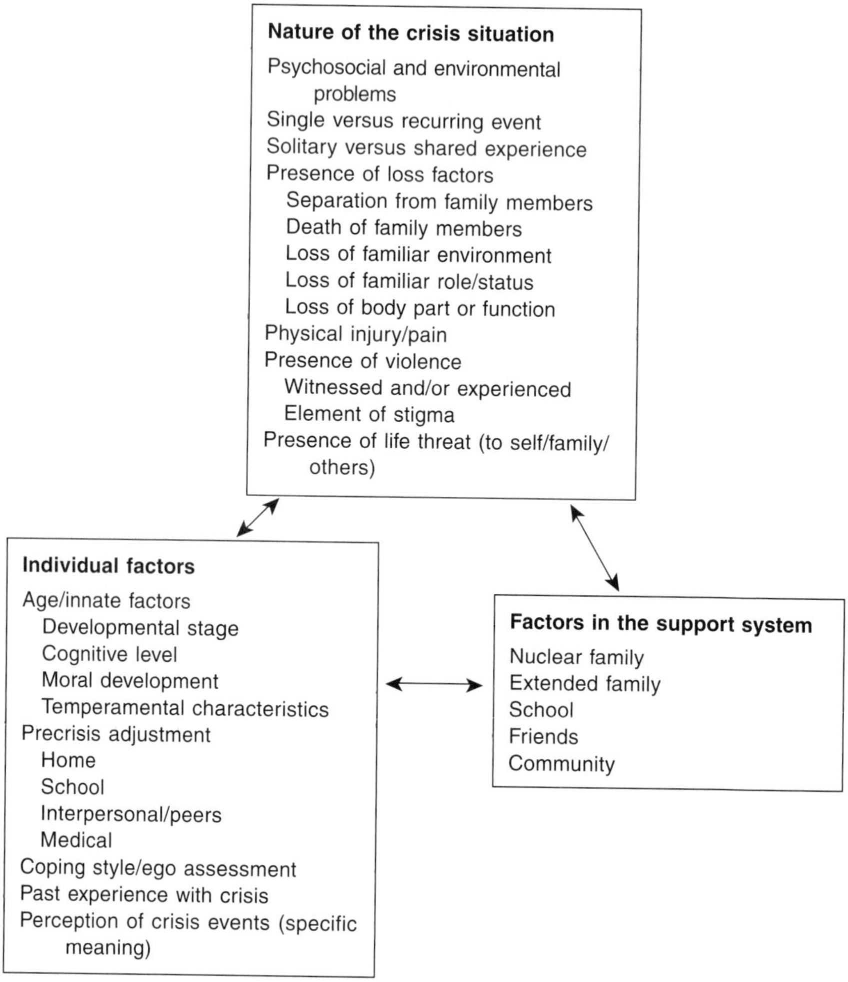

Figure 14.3 illustrates the various elements that must be considered in evaluating the impact of a specific crisis event, such as physical or sexual abuse in the family. (See Webb, 1999, for a full discussion of this assessment.) Two forms that can be used in recording the individual and situational components of the crisis assessment are provided in the Appendices. The eco-map (see Chapters 2, 3, and 4) is useful in assessing essential information about the support system.

When a child is being evaluated for abuse, special attention should be given to the child's history of loss, to recurring experiences of abuse, and to the possibility that the child believed that the abusive experience endangered his or her or another family member's or a pet's life. Fear of death or serious injury is an essential condition for the diagnosis of PTSD (see the next section).

In addition, a child's developmental and cognitive level will determine the child's interpretation of the abuse experience. For example, the preschool or early-latency-age child (up to approximately age 8) is still egocentric in his or her thinking and may believe that he or she is "bad" and therefore caused the abuse. Of course, a perpetrator, playing into a child's normal narcissism, often reinforces these feelings by using guilt and secrecy tactics to keep the child from disclosing the abuse.

THE ASSESSMENT OF THE TRAUMATIZED CHILD: PTSD IN CHILDREN

The symptoms of PTSD (American Psychiatric Association, 2013) may develop in children who have been exposed to actual or threatened death, serious injury, or sexual violence. It is important for child welfare workers and other social workers to be familiar with the signs and symptoms of this condition, because it is often confused with depression or conduct-disordered ("acting-out") behavior. Children with symptoms of PTSD require treatment from someone who is trained both in child therapy and in trauma counseling. Therefore, a referral to a child-trauma specialist may be appropriate once the diagnosis has been made.

Components of PTSD

According to the DSM-5 (American Psychiatric Association, 2013), a diagnosis of PTSD in children 6 years and younger can be made when the child exhibits the presence of specified intrusive and avoidance symptoms, together with some negative alterations in cognition and changes in his or her reactivity over a period of more than 1 month. Because the classification of PTSD originated with adult soldiers in the Vietnam War, its application to children is based on the work of child psychiatrists (Eth & Pynoos, 1985; Terr, 1983, 1988, 1989), social workers (James, 1989; Doyle & Bauer, 1989; Webb,

1999; Nader & Fletcher, 2014), and child psychologists (Gil, 1994; Nader & Fletcher, 2014). DSM-5 (American Psychiatric Association, 2013) contains criteria for the PTSD diagnosis that is specifically targeted to children.

Incredible as it may seem, only a fraction of individuals exposed to traumatic experiences demonstrate behavioral responses indicative of PTSD. As previously discussed in Chapter 8, McFarlane (1990) states that "even after extreme trauma, only about 40 percent of an exposed population develop PTSD" (p. 74). According to Nader and Fletcher (2014) "most research to date confirms the general conclusion that the diagnostic symptom clusters of DSM-IV apply to traumatized children of all ages, from preschool to adolescence, as well as they do to traumatized adults." However, children develop other responses to trauma as well.

Jenkins and Bell (1997, p. 17) have created a table that lists 17 trauma-related disorders other than PTSD in children and adolescents. Some other typical responses of traumatized children, in addition to PTSD, include aggressive or antisocial behavior (about 18% of the time) and regressive behavior (about 13% of the time; Nader & Fletcher, 2014). Whatever the responses, we must recognize the serious detrimental effects of traumatic experiences on children's normal developmental course, whether or not they develop full-blown PTSD.

The Distinction between Victimization and Traumatization

It is important to distinguish between victimization and traumatization. Gil (1991) points out that a person may be victimized without being traumatized. That is, the person who experiences trauma is a victim during the traumatic event, but not every experience of being victimized qualifies as a traumatic experience in terms of causing responses of intense fear, helplessness, or horror. Thus not all children who witnessed the New York World Trade Center attack or who have been sexually abused react with the intense fear that results in PTSD. Furthermore, resilient children may not exhibit any overt signs of disturbed behavior. However, the fact that children do not respond immediately and conspicuously to the experience of abuse and trauma does not mean that it has had no effect on them.

On an emotional level, child witnesses to family and community violence may experience a range of feelings, from fear to helplessness to violent revenge fantasies. It can be very helpful to them to draw and/or verbalize their wishes for revenge in a debriefing interview that "partially corrects the passive helplessness of the witness role" (Pynoos & Eth, 1986, p. 316).

Another typical reaction of children who witness family and community violence is posttraumatic guilt, connected to the children's imagined failure to intervene and prevent the violence. This response needs to be challenged with gentleness and reality testing, in terms of a child's size and dependent role in a family, in comparison with the size and controlling role of adults. Bevin (1999), in a case demonstration, illustrates how to permit a boy's *wish* for revenge on the man who raped his mother, while realistically questioning the possibility of a 9-year-old's being physically able to defend his mother against the attack of an adult male. Similar responses of gentle disbelief by a social worker can reduce a child's feelings of responsibility for somehow contributing to or failing to prevent a parent's death by not intervening in a situation of community violence, such as a drive-by shooting or a terrorist bombing.

A particularly terrifying experience for a child witness is the death of a sibling, especially when it occurs through the neglect or intent of a parent in a family that routinely uses battering and other forms of violence to settle marital disputes and to "discipline" children. The case of the siblings of Elisa Izquierdo (Bruni, 1995) illustrates the horror of alleged maternal homicide in families in which the deceased child was both physically and sexually abused by the parents.

Bereavement after homicide often generates a pathological response in survivors that is related to the nature of the death, which involves a combination of violence, violation, and volition, according to Rando (1993, citing Rynearson, 1987). The response of a child to a homicidal death in the family or community may be intensified by the "degree of identification with the victim" (Rando, 1993, p. 538). Thus, the closer in age and gender the child is to the victim, the more threatening the death. Steele (1998), in a video involving the three siblings of their murdered 16-year-old sister, used a drawing method to help each child deal with the traumatic memories by having them draw their mental picture of how their sister's body looked after she was dead. The children appeared to experience relief after completing the drawing, as this allowed them to mourn and to share their internalized trauma picture with the social worker, who supported and validated their feelings. The fact that this therapy occurred 1 year after the sister's death may have made the drawing exercise more feasible than if the therapy sessions were soon after the murder, when the children may have been reluctant to participate in such a review.

SELECTED HELPING METHODS

Most children in therapy would benefit from activities and exercises that help them learn to identify their own feelings. However, children with chronic abuse histories and associated attachment problems may be very deficient in this area and require a great deal of help in understanding their own feeling responses, as well as the reactions of other people. As previously discussed, these children are confused about the appropriate expression of feelings. The drawing exercises described here help children identify their own feelings and understand more fully how emotions lead to behaviors. The exercises can be used in individual or group therapy. Of course, the child's personal safety should be a number one priority, and the therapeutic exercises below assume that the child is no longer living in an abusive situation. Space does not permit discussion of treatment efforts geared toward the abusing adults, which must also be part of the comprehensive plan for helping the family.

Drawing Exercises to Identify Feelings

Because many abused children come from family backgrounds in which love and aggression were confused, and because this may create uncertainty about how to relate to peers and adults, it is often helpful to establish a therapy goal of naming and talking about a range of different feelings, such as "sad," "angry," "happy," "guilty," and "proud." The task of the social worker and others involved with such children is to help them "own" their emotional reactions to the events in their *present* lives, with the expectation that this will facilitate the gradual sorting out of the confused feelings related to their past experiences of abuse.

Feelings Faces and the Body Map of Feelings

One method to help children identify and talk about feelings is to ask them to draw faces with different emotional expressions. An exercise that will facilitate this is the Feelings Faces exercise (Heegaard, 1991), discussed in Chapter 12. Starting with a circle to represent a head and the word "happy" underneath, the worker invites the child to draw a happy face (see Figure 14.4). While the child is drawing, the worker asks the child about the kinds of things that make him or her happy and lists these on a separate piece of paper. Next, the Body Map of Feelings (Gregory, 1990; Heegaard, 1991), also discussed in Chapter 12, can be introduced. This is simply an outline of a human body (see Figure 14.5). The worker asks the child to close his or her eyes and think about a time when he or she was very, very happy, then to open his or her eyes and draw with a yellow marker the places on the body where the child felt the happiness.

This three-step process (Feelings Faces, the list of associated feelings, and the Body Map of Feelings) can be repeated in other sessions for other feelings, such as "sad," "angry," "afraid," "nervous," "guilty," and "jealous." I recommend that initially only *one* feeling be addressed in each session, especially with children who tend to confuse different emotions. Later the worker can introduce the idea of more than one feeling at a time by asking the child to pick two feelings that might coexist and then asking him or her to describe and draw a picture of a situation in which that coexistence happened. The child needs to understand that he or she can have different feelings toward a person simultaneously. This is especially important for abused children, who may have coexisting loving and angry feelings toward their abusing parents. This was definitely evident in the Barbie case, when she stated that just because her father hit her that didn't mean that he didn't love her.

FIGURE 14.4. Outline for drawing a happy face in the Feeling Faces exercise.

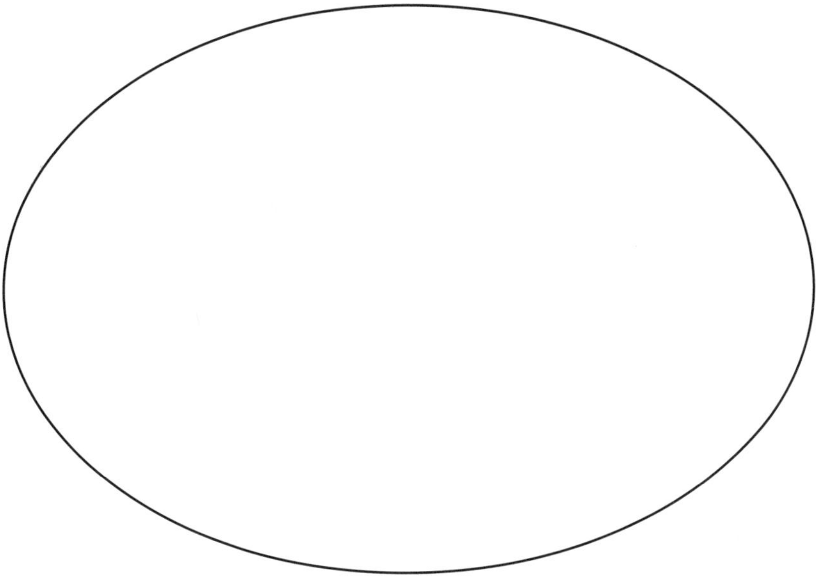

HAPPY

If all the child's drawings are kept in a folder, the child can later be invited to make "a feelings book" by stapling the separate pages together and creating a special cover for the book.

Stories and Workbooks for Children Ages 4–10

The Bureau for At-Risk Youth (located in Plainview, New York) has published a series of picture-story workbooks (Alexander, 1992) intended for traumatized children and children who have witnessed and experienced family violence. These story workbooks include sketches of children in frightening situations; one such sketch depicts a small boy listening at night in bed to his parents fighting (see Figure 14.6). On the facing blank page, the child is encouraged to draw and color what happened in his or her own house. Another sketch shows a child talking and playing with a counselor, who is pictured making helpful comments to the child, such as "Lots of people don't hit each other when they have angry feelings." The child, in turn, is pictured as saying, "I'm learning that I can use my words when I feel like fighting. I practice how with my counselor" (Alexander, 1992, p. 16). On the facing blank page, the child is invited to draw what he or she can do instead of fighting. These workbooks are available at discounted rates for bulk orders; they

FIGURE 14.5. The Body Map of Feelings. From Gregory (1990). Copyright © 1990 Family and Community Development Program, Lethbridge, Alberta, Canada. Reprinted by permission. (Although Gregory developed the Body Map of Feelings for use in working with children, neither she nor the Family and Community Development Program claims originality of the idea.)

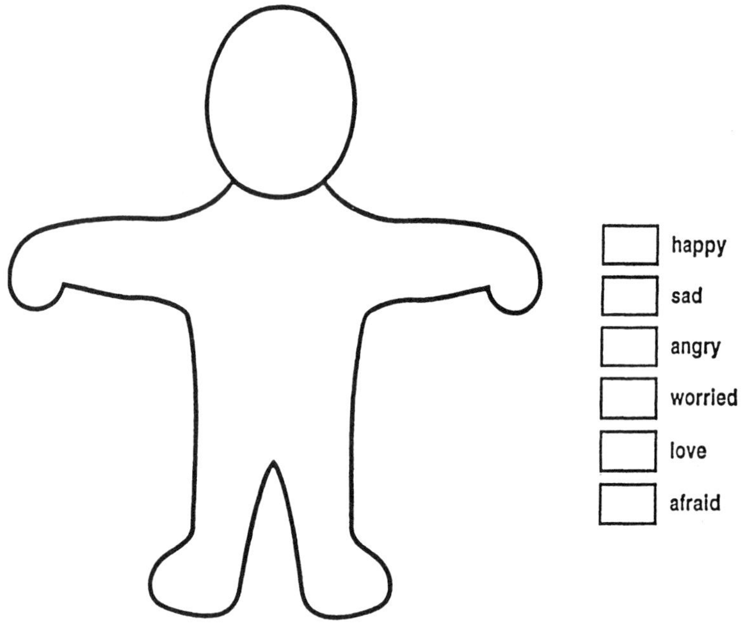

can be used in a group session a few pages at a time or by an individual child and counselor at the child's own pace.

Board and Card Games Dealing with Feelings

Therapeutic board games, such as the Talking, Feeling, and Doing Game and Feelings Playing Cards (both of which have been mentioned in earlier chapters; see Figure 3.3 and Table 4.1), may be especially useful in work with abused children. They provide structured activities that appeal to school-age children, while also offering excellent opportunities to talk about different feelings during the game.

Children who have problems with aggression may benefit from playing commercial board games such as Sorry! and Battleship which provide structured methods for "attacking" the other player while complying with the rules of the game. The worker uses the game to discuss aggressive themes during the play. Docker-Drysdale (1993) points out that children whose histories of deprivation and/or abuse contribute to severe developmental problems need appropriate outlets for their aggression.

FIGURE 14.6. Child listening to parents fighting. From Alexander (1992, p. 28). Copyright © 1992 Bureau for At-Risk Youth. Reprinted by permission.

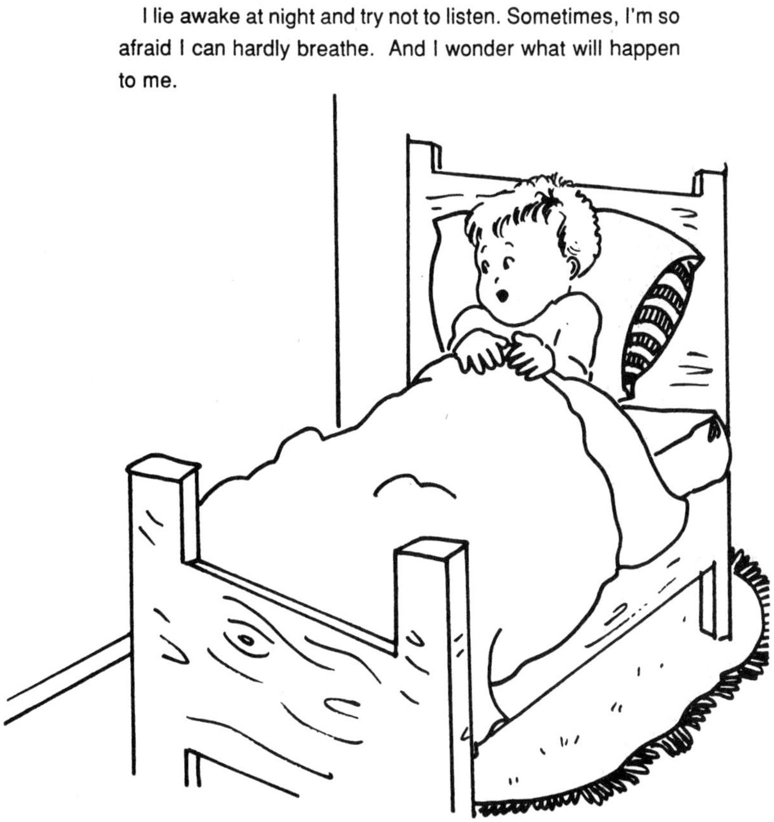

Animal-Assisted Therapy for Crisis Victims

The use of pets in therapy with children dates from the pioneering work of the psychologist Boris Levinson, whose 1969 book *Pet-Oriented Child Psychotherapy* describes his accidental discovery of the efficacy of his pet dog in stimulating the conversation of a difficult, previously noncommunicative child (see George, 1988, for a discussion). Levinson's work over the next decade convinced him and others that involvement with an animal helps children develop empathy, self-esteem, and autonomy, while also reducing their feelings of alienation (Levinson, 1978). He also emphasized the value of animal therapy for abused children who are afraid of human contact (Levinson, 1962).

Note. I acknowledge the contribution of Kay Scott, ACSW, in this section and in the Marta case.

Over the years, animal-assisted therapy has been used effectively, employing horses, dogs, cats, and other animals. For example, teaching physically disabled children to groom and ride horses gives the children a sense of efficacy, empowerment, and improved self-esteem (Pegasus Therapeutic Riding, 2001). In animal-assisted therapy, the mental health specialist uses the animal in a deliberate way to communicate with the child and to help the child express a range of feelings.

Treatment of Attachment Disorder

In the first edition of this book, I presented the case of a girl, Dorinda, who had a history of parental neglect and physical, emotional, and sexual abuse and who, in addition, witnessed the violent death of her 18 month-old sister (Webb, 1996). After failing to adapt in five different foster homes, Dorinda was placed in a residential treatment center that employed animal-assisted therapy. There she learned to identify a range of feelings and develop empathy with a pet rabbit. Counseling sessions with a social work student using the rabbit as a "cotherapist" over the course of 11 months contributed to substantial improvements in this girl's ability to relate to her peers and to adults.

In Situations of Crisis or Trauma

Therapy animals, in collaboration with an animal handler and a trained mental health professional, can also assist in situations of crisis or trauma (see Figure 14.7). This collaboration was used very effectively to engage and help many families following the New York World Trade Center and Pentagon terrorist attacks on September 11, 2001. The goals in this form of crisis intervention

FIGURE 14.7. A therapy dog named Diamond, who is trained to interact with children and adults in crisis situations under the guidance of an animal handler. Photo: Barry Rosen.

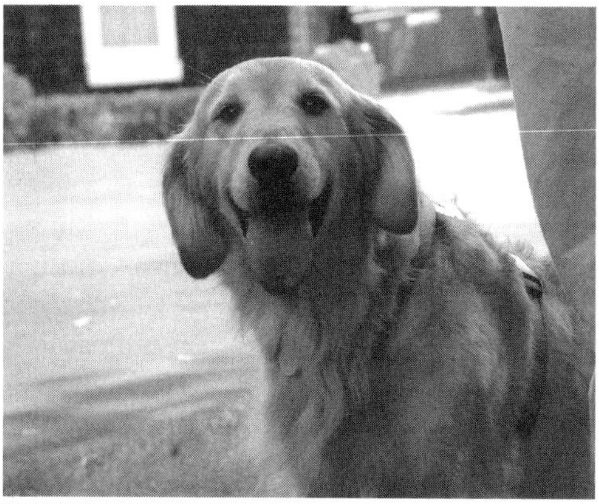

work depend on the specific situation and the needs of the affected individuals. These may range from providing comfort and pleasure through physical contact with the animal to interactions that are deliberately focused on helping children express their feelings.

THE CASE OF MARTA, AGE 5, WHOSE FATHER DIED IN THE NEW YORK WORLD TRADE CENTER TERRORIST ATTACK: AN EXAMPLE OF COMMUNITY VIOLENCE

(This case is a fictionalized composite of several similar family situations. Any similarity to real persons is purely coincidental.)

Family Information

Marta is a 5-year-old Puerto Rican child whose father worked in a restaurant in the New York World Trade Center. She is an only child. The family is bilingual, and Marta has extended family in the metropolitan New York area.

Following the attacks, Marta's mother would sit for hours watching the television replays of the events and the people escaping from the buildings. Holding Marta in her lap, Marta's mother would cry and say, "Watch for Papa. Is he there? Where is he?"

Presenting Problem

Marta's mother had explained to the child that her father was in the towers when they fell. They were waiting for some news about whether he had escaped or was in a hospital or if his body had been found. Marta saw her mother crying and heard the whispers of the relatives and friends who visited them. Marta tried to pretend everything was all right, and she refused to talk about her father. A few days after the attacks, when Marta's mother told her that her father was not coming home again, she began wetting the bed and having bad dreams.

Two weeks later Marta's mother went to the Family Assistance Center with Marta to obtain a death certificate in order to qualify for financial aid. She had been there earlier with Marta to register her husband's name and to leave his razor and comb for DNA samples. Marta's mother told the child that she now believed that her father had died and was not coming home.

Marta's mother spoke to a social worker at the Family Assistance Center, explaining her concern that her daughter had not accepted the fact that her father was not coming home. Despite several attempts by the social worker to engage Marta, the child refused to talk. She was playing on the floor next to her mother, ignoring the other children and the social worker, when several therapy animals and their handlers walked by. Marta noticed the large red golden retriever. The social worker asked Marta's mother if it was all right for her to introduce Marta to the animal; the mother nodded her agreement. The social worker then motioned to the therapy dog's handler to bring the dog over. The following interaction occurred:

SOCIAL WORKER: Marta, I saw you looking at the dog; would you like to pet him?

MARTA: (*Looks up and nods.*) *Sí.*

(The handler and the dog come over.)

SOCIAL WORKER: (*to handler*) What's your dog's name?

HANDLER: This is Tucker. (*to Marta*) Would you like to pet him?

MARTA: (*Nods "Yes."*)

(The handler puts Tucker in a down position beside Marta and places one of Marta's hands on Tucker. Marta runs her hand over the dog's fur. The handler shows Marta how dogs like to be rubbed under the ears and along the sides of the body. The handler and the social worker talk to Marta for a moment about the softness of Tucker's fur.)

SOCIAL WORKER: Marta, you really seem to like the dog and you're very gentle with him. Do you have a dog?

MARTA: (*Looks up and answers softly.*) *Sí.* (*Begins to talk about her dog—a boxer named Tia who is home in their apartment. She says that her father got the dog for her. She says that he taught her how to give Tia fresh water.*) He loves Tia. (*Hugs Tucker.*)

SOCIAL WORKER: He??

MARTA: *Mi papa.* My dad.

SOCIAL WORKER: So, what do you think Tia feels about your dad not coming home?

MARTA: I know she's sad. She cries at night. I hear her crying.

SOCIAL WORKER: Crying?

MARTA: *Sí.* My papa told me that dogs dream. Tia's having bad dreams. She cries like me, like my mama. (*Grows quiet and continues to stroke Tucker's fur.*) She misses my papa.

SOCIAL WORKER: Who misses your papa?

MARTA: Mama.

SOCIAL WORKER: And I bet you miss your papa too. (*Marta nods.*) Can you tell your mama that you miss your papa?

MARTA: (*Looks down.*) She's sad. I don't want to make her sadder.

SOCIAL WORKER: And she'll be sad if you say it to her? (*Marta nods.*) What if you told Tucker? Could you tell Tucker?

(Marta nods and puts her head against Tucker. She whispers to Tucker, then begins to cry. Her mother puts her arm around Marta and they cry together. They talk softly in Spanish.)

The social worker decided to refer Marta and her mother to a mental health agency that uses animals as adjuncts in longer-term therapy. She considered the possibility that Marta could be diagnosed with PTSD if her symptoms continued another week, and she wanted to be sure that the child would receive some specialized assistance for her traumatic bereavement. Marta's mother would also be invited to attend a bereavement group at the agency.

Considerations in Animal-Assisted Therapy

Whenever possible, parental permission should be obtained prior to involving animals in an interaction with a child. Because various cultures have different views about companion animals, some clients would neither understand nor approve their use in a therapy situation as just described. For example, most Jamaicans keep animals outside and do not consider them as "indoor pets" or as part of the family, in contrast to many families in the United States. And many Muslims consider dogs to be unclean. Therefore, the worker must show cultural sensitivity toward the family's beliefs about animals, ask about these beliefs, and always obtain permission prior to beginning animal-assisted therapy.

Social workers interested in using animals as adjuncts in their treatment of children should inquire about the training and screening of the animals and the handlers before involving them in the work. Untrained and unscreened animals should never be used. Training and/or screening for animal–handler teams is conducted by various national, regional, and local animal-assisted-therapy organizations and registries. For example, Delta Society (*www.deltasociety.org*) offers a publication detailing standards of practice for animal-assisted therapy and activities. Other organizations and registries include Therapy Dogs International (TDI), Hudson Valley Animal-Assisted Crisis Response Coalition (*www.k9crisisresponse.org*), and HOPE Crisis Response (*www.hopeaacr.org*). The latter two organizations provide animals trained for a variety of disaster and crisis situations, including work with rescuers.

GROUP APPROACHES

For Abused Children

According to the *Harvard Mental Health Letter* ("Child Abuse: Part III," 1993),

> there is no accepted formula for treating children and adults who are victims of incest or physical abuse. Since the symptoms vary a great deal, many kinds of psychotherapy and medication may be appropriate, and there are no controlled studies of outcome. . . . Surveys indicate that professionals experienced in treating victims of child abuse prefer group therapy above all other kinds of treatment, especially for adult female survivors but also for men, adolescents, and children. . . . Group members with similar experiences are an ideal audience, certain to understand or sympathize. (pp. 2–3)

The many advantages and types of therapy and activity groups were discussed in detail in Chapter 8. This section focuses on using a group intervention to help children who had experienced violence and/or abuse. A time-limited, school-based group can help the participants deal with their feelings of shame and vulnerability, while also enhancing their feelings of self-esteem and their understanding of how to use appropriate limits in relationships.

Details of a 12-session group for children who had witnessed violence was presented by Nisivoccia and Lynn (1999). This group consisted of nine girls between 9 and 11 years of age. The goal was to help the youngsters develop new patterns of interaction through other means than dominance and abuse. All were experiencing some difficulties in school and had been given parental permission to attend the group.

The group sessions included a variety of activities to deal with the following topics:

- Identification and expression of feelings.
- Issues of isolation and shame.
- Establishing responsibility for the violence.
- Conflict resolution.

Although the authors recognize that a group intervention cannot change a child's home or neighborhood environment, they emphasize that the group experience did help the children to feel less alone and to experience a trusting relationship with an adult (the leader), as well as meaningful peer relationships.

For Children Exposed to Family and Community Violence

Another elementary-school-based intervention program used a combination of individual and group psychotherapy and mentorship in an effort to help children exposed to violent behavior in a community with a high rate of crime and violence (Murphy, Pynoos, & James, 1997). This comprehensive mental health program for children and their families targeted children who had been exposed to violence in their homes and in the community. Many of these children lived with daily exposure to violence in their communities and were preoccupied with aggressive, retaliation/revenge fantasies. The program included specific interventions designed to address these directly, while also promoting more constructive responses through activities, discussion, and ongoing mentorship with adults who offered examples of nonaggressive and constructive responses to community violence.

As a method for dealing directly with children's exposure to horrific events during the course of the school year, the staff used Pynoos and Nader's psychological-first-aid classroom consultation format (1988, 1993) to open a discussion with the class about their experiences, after which they involved the children in two drawing exercises: one to permit the children to show their feelings about what happened, and the other to show how they wished things could have been different. During this trauma-focused drawing and storytelling activity, each child was seen individually, with referrals to a crisis trauma group for children most affected by exposure to the violence. This intensive, comprehensive mental health program recognized the detrimental effects of exposure to all forms of violence on children and targeted intervention in an elementary school, based on the belief that schools provide the most accessible, functional, and efficient setting in which to provide these services. A similar point has been made by Garbarino et al. (1992), who state that teachers who let children play out their fears of danger serve as psychic healers for children who are living in a state of "chronic, not posttraumatic stress" (p. 221).

PREVENTIVE APPROACHES TO FAMILY AND COMMUNITY VIOLENCE

Helping children cope with their confused feelings related to family and community violence does not deal with the problem at its roots. Unfortunately, U.S. society condones and even glamorizes (in movies and on television) the aggressive, abusive behavior of the strong toward the weak. The stage is set for violence when social values sanction the use of force against women and children and between adults who decide their differences with their fists and weapons, rather than through their brains.

The problem of family and community violence must be confronted on many levels. My emphasis in this chapter on the child witnesses and victims does not imply disregard for essential interventions on the familial, societal, and community levels. Chapter 17 discusses the need for clinicians and advocates on behalf of children to join forces and work toward common goals. Perhaps nowhere is this joining of purpose more essential than with reference to the child's right to grow up in a safe and nurturing home and community environment. It is therefore undeniable that to help children *in the long run,* we must focus on improving the life conditions of their parents, families, and communities.

SELF-CARE STRATEGIES TO HELP PRACTITIONERS AVOID VICARIOUS TRAUMATIZATION

It is difficult and emotionally draining for social work practitioners who are involved in helping child victims of family and/or community violence. Listening to accounts of abuse and witnessing its impact on helpless children can make any adult feel angry. Empathic social workers are particularly vulnerable to these feelings because their responsibility is to help the child. When the helping involves removing the child from his or her home, the experience can be gut-wrenching, both for the child and the worker! Although the worker knows that removal is in the long-term best interests of the child, carrying out this function can take a toll, because the child is terrified and angry about the unknown future.

Social workers who deal with children who have endured physical and sexual abuse must find ways to cope effectively with their own painful responses to the realities of their work. Without attention to necessary self-care methods, social workers can become overwhelmed by their responsibilities and unable to function at their best. These reactions have been labeled "vicarious traumatization," "secondary traumatization," and "burn-out." This can lead to ineffective practice, or, at the extreme, to job loss. Methods for confronting these negative outcomes include the following:

- Regular clinical supervision in which the worker discusses his or her feelings about the work and receives validation and support.
- Self-awareness and a commitment to maintaining balance in one's life.
- Engaging in mindfulness and/or spiritual meditation.
- Utilizing daily relaxation and recreational practices.

Space does not permit further discussion here; readers may consult Maschi (2015) for a full discussion of this topic.

CONCLUDING COMMENTS

Most social workers whose practice puts them in contact with children will sooner or later become involved with a case of physical or sexual child abuse; many also will be called to help with conflicts at schools or between neighborhood gangs. Because of the magnitude of the problem, it is unavoidable. Some workers find it impossible to accept the evidence of parental abuse of children, joining in society's denial of the fact that parents, who are supposed to protect their children, can instead sometimes behave in a manner that threatens their children's physical, mental, and emotional health.

A frequent consequence of violence and abuse is an increase in aggressive behavior in the victim (Englander & Lawson, 2007; Jenkins & Bell, 1997;

Nader & Fletcher, 2014). Of course, there are many intervening factors, and other influences besides abusing parents and bullying peers contribute to violent behavior. Perhaps the ultimate question, however, is *why* parents feel the need to resort to hurting their children, or *why* bullies feel the need to persecute and demean their peers. This topic is explored further in the next chapter.

The problem can be addressed on a macro level, recognizing the stresses on parents due to poverty, substance abuse, and ignorance. A wide-angle view focused on social factors clearly has merit. Meanwhile, on a micro level, the children are learning that parents who love them can also hurt them. Children are also learning that when our country is attacked, we fight back with weapons of destruction and that we have reasons to fight wars in different parts of the world. Violence is pervasive in our society, and it is difficult to counteract the lessons learned at home, in the community, and on a global level.

DISCUSSION QUESTIONS

1. Outline a treatment plan for the five siblings of Elisa Izquierdo, ages 2–9, who were placed in custody following the imprisonment of their mother for the murder of their sister (Bruni, 1995).
2. Consider the probable reaction of a 4-year-old who witnessed the sudden, violent death of a sibling. What interventions would be appropriate to help the preschool-age witness?
3. What are some methods for helping children with their revenge fantasies after they have witnessed the death of a neighborhood friend in a drive-by shooting? Do you think there is a danger that permitting a child to express these feelings in play therapy may stimulate him or her to act them out? What can the worker do to avoid this possibility?
4. Discuss the effect on the worker of interacting with a child who has witnessed or experienced severe abuse. How can the worker deal with his or her own reactions?

CHAPTER 15

The Interpersonal Violence of Bullying

Its Impact on Victims, Perpetrators, and Bystanders/Witnesses

Interpersonal violence in the form of peer abuse or bullying is not a new problem, but there has been growing interest in the topic, as demonstrated in a 200% increase in published articles and books on bullying in the years from 1997 to 2007 (Swearer, Espelage, & Napolitano, 2009). The aggressive behavior of bullying involves an imbalance of power between the perpetrator and the target and may include face-to-face or covert confrontations in the form of intimidating physical, relational (i.e., between two people), or online attacks (cyberbullying). Nationwide statistics report that between one in six and one in four students are frequently bullied in school (Englander & Lawson, 2007, citing Nansel et al., 2001). Studies have shown that bullying begins in elementary school, peaks in middle school, and is somewhat less frequent in high school (Banks, 1997). Schools can feel like dangerous places because of the taunts of bullies and the existence of gangs and their accompanying violence in and around the school buildings. Furthermore, bullying behavior is now spreading to new locations. Whereas it used to occur in the schoolyard, the school bus, bathrooms, or hallways, technology now makes possible the anonymous dissemination of insulting and hurtful messages and photographs on the Internet, thereby making the child victim's life full of ongoing torment, with no place to hide.

Several high-profile suicides of adolescent victims of bullying have drawn public attention to this problem. As tragic as these cases are, this chapter focuses on violent interpersonal behavior in the *elementary schools* because the focus of this book is on children up to preadolescence and also because there has been less attention given to early incidences of bullying behavior and to some possible methods of dealing with it. According to Olweus (1993), bullying happens most frequently in grades 4–8, but potential bullies can be easily identified as early as preschool if we recognize the warning signs (Weinhold, 2003). One study found that approximately 20% of kindergarten children reported being frequently victimized (Kochenderfer & Ladd, 1996). It is notable also that aggressive students in elementary schools tend to be the same students who are aggressive in middle and high school (Harachi et al., 2006). In studying bullying behavior, our concern and focus must be multifaceted and include the repercussions for the victim, the perpetrator, and the bystanders and the serious implications for the school community and the family members of those involved.

DEFINITIONS AND IMPACT OF BULLYING

As indicated previously, bullying consists of aggressive behavior characterized by an imbalance of power that occurs repeatedly and is intentionally harmful (Olweus, Limber, & Mihalic, 1999). In its simplest form bullying occurs between one person and his or her identified victim. An example may involve a verbal threat to do some harm to the person or a negative statement about the youth's appearance, walk, manner of speech, or school performance. The aggression of bullying includes three key features: (1) the *intent* to harm the victim, (2) the occurrence of the bullying *repeatedly* over a period of time, and (3) *imbalance of power* in the bully–victim relationship (Green & Myrick, 2015, citing Nansel et al., 2001). My husband, a retired college professor, still remembers being threatened by a boy in fourth grade who said that he was going to kill him. He doesn't remember what precipitated this threat, but he took it very seriously and changed his usual route for several days when walking home after school. He never had another confrontation with this aggressive boy, but the fact that he still remembers this experience more than 60 years later attests to the anxiety and fear that the threats of bullies can arouse. This is not a typical case, since bullying behavior usually persists, repeats, and escalates over time. Frequently the bully is accompanied by two or three "henchmen" or followers who give him or her psychological and physical support by serving as backup and whose presence adds further weight to whatever the bully says or does to the victim. The problems associated with this behavior are long lasting for both the bully and the victim, as described below (Englander & Lawson, 2007).

Effects on Victims

The lingering memories of childhood experiences with bullies are confirmed in a front-page article in the *Boston Globe* (Russell, 2010) that gives lengthy examples of adult men who still recall with great trepidation their experiences of being bullied as boys. The *Globe* interviewed more than 100 adults who were victims of bullies and who shared their stories. Their reported reasons for becoming victims ranged from having a physical deformity or an "effeminate" voice to being overweight or just new to the school. Unfortunately, the victim often internalizes some of the bully's cruel criticisms and begins to feel shame, self-loathing, and greatly diminished self-esteem. Feelings of estrangement from peers continued to permeate the lives of many of the self-identified victims in the *Globe* article throughout their adulthood, even into retirement! This confirms other reports indicating that many victims suffer from depression, including suicidal thoughts and behaviors (Fox, Elliott, Kerlikowske, Newman, & Christeson, 2003). The seriousness of these outcomes belies the traditional tendency of parents and teachers to minimize bullying behavior and counsel children to "just forget it." One man in the *Globe* article still recalls seeing his gym teacher watching with a "disgusted look" (but doing nothing) as he was beaten by several bullies in the locker room. In cases like this adults tend to blame the victim, rather than the perpetrator.

Effects on Perpetrators

Research has shown that children who bully usually become more violent over time (Garbarino & deLara, 2002) and are at high risk of ending up in the criminal justice system (Englander & Lawson, 2007). In fact, one study of boys classified as bullies between the sixth and ninth grades found that nearly 60% were convicted of at least one crime by the age of 24 (Fox et al., 2003). Obviously, this behavior should be taken very seriously, both for its effects on the victims and bystanders and for the negative impact on society in years to come.

The bully's accomplices may not actively engage in attacking, but they nonetheless bask in the status of being associated with the powerful bully. According to Englander and Lawson (2007), these "henchmen" may have poor self-esteem and poor social skills themselves, and they befriend the bully to avoid being victimized themselves.

Effects on Bystanders

Many bystanders simply watch bullying episodes and do nothing to try to stop them. Garbarino and deLara (2002, p. 2) state that "most children watch the bullying of their peers with a sense of helplessness, frozen in fear, with guilt and, ultimately, shame for doing nothing to help." The inaction of bystanders gives the bullies an audience and peer attention for their mean, abusive, and dominating behavior. The fact that no one openly disapproves or tries to stop the bully ultimately makes the aggressor more confident in his power, and the behavior continues unpunished.

Crossover Behaviors

As if to complicate matters further, experts who have studied bullying behaviors in schools point out that some students both bully others and are victimized themselves (Swearer et al., 2009). Especially in elementary school, students may move from bully to victim and vice versa (Dempsey, Fireman, & Wang, 2006).

Gender Considerations

Boys who are bullies tend to use direct physical and verbal attacks and are more likely to bully other boys (80%). Boys also are more likely than girls to be both perpetrators and victims of aggression. On the other hand, girl bullies tend to use more subtle and social methods such as ostracism, manipulation, and spreading rumors. Girls tend to bully only other girls using relational aggression (Nagin & Tremblay, 2001) and to bully in groups (Weinhold, 2003).

CAUSES OF BULLYING

Although every situation is unique, there are many different risk factors that seem to contribute to bullying behavior. As with any assessment of risk factors (and as discussed in Chapter 4), *no one factor* will determine a specific outcome because of the complexity of human nature and the varying influence of compensating protective factors. Nonetheless, Weinhold (2003) lists certain risk factors pertaining to bullies and organizes these according to *family factors, personality factors, school factors,* and *community factors.* These include the following:

- Violence directed at young children in the home (often by the mother and older siblings).
- Parents and older siblings who accept and model aggressive and/or bullying behavior.
- Desensitization caused by the prevalence of violence in the media.
- An impulsive, aggressive temperament, which makes a child more likely to develop into a bully (Olweus, 1993).
- Lack of empathy for others (Olweus, 1993).
- The belief, or rationalization, that the victim provoked the attack and deserves the consequences.
- Reduced adult supervision, which directly affects the frequency and severity of bullying in schools (Saunders, 1997).

A quick perusal of these selected factors possibly contributing to bullying makes it clear that intervention efforts intended to prevent or reduce bullying will have to encompass the home, the school, and the wider community, in addition to interventions focused on the individual.

Children's Exposure and Desensitization to Violence

Anyone who doubts that we live in a "culture of violence" only needs to watch daily TV news broadcasts to see the array of robberies, murders, and other violent events that children will see, even as they may observe their parents' positive, negative, or neutral responses to this highly publicized behavior. Of course, children's cartoon programs are also full of violence, and up until the middle elementary school years, children may not distinguish between the fantasy on the TV screen and the reality of their own everyday lives. Nader (2010, p. 216) states that "well-designed research has repeatedly shown that watching violence on electronic media increases the risk of behaving aggressively right after viewing and years later."

Unfortunately, the violence many children observe on TV also replicates what happens in their own families, in which disagreements may be routinely settled with verbal or physical abuse, and in which the strongest person usually ends up controlling the weaker ones. When a young child repeatedly witnesses or experiences marital discord, parent–child abuse, or sibling abuse, this can cause insecure attachment to the caretaking adults and a tendency for the child to model the seemingly powerful aggressive and bullying behaviors of parents and older siblings. According to Weinhold (2003), children who are constantly exposed to abuse or witness the abuse of others are likely to become hyperaroused due to adrenal stress reactions in their brains that keep them alert and ready to face any future conflict (Perry, 1996, 2006). It is as if they are persistently on guard and expecting trouble, and because of the subtleties of human motivation, they may decide to attack first before someone attacks them. Their identification with the behaviors of the abuser gives them a sense of mastery instead of helplessness. We know that children who are aggressive in elementary school tend to be the same students who are aggressive in middle and high school (Harachi et al., 2006). This behavior does not dissipate with time.

Sometimes children who are exposed to or are victims of violence in the home become traumatized and develop symptoms of PTSD. Often their anxiety is not recognized as such, and it may be mislabeled as oppositional defiant disorder or conduct disorder. A school social worker who understands the possibility of these dynamics can advocate on behalf of mental health services rather than punitive interventions for the bully. Approaches to help the families, the school community, and the children are discussed later in this chapter.

Children Who Are Different

Children strive to be like one another, and they feel uncomfortable when something about them makes them seem "different" from their peers. This difference can stem from anything out of the ordinary, such as the fact that they live in a home with two mothers, or that they lost their hair due to radiation treatments for cancer. Whereas most mature adults subscribe to a "live and let live" attitude and accept people who are or look different, children may feel threatened by kids who wear atypical clothes or who don't know how to fit in with the mainstream. Although the United States is composed of people of diverse nationalities and backgrounds, children who stand out from the majority risk becoming the target of bullies. Brown (1999), who conducted school workshops on bullying, lists over 25 qualities or features named by schoolmates that could cause students to be bullied. Minority kids are on the list, as are lesbians and boys who act like "fags."

Children with physical disabilities are twice as likely as nondisabled peers to be victims of bullying (Dawkins, 1996)

Because of the high-profile suicides of some gay adolescents who were bullied, this section discusses the specific pressures on lesbian, gay, bisexual, and transgender (LGBT) students in their struggle to form their own gender identities and to find a path toward acceptance among their straight peers in school.

Although there is controversy about when gender identity develops, numerous anecdotal accounts testify that some children feel uncomfortable about their biological gender as early as 5 years of age, and many LGBT adolescents who have come out maintain that they knew from a very early age that they were "different," but they did not speak up about their feelings because of fears of rejection or discrimination. (See Chapter 6 for a detailed discussion of issues related to gender development.) These children may reveal their nonconformity through their gender-atypical interests (e.g., a boy might feel attracted to female clothes or enjoy participating in art classes and be uninterested in sports and in other "masculine"-type activities). Reactions by the families of gender-atypical children vary from denial to quiet acceptance. Most families struggle to help the gender-atypical child "fit in," partly because of their own discomfort over how to handle the situation and also because they fear that their child will be ostracized if he or she renounces expected gender-specific behavior. However, often the child's physical gestures, manner of speech, and walking style may reveal some subtle gender identity issues that are noticed by peers and others. This can result in bullying of the child who is different, and even elementary-school-age children are familiar with pejorative terms such as "queer," "gay," "dike," "sissy," "tomboy," or "faggot." Obviously, this extreme scorn can have serious effects on a growing child's identity formation, especially when the young person senses that his or her parents do not understand or sympathize with him or her.

Many LGBT youth feel unsafe in school and unsupported at home, with the result that they grow into adolescence with a sense of alienation and isolation from their peers and their families. The victims of such verbal abuse soon learn that it is unacceptable to reveal any of their atypical interests or inclinations to others, so these youngsters try to hide their gender issues until adolescence, when they may find support groups or other ways to express their preferences. The point is that elementary-school-age children who are not comfortable with their biological gender have few, if any, supports either in their schools or elsewhere. These children may be bullied because they are different, and they may spend many of their growing years feeling cut off and estranged from their peers. Similar feelings of isolation and vulnerability also occur in children who are immigrants or refugees, in children who are disabled, or children who in some manner present as different from "the norm" and therefore are ostracized and/or bullied by their peers.

CYBERBULLYING OR INTERNET AGGRESSION

We live in an electronic world in which many schools expect and/or accept students' homework online and in which students as young as 8 or 9 years old have their own cell phones with Internet access. Children learn about social media, such as Facebook and Twitter, either through older siblings or peers, and they quickly become aware of the possibility of writing and sending insulting and personal messages about unpopular classmates.

Cyberbullying refers to intentional acts of aggression toward another person online (Ybarra & Mitchell, 2004). A unique feature of this type of bullying is that it can be done anonymously, and thereby it permits children who otherwise might not participate in bullying behavior to engage in it. Furthermore, unflattering or humiliating pictures or statements about an individual can be sent to hundreds of viewers, thereby multiplying the victimization experience and increasing the sense of helplessness of the victim. The youth rightly feels that there is no escape and that the entire world has been informed of his or her weaknesses. Several instances of suicide have occurred following such bullying behavior in which the victim felt desperate and humiliated. This form of bullying is difficult if not impossible to control, since it may occur in any location in the home or community and is not limited to the school environment.

The secrecy of cyberbullying permits groups of children to acquire and send humiliating pictures or insulting comments about a person without the knowledge or consent of the individual involved. Because of their immaturity and poor judgment, most young children often do not think or worry about the consequences of their actions, and therefore a "silly" photo of a former friend who was pretending to have large breasts by stuffing her bra can become a laughingstock for scores of classmates in the fifth grade and elsewhere. Although parents may complain to the schools when they learn about an escapade like this, the school really has no jurisdiction over what pupils do on weekends when they are meeting in small groups on their own.

ANTI-BULLYING INTERVENTION PROGRAMS

Helping approaches to prevent bullying must be multifaceted, because bullying does not occur in isolation, but rather results from a complex set of interactions between the individual and his or her family, peer group, school, community, and societal norms (Swearer & Espelage, 2004). As of April 2015, anti-bullying legislation has been passed in all 50 states (Temkin, 2015), with the requirement that all schools adopt a bullying prevention policy. However, as Temkin points out, passing a law is not enough, because resources must also be provided, with obligations to offer staff training and a comprehensive approach that includes bullying-prevention policies and programs.

The 10 best policy practices to help schools prevent bullying (from Swearer et al., 2009, p. 50) are the following:

1. Change the school climate.
2. Assess bullying/victimization.
3. Train *all* staff.
4. Create an anti-bullying advisory team.
5. Actively include staff, parents, and students.
6. Disseminate clear rules and consequences.
7. Increase adult supervision.
8. Provide consistent individual intervention.
9. Allow class time to focus on social-emotional learning.
10. Make these efforts ongoing.

A multitude of different programs have been implemented in various parts of the country to combat bullying (Espelage & Swearer, 2011; Zins, Elias, & Maher, 2007; Swearer, Limber, & Atley, 2009). These programs generally involve developing school rules prohibiting bullying, procedures for reporting and responding to bullying, and psychoeducation for students, school personnel, and parents (Swearer, Schwartz, & Garcia, 2015). Most of these incorporate the principles listed above.

Examples of research-based schoolwide programs for elementary students include:

- The Olweus Bullying Prevention Program (Olweus & Limber, 2002)
- Bully Busters (Horne, Bartolomucci, & Newman-Carlson, 2003)
- Steps to Respect (Committee for Children, 2011), and
- The Peaceful Schools Project (Twemlow et al., 2009)

Details of some additional programs are discussed briefly below.

Massachusetts Aggression Reduction Center Anti-Bullying Program

An innovative anti-bullying program in Massachusetts aims to raise schoolwide awareness about bullying through involving trained college students working with high school students to help them lead anti-bullying programs in their schools (Englander & Lawson, 2007). This use of high-status peers as educators and mentors holds promise for effective results, since younger students look up to the older college students as role models. This program targets high schools and does not have a component for use in elementary schools.

Kindness Campaign to Curb Bullying and School Violence

Begun in 1994 at the University of Colorado at Colorado Springs, this program was designed as a primary prevention program to deal with violence among youth in families and schools (Weinhold, 2003). The campaign is based on the concept of substituting kindness for the aggressive behavior of bullying.

The program includes an activity guide for preschools (with 36 field-tested activities), a curriculum guide for elementary schools (with 54 activities), and a peer mediation/conflict resolution program for middle and high schools. It also has components for teachers, for parents, and for local businesses who arrange for employees to volunteer at schools as tutors or classroom aides. This comprehensive program, which has spread to at least 12 other U.S. cities, received an award in 1997, naming the city of Colorado Springs a Community of Kindness.

Comment

This program is exceptional for its broad view of bullying and human rights and its recognition of the possible trauma-related effects of violence and aggressive behaviors on young people. It includes the family and the community, in addition to the school.

Expect Respect Elementary School Project

Sponsored by a grant awarded by the Centers for Disease Control and Prevention in 1997, this 3-year project (Sanchez et al., 2001) in Austin, Texas, was designed to help schools address bullying and sexual harassment on their campuses. It sought to reduce sexual harassment by focusing on staff training, classroom education, parent education, policy development, and support services in the elementary schools so that students would not come to accept mistreatment as the norm in their peer relationships.

The project consisted of 12 weekly sessions with fifth-grade students using a guide (Stein, 1996) that was intended to help students distinguish between playful teasing and hurtful teasing/bullying. The lessons included writing assignments, role plays, and class discussions. The staff training component encompassed all adults, including teachers and even bus drivers, and focused on the research on bullying and strategies for response. Newsletters were addressed to parents to keep them informed about this project, and periodic seminars were offered for parents as well.

After a year, staff and students all reported that there had been a reduction in bullying behavior. The conclusion was that a project such as this can succeed when it has the full support of administration and staff, as well as a schoolwide commitment to the project's goals.

Comment

This project is commendable for its comprehensive inclusion of the entire school community, based on its philosophy that the students alone cannot change aggressive behavior that has been allowed to continue. It is logical that intervening at the elementary-school level with the goal of increasing awareness about bullying can bring about a significant reduction in this behavior.

The question for future research is whether a 12-week program will have long-term results or whether there must be ongoing educational efforts to continue the reduction in this behavior.

Teaching School-Age Children Conflict Management Skills

Children learn from examples at home, and what they learn is repeated in their own interactions with their peers. A school-based peer mediation program (Gentry & Beneson, 1993) attempted to teach anger management in fourth to sixth grades in the hope that this learning would transfer to the home. This approach to conflict management helped children understand that tensions and disputes can be resolved through the following specific rules of mediation:

- Agreeing to solve the problem.
- Not interrupting.
- Telling the truth.
- Avoiding name-calling or putdowns.

Trained peer mediators helped students deal with problems. The rationale for this program rested on the belief that the behaviors of children in one setting would transfer to another. This proved to be the case when conflict management was learned and practiced in the school: The skills appeared to generalize to the home setting for use with family members, particularly siblings (Gentry & Beneson, 1993, p. 72).

Comment

Because all children go to school, the potential of this setting for interpersonal learning must be recognized and used to the fullest. Attempts to teach children constructive ways to deal with intense emotions constitute a rich opportunity to interrupt the intergenerational transmission of family and community violence. It is gratifying to know that more than 8,500 of the approximately 85,000 schools in the country teach conflict resolution to all students (National Institute for Dispute Resolution, 1999). An update on these statistics was not available.

Bullying Intervention Program

This program (Swearer & Givens, 2006) is an alternative to school suspension or expulsion for aggressive bullying behaviors. It has been implemented in several elementary and middle schools in Nebraska. The program involves school counselors and school psychologists working one to one with bullying students for a 3-hour cognitive-behavioral intervention. In this, an assessment is completed, a 2-hour psychoeducational session is given, including a video, and the conclusion focuses on the student's reflection about the material and its relevance to his or her own experience. This program involved children ages 8–14 years in grades 3–8. No empirical data were available, but the authors believe that the program is effective in helping students better understand the effects of bullying.

INTERVENTIONS WITH THE INDIVIDUAL CHILD

In addition to the large-scale approaches reviewed above that target the entire school in bullying prevention programs, interventions that involve the individual aggressive child who employs bullying behavior may be helpful. We know that aggressive children and adolescents are at risk for numerous negative outcomes, such as academic, social, and behavioral difficulties (Crick & Dodge, 1996), and therefore schools should either make referrals to mental health clinics or offer individual treatment in the school setting to help bullying children learn to reduce their aggressive behaviors. Swearer and colleagues (2015) give examples of play therapy interventions for aggressive children, including the use of bibliotherapy (with an extensive list of books about bullying to use with elementary school children; Swearer, Espelage, & Napolitano, 2009), and the inclusion of parents in therapy with children to encourage increased use of positive parental practices (Davenport & Bourgeois, 2008).

CONCLUDING COMMENTS

Bullying is a complicated interaction that involves not only the bully and the victim, but also all those who know about the act of intimidation and who may experience fear and anxiety related to witnessing the deliberate cruelty of one or more persons against another. Some people maintain that we live in a culture of violence and that bullies are simply replicating what they witness at home or in their community or the media. But all children who are exposed to violence in their homes and communities do not become bullies. Maybe someone in their lives expressed admiration and respect for them. Maybe they have some religious training that provides a meaningful foundation for a positive view of others. If schools, parents, and society can find ways to nourish children's spiritual and emotional needs, they are more likely to develop respect for the rights of others and learn to tolerate differences.

This chapter has presented several intervention models aimed at sensitizing individuals in the schools, the home, and the wider community to the need for respect for others' rights. Let us hope that with more attention to this topic and with efforts to intervene in the elementary schools, children will no longer have to fear aggressive assaults that threaten their safety and basic identities.

DISCUSSION QUESTIONS

1. Were you ever bullied in elementary school? If so, please discuss with a partner the circumstances, and whether you told any adult about this, and if not, why not. Did you have any thoughts at the time about what you would like to have an adult do? In retrospect, how do you think it should have been handled?
2. If you learn that a sixth grader is being bullied on the Internet, how would you handle this? How would you help the child make a decision about whether and to whom to report this?
3. If you are a school social worker in an elementary school and you become aware that there are some "cliques" or "gangs" of third- or fifth-grade students who routinely pick on peers who do well in their schoolwork, how would you respond? What steps would you take first? Set up a plan for a gradewide anti-bullying intervention. How would you structure this? Would you include the parents? Why or why not?

CHAPTER 16

Immigrant and Refugee Children

The United States is a country of immigrants and refugees. Except for Native Americans, the ancestors of *all* U.S. citizens came from other countries. However, after several generations are born and grow up in the United States, many people tend to downplay their countries of origin; they identify themselves only as Americans, and this conviction sometimes is tinged with a coating of superiority over recent immigrants and refugees. Furthermore, the political climate of 2018 has uncovered a marked suspicion and hostility among many people toward immigrants or refugees who have entered the United States without documentation and who subsequently have given birth to children who, by law, enjoy all the rights of citizenship. Although the children of these undocumented immigrants/refugees have legal status, their parents do not, which means that the parents live in constant danger of being deported. When a parent is apprehended and deportation is threatened, he or she must contemplate the alternatives of either taking the children with him or her or leaving them in the United States in the care of relatives or friends. The ever-present possibility of deportation causes these families to live in constant states of uncertainty, anxiety, and fear, even for the children who have citizen status.

The dictionary defines the term "immigrant" as a person who migrates to another country, usually for permanent residence, whereas the term "refugee" applies to someone who has been forced to leave his or her country to escape war, persecution, violence, or natural disaster. Immigrants typically apply ahead of time for legal documentation (a visa) that permits them to enter the country for a designated period with the option to later seek permanent residence; in contrast, refugees usually relocate under the pressure of great fear and anxiety, without the opportunity to obtain the necessary papers to give them legal status.

This chapter discusses the numerous challenges facing immigrant and refugee children and their families and the role of social workers in facilitating the assimilation process and helping the children grow and develop into productive citizens. Social workers may interact with immigrants and refugees in various locales in the community, ranging from medical settings to shelters, religious institutions, or schools. Often the illegal immigrants are hesitant to seek professional help because of their fear that this process could reveal their status and put them in danger of being identified as illegal. This, obviously, makes the practitioner's job very sensitive. The task of helping is, by necessity, facilitated or hampered by existing legal regulations, because without legislation that supports the immigration process, well-meaning efforts to help children and families will be severely handicapped.

CATEGORIES OF IMMIGRANTS AND REFUGEES

The specific circumstances that propel an individual or family to leave their own home country are varied, but it is a decision that usually is grounded in a desire for a better life, with hopes for a safe environment with economic, educational, and personal opportunities and an improved standard of living. The process of legal immigration takes time and patience, as there are limited numbers of visas or "green cards" available in the United States for immigrants who apply for them. The lengthy process includes a waiting period and requires a lot of paperwork. Some immigrants get visas as tourists or students and may stay after their visas expire. When people are under great duress because of danger and violence that is threatening their personal safety, they may decide to try to immigrate without the necessary papers that would permit them to enter the country legally. Illegal entry into the United States can occur by foot, boat, train, car, or truck and often involves smugglers who demand high prices for their services. These arrangements usually are complicated, and one or both parents may decide to leave their home countries without their children, with the intent to obtain employment, establish a residence, and later send money to cover the expenses for the remaining family members to join him or her. Sometimes this plan can take years to execute, and sometimes the plan fails because the refugees do not survive the dangerous and severe conditions of the long, difficult journey. Other times, refugees who lack documentation to enter the United States are apprehended at the border and sent back to their countries of origin. This is a risky and arduous process in which children may either accompany a parent or relative or may attempt to cross the border unaccompanied by an adult.

Immigrants and refugees enter the United States from many countries, with approximately 81% of unauthorized immigrant populations coming from Latin America, primarily Mexico (Hoefer, Rytin, & Baker, 2011; Zayas, 2015, p. xii). Because of their statistical majority, this chapter focuses on immigrants and refugees from Latin America. A report in *The New York Times* (Gladstone, 2016, p. 9) states that nearly 50 million children worldwide have migrated across borders, with more than half (roughly 28 million) fleeing from situations that were considered violent and insecure. Zayas (2015, pp. 2–3) distinguishes between the following different categories of immigrant/refugee children in the United States:

- Children born in the United States of undocumented immigrants; these children become U.S. citizens at birth, a right given to them through the Fourteenth Amendment (they number approximately 4.5 million; Wessler, 2011; Dreby, 2012). Although these "citizen-children" have all the accompanying rights of citizens, their parents remain illegal and may be in danger of deportation if they are identified and reported. These families live in constant fear that their undocumented loved ones will be discovered and taken into custody.

- Undocumented children who were born elsewhere and brought to the United States at a young age; these number approximately 800,000 (Shear & Yee, 2017). In 2012 President Obama signed an executive order permitting these children to remain in the United States and to work and/or attend universities as a pathway to earned citizenship. The legislation, known as DACA (Deferred Action for Childhood Arrivals) is currently being threatened by President Donald Trump, thereby creating fear and concern among the young "dreamers," to whom it applies (Robbins, 2017; Shear & Yee, 2017).

- Undocumented, unaccompanied minors. These are children under the age of 18 who travel to the United States without an adult and possibly with other young people. In the first 6 months of 2016 agents apprehended 28,000 unaccompanied children trying to cross the border, which was a 78% increase from the previous year (Phippen, 2016). They attempt to cross the US/Mexican border with the goal of reuniting with family members who are already in the United States or because of intolerable conditions of violence in their home communities. Recently, most unaccompanied minors come from El Salvador, Guatemala, and Honduras.

Other terminology related to the above categories includes the term "mixed-status families," which refers to families in which parents and children have different types of legal status, and the terms "exiles" and "orphans," which apply to children who are taken from the United States with their deported parents ("exiles") or children who remain in the United States, while their parents, still alive, have been deported and live elsewhere ("orphans").

THE PROCESS OF LEGAL IMMIGRATION AND DEPORTATION

Legal immigration involves a process that grants a "green card" to individuals who meet certain requirements and who apply for permanent residence in the United States. A "green card" is the colloquial term for the official designation, which is "legal permanent resident" (LPR). In contrast to a visa, which is time-limited, a green card grants the individual permanent residence, although it does not automatically confer citizenship. Eligibility to obtain a green card can occur through having family members who are U.S. citizens (the most common method) or through employment or a job offer, or it can be conferred because of refugee or asylum status. There are several required documents for obtaining the card, such as a medical exam to rule out HIV, tuberculosis, and other illnesses, plus an affidavit of support indicating that the person has sufficient finances to live in the United States without requiring welfare or financial support from the government or public resources (U.S. Citizenship and Immigration Services, 2013). Persons who meet these stringent requirements can live in the United States indefinitely, with no threat of deportation unless they are convicted of engaging in an illegal act. Obviously, these people and their families function without fear and anxiety about the possibility of deportation.

In contrast, families of mixed legal status, or with undocumented children, live with the constant threat that their illegal status will become known and that deportation will occur. When this happens, the individuals typically will be sent to "detention facilities" where they may be held for an unspecified amount of time (Snyder, Bell, & Busch-Armendariz, 2015). The options for relief from detention are (1) applying for asylum, (2) requesting a formal legal hearing, and (3) agreeing to being deported. During the time that these matters are under review, the individual usually is placed in mandatory detention, which potentially can last a few days or many months (Zayas, 2015). A cover article in *The New York Times* magazine section (Hylton, 2015) describes the harsh conditions in some of these facilities, which are privately run and which resemble a jail.

In 2016 the Immigration and Customs Enforcement Agency (ICE) was responsible for apprehending and removing a total of 240,255 illegal "aliens," which was a 2% increase over the previous year but a 24% decrease from the deportations in 2014. Approximately half of these detentions occurred at or near the border; approximately 58% of those detained had been previously convicted of a crime, and about 2,000 were classified as suspected or confirmed gang members (U.S. Immigration and Customs Enforcement, 2016). This chapter does not discuss all the details and implications of these removals, but we certainly can imagine the ramifications in the lives of the family members of those who were detained and deported. Zayas (2015), citing Capps et al. (2007), refers to an estimate that for every two undocumented immigrants deported, one citizen-child is directly affected. Sometimes one or both parents may be detained at the border with their children, and other times, a mother without documentation is removed from her home or arrested because of a traffic violation and sent to one of the detention facilities to await processing of her status.

A total of 34,000 beds were designated for detainees in facilities across the United States in 2015, with most of these in facilities in the southwest

(LA Times, as reported by Zayas, 2015). In Texas, The state of Texas has three family detention centers that hold migrant children and their mothers as they await the granting of asylum status; together these centers have about 3,500 beds (Phippen, 2016). There have been multiple efforts by family protective services and others to close these facilities, which have been described as "prisons" and in which the migrants went on hunger strikes twice in 2015. Half of the population is composed of children, with an average age of 9 years. The length of stay ranges from 22 days to a year (Phippen, 2016). However, because of the considerable backlog in immigration courts and the limited number of immigration judges, the hearing dates to decide the cases under consideration sometimes can stretch to 5 years ("Immigration report hits home," 2017). For reasons that are unclear, the length of stay in detention for women is 10–18% longer than that for men (Brané & Wang, 2013). Because ICE prohibits the mingling of men and women, parents are often separated, and it can be extremely difficult for mothers and fathers to maintain communication with each other (Brané & Wang, 2013). Several studies have demonstrated that the disruptive effects of a parent's detention and removal can have serious consequences on the psychosocial functioning of their children (Allen, Cisneros, & Tellez, 2015; Zayas, Aguilar-Gaxiola, Yoon, & Rey, 2015).

THE MULTIPLE TRAUMAS OF IMMIGRANT AND REFUGEE CHILDREN AND TEENS

We must acknowledge the ever-present reality of multiple losses and traumatic events in the lives of immigrant and refugee children and adolescents. In the first place, they have left a familiar home environment in which everyone spoke the same language and where they attended school. Their parents typically were experiencing mounting anxiety and fear due to being in a dangerous environment in which drug wars were rampant, and the children certainly knew about the threat of violence from gangs. Some children may have been very young when their parents decided to flee, whereas older children and teens probably helped to carry bags of the family's possessions as they endured the numerous hardships that typically occur during the dangerous trip to the United States border. This journey often occurs in several stages, with different means of transportation and with different groups of migrants and smugglers. Conditions may be crowded, hot, and very unpleasant on a bus, truck, or train, and food and water may be scarce. People under extreme stress often are unpleasant and hostile toward one another, and some may steal and fight, resulting in injuries, which the youth observe as they worry about their parents' and their own safety. For these young people, their world appears to be full of lurking danger and trauma. Fong and Earner (2015) emphasize that it is very important for mental health practitioners in the United States who are working with immigrant families to know the details of the conditions that propelled them to leave home as well as the circumstances of their migration.

The Case of the Rivera Family

(The details of this immigrant family were printed in *The New York Times* (Otis, 2017). The report clearly describes the numerous crises of this family that fled from El Salvador in search of a safer life in New York City. Names are as printed.)

Family Information (at the Time of the Mother's Migration):

Mother	Flor de Maria Rivera, native of El Salvador, where she was an elementary school teacher.
Father	Abandoned the family after the younger son's birth.
José	Age 6, attended school in San Salvador.
Juan	Age 1, in care of his maternal grandmother while his mother worked.

History of the Family's Immigration

The mother left her children in the care of her mother when she immigrated alone to the United States, where she obtained a full-time job in New York as a waitress and, in addition, worked part time cleaning apartments. She sent money back to her mother to pay her sons' expenses for approximately 10 years. The mother kept in touch with her boys via Skype several times a week, but there were no visits over her 10-year absence.

The circumstances of the mother's initial leaving are not reported in the article, but she is quoted as saying that she never intended to remain in New York permanently and that it was very difficult for her to be without her boys.

When the mother learned that José was receiving threats from gang members who wanted him to traffic drugs, she made the decision to arrange for the boys, now ages 17 and 12, to join her, despite her worries about their making the perilous 2-week journey by car and foot, with the assistance of a smuggler.

The boys traveled from El Salvador to Guatemala, then from Guatemala to Mexico, and finally from Mexico to the United States. One time they had to cross a river with frightening rapids, and another time they were robbed at knifepoint. Their journey ended when they were apprehended by the U.S. border patrol in Texas and sent to a refugee center. At that point Catholic Charities became involved and arranged for them to be sent to New York and reunited with their mother.

The Current Situation

The boys do not know much English, and they are now struggling in school. They report being bullied because of their immigrant status, with some kids threatening to report them to officials. In fact, the brothers hold special immigrant juvenile status, and they have applied for permanent residency. Their mother's legal status is not reported in the article, but it is unlikely that she would have agreed to this publicity had she not been confident about her own legal status.

Discussion

The following analysis of the boys and this family is based on my review of the facts, as reported in the article and repeated here, and my professional opinion about how other children under similar circumstances might react. My analysis is not based on any personal contact with the family. My intent is to project some probable outcomes and possible treatments for refugee children who have endured similar traumatic histories. My purpose in doing so is to inform and educate practitioners about the experiences of refugees such as this family, so that they will be better prepared to help children with similar backgrounds in the future.

Although the article reports the happy reunion of these two young boys with their mother after a 10-year separation, it is very clear that both boys have been exposed to numerous traumatic events over the years, and it would be quite possible for one or both to be experiencing symptoms consistent with the diagnosis of PTSD, although the article does not give any details to support this speculation. Hopefully, the religious organization that helped to reunite the family has the capacity to offer mental health counseling that would be appropriate in this situation. The mother openly refers to current adjustment problems with the boys because of the differences in her parenting style, which is stricter than that of her mother, with whom they lived previously. Some family counseling sessions could help mediate the adjustment of each person to this new family situation.

In addition to the current family issues, it is very important to review the numerous losses these boys have endured so that we can formulate an assessment of their present status and develop an appropriate treatment plan for each of them. The losses began with the absence of their father (from age 5 for José, and from age 1 for Juan). The fact that the father abandoned the family suggests that the parents were not getting along well, and, therefore, José probably witnessed tension and arguments between them. Schore (2001) writes about the effects of unfavorable attachments in the early years of life as possibly resulting in future emotional instability and impaired relational capacity. Clearly the father does not appear to have been a positive factor in the lives of these boys, and they seem to lack any other male role model. Equally important, their mother's absence for a decade must have been a major wound, which would be difficult for young children to understand and accept, despite the weekly contacts via Skype. Furthermore, since their immigration they are now without contact with their grandmother, who served as their primary caretaker over more than a decade. Clearly and sadly, the history of these boys indicates that *all* their important family relationships have suffered significant ruptures, and we could understand if they now would approach any new relationship with feelings of insecurity and mistrust. This would, of course, apply both to the reunification with their mother and to the development of a relationship with a therapist. Therefore, it would be important for any therapist to understand the need for time and patience to build a positive relationship with these boys in view of this history.

Other losses endured by these boys include that of their familiar environment at home and school in El Salvador and that of their native language, Spanish. The world of New York City is vastly different from the rural setting of El Salvador. In New York City, for example, they may have had their first elevator or subway ride. They have experienced profound changes in their physical environment. Furthermore, they have experienced frightening threats to their physical safety from gangs who tried to intimidate José in El Salvador and from the bullies in New York who make fun of both boys' limited English. In addition to these losses, the boys experienced multiple traumas that probably remain embedded in their memories associated with the grueling journey they endured over the 2 weeks of travel, with the crisis of the river crossing and the robbery at knifepoint. Can we expect young children to simply "forget" these traumatic events and move on with their lives? It has been reported that only about 5–13% of individuals exposed to a traumatic event will develop PTSD (Breslau, 2001). However, these boys experienced *multiple* traumas over the course of the formative years of their lives, and therefore I maintain that the cards are stacked against them unless they receive some form of mental health treatment. Blaustein and Kinniburgh (2019) state firmly that "it is without question that chronic early trauma exposures may seriously and significantly derail and alter children's developmental pathways" (p. 32).

Individual assessments would probably reveal the existence of some or many of the symptoms consistent with the diagnosis of "complex trauma" (Herman, 1992). This term refers to trauma that is repeated and chronic, instead of a single traumatic event. Other terms that seem to apply to the experiences of Juan and José are "developmental trauma," which refers to the adverse effects of trauma on a child's development (van der Kolk, 2005) and "relational trauma," which identifies the role of the primary caretaker in the formation of a deleterious traumatic relationship (Schore, 2001). The fact that these boys are brothers does not assume that their individual responses to this chronic trauma would be the same. Clearly the older boy had the benefit of being with his mother for the first 6 years of his life and therefore could have formed a positive attachment to her during this period. Nothing is known about the quality of either boy's relationship with their grandmother, but is it probable that the younger boy developed an attachment to her, as she was his caretaker for most of his younger years. The boys' current move has ruptured whatever relationship they may have had with the grandmother. Each boy should have a separate evaluation to determine the specific effects their life experiences has had on them.

TREATMENT FOR TRAUMATIZED IMMIGRANT ADOLESCENTS

Possible Helping Interventions

Once an assessment has been made, the next step in determining recommendations for a specific treatment method involves establishing some treatment goals. In the example under discussion, most practitioners would agree that it would be important to try to help each of the boys deal with whatever traumatic memories might be intruding and interfering with their present lives. A second important goal would be to help them establish a secure relationship with their mother and to be able to replicate this subsequently in a relationship with the therapist. Both goals would need to consider the boys' limited facility in English and their lingering worries about their immigrant status.

Possible treatment interventions include the following modalities:

- Individual therapy
- Family therapy
- Group therapy

With the above-mentioned considerations about the boys' discomfort with their limited language and their concerns about their immigration status, the preferred helping method for these boys would be a therapy group of young Spanish-speaking immigrants like themselves. Whether it would be possible to convene such a group in New York City is not known, but the group size would not need to be larger than eight, and there is a large Spanish-speaking population in New York, so it is probable that a group could be readily assembled. If possible, a school setting would be preferred for such a group, as the youth are already enrolled and attending school and there would be less "stigma" associated with participating in a group in a school setting than in a mental health clinic. The age difference between the brothers in the case under discussion constitutes a wider spread than some group leaders might prefer, but in this situation the shared experiences of chronic trauma would take precedence over the few years of age spread.

There are many choices regarding the focus and content of groups for trauma-impacted adolescents. Although much of the literature focuses on the use of TF-CBT in working with trauma survivors (Cohen et al., 2012) and on working toward creating a "trauma narrative" about the traumatic experiences, adolescents may be reluctant to talk about their experiences, and for this reason the use of creative arts in a group format permits the release of tension and provides relief through *symbolic* reenactment of difficult emotions and experiences (Haen & Aronson, 2017). Malchiodi (2014a, p. 6) states, "For some individuals, conveying a memory or story through one or more expressive modalities is more easily tolerated than verbalization."

What kind of activities could be included in a creative arts group for immigrant adolescents? The choices include various art and drawing exercises, writing or journaling or poetry activities, or dramatic and/or musical participation, which could be utilized in a directive way to help the group members gradually and symbolically express some of their feelings about their past and present experiences. It merits recognition that the field of play therapy incorporates all these expressive modalities, but adolescents often believe that "play" therapy is appropriate for younger kids, and therefore most play therapists who use creative arts with adolescents avoid the term "play therapy" and instead refer to the activities as "art therapy" or "music therapy."

Dealing with traumatic experiences in groups requires sensitivity and caution on the part of the therapist to avoid moving too quickly or to risk retraumatizing some group members. Blaustein and Kinniburgh (2019) provide many detailed examples of methods to help youth both review some of their traumatic memories and balance this review with a focus on the positives in their present lives. One example features the creation of a lifebook that contains both happy and frightening memories. Dean and Landis (2017) also use various creative arts methods as ways to help youth express a broad selection of positive and negative feelings. An example (p. 133) explored the range of possible human feelings by having each group member write a feeling on a piece of paper, and after these all are placed in a box, each member selects one and then tries to express that feeling through using a drum. The other group members then try to guess the feeling being expressed through the drumming, and after all group members have had a turn, a group discussion follows about these various feelings. The discussion provides the opportunity for the leader to emphasize the universality of both good and bad feelings. The intrinsic value of the group modality over individual therapy rests in shared experiences such as this that inevitably combat any individual's painful feelings of isolation and loneliness. Singing songs from the country of origin also can result in a strong sense of bonding among the group members.

Groups typically have time limits of several weeks, with the option to permit members to continue. In some cases, it may be appropriate to refer a child or teen for individual therapy, once it becomes evident that the group setting cannot adequately meet his or her needs.

This chapter cannot discuss the numerous other examples of the use of creative arts in helping traumatized youth, but the possibilities are many, and readers are encouraged to consult this book's reference list for descriptions and guidance about applying various creative arts methods in a sensitive manner that will not retraumatize sensitive adolescents. Malchiodi (2014a) refers to this method as "trauma-informed creative arts therapy," and she has coedited a book demonstrating the use of this approach for attachment problems. Thus it appears that the same type of therapeutic intervention that is recommended to help deal with traumatic memories may also be appropriate for attachment problems (Malchiodi, 2014b).

The previous discussion of goals in the case example identified the need to work and repair the boys' attachment relationship with their mother, who had been absent from their lives for more than a decade. This goal would be best served through parent–child therapy with a therapist who understands the aftermath of insecure and relational attachments and who can engage the parent and children in creative activities that will attempt to mend their relationship and draw them closer together. This method relies on having the therapist deliberately model appropriate responses to the child's and parent's creations, thereby enhancing a sense of positive regard and mutual respect for each participant. The assumption is that the parent will learn through the therapist's examples and that the resulting positive interactions will help to heal a broken relationship. Once again, readers may wish to consult Malchiodi and Crenshaw's edited book (2014) for more examples of how to effectively use creative arts methods to help with attachment problems.

CONCLUDING COMMENTS

Social workers and other practitioners have the knowledge and skills to help refugee and immigrant children and families recover from the trauma of migration and to facilitate their adjustment to a new country. However, it is critical for new arrivals to feel safe and welcomed in their new setting. Unfortunately, at the time this chapter is being written, President Trump is issuing executive orders to restrict immigration and to increase the monitoring and detention of immigrants in the United States. Parents and children are being separated, with very limited telephone contact, and uncertain plans for reunification. This impacts both those trying to enter the United States and those who may have been here for many years. Families of mixed status are living in more fear than ever that they will be sent back to the countries from which they fled because of intolerable living conditions. Many issues have yet to be resolved, such as how this process will be enacted and how the proposed deportations will occur. If legal reviews will be conducted, then many new facilities would need to be built and many more officers and court judges would need to be appointed. Congress would need to approve the considerable associated expenses. Meanwhile, the disruption of families and the future healthy development of the children would be severely compromised. This chapter therefore concludes with a sincere hope for a reversal of the proposed policy and a return to sensible legal efforts to facilitate the immigration process for the thousands of families who are relying on American's historical role to welcome and admit refugees who are fleeing persecution and violence.

DISCUSSION QUESTIONS

1. Consider the psychological effects on the therapist of working in a political environment that threatens to return refugees to the dangerous environment from which they fled. How can therapists deal with their personal sense of frustration and helplessness?
2. Discuss the role of the school social worker in dealing with reports about the bullying of immigrant children. How might this be addressed? Do you favor a schoolwide intervention or a targeted personal one, or both?
3. Do you think that the mother of the refugee boys should be offered individual counseling? Why or why not?
4. How could the lack of a male role model in these boys' lives be addressed?

CHAPTER 17

The Impact of a Changing World on Practice with and for Children

The numerous challenges of practice in the 21st century compel social workers and other practitioners involved with children to review their past and current efforts, as well as their plans of action for intervening helpfully in children's lives. The 20th century has been referred to as the "century of the child" (Aries, 1962), because acknowledgment of childhood as a distinct developmental phase occurred during this time, and children began to be treated as *children,* not as small adults. Certainly, we would like to believe that in the second decade of the 21st century we know more about children and how to help them and that we are doing better as a society and as helping professionals than we did in the early 1900s.

However, our enhanced knowledge and desire to help has not prevented the fragmentation of the family and kinship network; nor has it countered the debilitating influences on children of poverty, substance use disorders, violence, and child abuse. There is a disturbing contradiction between the United States' view of itself as a child-centered nation and its fiscal policies, which suggest a weak commitment to children (Edelman, 1998). In 2017, spending for children's programs was drastically cut, as were many school budgets. Practitioners committed to working on behalf of children must avoid becoming demoralized by these harsh realities as they make decisions about how to respond to the needs of children in today's world.

This chapter reviews some of the pivotal challenges facing practitioners who are working with children who have a variety of problems at home, in school, and in the community at the end of the second decade of the 21st century. The following topics are addressed as they apply to children:

- Poverty and homelessness.
- Family breakdown and parental absence due to military deployment, imprisonment, addiction, and/or abandonment.

- Exposure to violence, trauma, and interpersonal bullying either first-hand or electronically.
- The stresses on children and family related to gender issues in child development.
- The stresses of noncitizen status and fears of deportation.

THE IMPACT ON CHILDREN OF POVERTY AND HOMELESSNESS

Poverty

Children who grow up in poverty often suffer the associated problems of poor nutrition, inadequate health care, and substandard housing. Furthermore, race and ethnic minority membership often coexist with poverty, thus presenting additional obstacles to children's optimal growth and development. "When children are both poor and members of ethnic minorities, the negative and long-term impact of poverty increases significantly" (Gibbs, Huang, & Associates, 1989, p. 6; Allen-Meares et al., 2000).

Pronounced changes are taking place in the demographic composition of the United States. As reported by the Pew Research Center (Cohn, 2016) the U.S. Census states that just over half (50.2%) of U.S. children younger than 1 year old in 2015 were racial or ethnic minorities (Cohn, 2016). By 2055 it is projected that the United States will not have a single racial or ethnic majority. In 2016, about 14% of the country's population was foreign born, compared with just over 5% in 1965 (Cohn & Caumont, 2016). This is due to the nearly 59 million immigrants who have come to the United States in the past 50 years, mostly from Latin America and Asia.

Social workers will need to employ a multidimensional framework of assessment and treatment to include cultural, together with developmental, familial, and environmental factors as the basis for understanding and treating children from diverse backgrounds.

Homelessness

It is difficult to document the precise number of homeless individuals or children in the United States. However, a serious lack of medical care and inconsistent schooling are problems that seriously affect children in homeless families. As demonstrated in the case of Barbie Smith (Chapters 3–5), many homeless children fail to attend school while they are temporarily housed in shelters, motels, and welfare hotels.

The acute shortage of low-income housing, combined with fiscal constraints and restrictions on welfare benefits, does not bode well for homeless families who also are confronted with the threats their children face of violence and exposure to substances in their unsafe neighborhoods. The case of Barbie Smith illustrates the interweaving of environmental and psychological stressors in a homeless family, as well as the limitations on what practitioners can do in the absence of potentially helpful programs.

FAMILY BREAKDOWN AND PARENTAL ABSENCE

Approximately 60% of children living in mother-only families are impoverished, compared with only 11% in two-parent families (Kirby, n.d.). This means that many children in families with only one parent suffer not only the loss of that person but also the ongoing hardship and resentment from the associated economic repercussions. A parent's absence may create ongoing stress and worry for the child and other family members, for example, when a parent is deployed to a combat zone and his or her physical safety is at risk. Children in a divorced family may have witnessed years of marital tension and possible open conflict culminating in the departure of one parent (usually the father). Yet other scenarios involve imprisonment or parental substance abuse, which, as discussed in Chapter 13, may result in neglect, abandonment, or even abuse of the children.

An integral part of a social worker's responsibility is to be aware of the stresses in a child's family that may be contributing to the youth's own difficulties. Certainly not all single-parent families are problematic, and some function well and demonstrate strength and resilience. However, many times this is not the case, and children may suffer when a single parent is struggling to raise a family with few resources. In situations such as these, helping the child may include, of necessity, helping the family.

EXPOSURE TO VIOLENCE, TRAUMA, AND BULLYING

The world today seems to be full of violence, both in faraway wars and on our city streets. The media bring details of rapes and murders into our living rooms with the nightly news, and even young children may know about the self-inflicted death of a classmate who became depressed and desperate due to relentless bullying.

There is growing awareness among the general public about the possible occurrence of PTSD following a traumatic event such as a fire or a vehicle accident. We also are learning that prolonged or repeated watching of traumatic events on TV can contribute to PTSD, anxiety, depression, conduct disturbances, and other symptoms (Nader, 2010). Although closer proximity to the traumatic event increases the likelihood of a serious reaction, we know that individuals far from the actual location of the disaster/tragedy can also suffer serious repercussions because of their capacity to imagine the scene and to empathize with those who were trauma victims.

This information underscores the necessity for helping professionals to routinely ask about typical television viewing, as well as about firsthand exposure to violent events that might have been upsetting to a child or youth. As discussed in Chapter 15, many students witness repeated episodes of bullying behavior among their peers, and most do not report this or do anything about it (Englander & Lawson, 2007).

This problem is receiving considerable attention because of a growing number of suicides connected to bullying experiences. Many states are enacting anti-bullying legislation, and schools increasingly will be expected to have a specific intervention policy for dealing with the perpetrators and the victims and the entire school population.

STRESSES RELATED TO GENDER ISSUES

As discussed in Chapter 6, the issue of gender dysphoria is receiving attention in families with children who believe that their bodies are the wrong sex/gender. Social workers need to help families and schools in dealing with this sensitive issue.

THE STRESSES OF NONCITIZEN STATUS

Many children who are new arrivals in this country come from a background of political upheaval and family displacement related to their status as refugees. The child immigrant to the United States brings with him or her the "excess baggage" of family crisis associated with the often stressful reasons that led to their emigration from their countries. There can be many motives for immigration, but it seems obvious that families would not willingly leave an environment in which they felt safe and optimistic about their future. Moving a family to a new country may be the "least detrimental alternative" (i.e., better than remaining home in the middle of a war zone), or it may represent the father's or mother's wish for better economic opportunities (Bevin, 1999; Crawford-Brown & Rattray, 2001; Wu, 2001; Zayas, 2015; see also Chapter 16, this volume).

Children who leave one country to establish residence in another, regardless of the reason for the major family move, have to cope with numerous losses. Although a refugee child's vulnerability to stress is greatly increased by such losses, these negative effects can be reduced by a supportive family milieu and a supportive community (Ajdukovic & Ajdukovic, 1993). The ability of the family members to adjust in a new environment, moreover, relates to the degree to which the rules and norms of their own culture remain the same and the extent to which role expectations, morals, and values are different and clash with the prevailing norms in the new locale (Crawford-Brown & Rattray, 2001; Webb, 2001; Zayas, 2015). Unfortunately, the political environment in the United States in 2018 is not welcoming to immigrants and refugees, and the threat of deportation adds a terrible weight to immigrant families who are already in the United States.

The school is often the place in which difficulties in adjustment become evident, because the child is thrust into a new situation that expects certain behaviors even as the child is attempting to learn a new language and to establish some peer contacts (Allen-Meares et al., 2000; Openshaw, 2008; see also Chapter 16, this volume). The role of the school social worker in serving as a bridge between two sets of values is illustrated in the case of Alexa, an adopted 8-year-old Russian refugee with special needs.

THE CASE OF ALEXA, AGE 8

(This case is a composite of several different cases.)

Presenting Problem

Alexa, an 8-year-old Russian child in the second grade of a public school, was referred to an early intervention program (staffed by a local mental health agency) because of her aggressive behavior with other children, her failure to follow directions, and her immature behavior. She had been a student in the school for 2 years, and in first grade she had been suspended twice—once for slapping another student and once for hitting a teacher. At the time of intake, she spoke English fluently, but when she arrived in this country she knew no English.

Family Information

Alexa was adopted when she was 4 years old. She had been orphaned during the first year of her life, when both of her parents died as a result of civil unrest in the Ukraine. She was placed in an orphanage with other displaced children at that time.

Alexa's adoptive parents are of Russian backgrounds; they decided to adopt a Russian child when they were unable to conceive a child of their own. Both parents are employed in international business organizations. At the time of intake, the father was 42 years old, and the mother was 37. Alexa is their only child.

Biopsychosocial Assessment

No developmental history is available regarding the first 4 years of Alexa's life. We know, however, that loss of the parents during the first year of life creates a sense of abandonment in the child, with resultant problems in lack of trust and attendant attachment difficulties (Shapiro et al., 2001a; Bruning, 2007). We do not know the details about Alexa's parents' deaths or whether she witnessed one or both of them. These facts may never be known, as the preverbal child lacks the language to convey traumatic experiences, which nonetheless may be imprinted on his or her visual memory (Terr, 1988).

We also do not know the conditions in the orphanage in which Alexa lived until her adoption at age 4, or whether she had any opportunity to form attachment bonds to one or more staff members there. It is likely that this child did receive enough attention and care from *someone* to benefit her development sufficiently that a couple seeking to adopt a preschool child found her to be appealing. However, we know that many children adopted from institutions suffer from various forms of attachment and affective disorders (Shapiro et al., 2001a; Bruning, 2007), and they may continue to show difficulties for many years following adoption.

Alexa's anger and frustration when she was uprooted from the orphanage at age 4, brought to the United States, and enrolled in school are understandable in view of her isolation, caused by her not knowing the language. Another possible factor contributing to Alexa's aggressiveness could be related to this child's sensitivity to change and to her depleted ability to adapt to the loss of a familiar environment. Shapiro et al. (2001a) point out that, even when institutional life is hard, it constitutes a familiar "home" for the child, and the prospect of leaving and going to a new country with strange parents who spoke a different language could have been very frightening.

The facts that Alexa learned English in 2 years and that she was able to make some friends reflect her strengths and resilience. Her ongoing adjustment, however, required close monitoring.

Treatment Summary

Individual weekly play therapy sessions provided a range of nonverbal methods by which Alexa could express her frustrations symbolically, without the pressure to put them into words. Paper and markers offered a nonstructured method for Alexa to "draw out" her feelings in a safe environment. She sometimes referred to "a faraway place" in her drawings, which seemed to allude to some of the shadowy memories of her past. A dollhouse and family dolls were also available to the child, in addition to a variety of puppets and clay.

Group therapy was also an important part of Alexa's initial treatment, in order to offer her a socialization experience. She participated in a group of four children, two girls and two boys. Other members of the group also had difficulties with peer relationships. The goal for Alexa in this experience was to help her become aware that the other children also had to struggle to control their behavior. A second goal was for Alexa to receive a sense of being accepted by the group.

The involvement of Alexa's adoptive parents in counseling was crucial in promoting the optimal development of their child. It is essential for the child's therapist to meet regularly and work closely with the parents, in order to guide and coach them so that they can support their child most effectively. The school initially focused on Alexa's troublesome behavior, which the social worker "normalized" with the parents in view of this girl's traumatic life experiences. Until the worker presented this perspective to them, the parents were joining with the teacher in viewing Alexa as a "bad" child and responding to her punitively.

Another important goal in ongoing parent counseling was to help Alexa gradually understand her traumatic past. It is quite likely that she remembered some details of her experiences in the orphanage. Both the parents and the therapist must encourage and be willing to listen to the child's memories. Ideally, this recollection will first occur in individual therapy, with later family sessions to sensitize the parents to the ongoing influence of their daughter's early experiences in her present life. Eventually Alexa can be encouraged to construct a lifebook (see Chapter 10) in which she records the significant events of her life—both as she actually remembers them and as her parents help supply missing information.

Discussion

Alexa has experienced multiple traumatic events in her short life. However, the impact of Alexa's major losses during the first year of her life may be underestimated even by trained practitioners who are unaware of the impact of a child's preverbal experience. Terr's (1988) studies of children traumatized during their preschool years confirm that traumatic events create lasting visual images that "seem to last a lifetime" (p. 103). "When a trauma or series of extreme stresses strikes well before the age [of] 28 to 36 months, the child 'burns in' a visual memory of it, sometimes later becoming able . . . to affix a few words to the picture" (p. 103).

Terr's comments have direct treatment implications for Alexa and for other refugee children who may have witnessed multiple frightening events during their preverbal years. The recommended method of helping is to facilitate gradual recollection of the experience, in the belief that this recollection (in the context of the safety of the child's present reality and the support of a warm helping relationship) will reduce the child's anxiety about the trauma. This process should enable the child to locate the experience in the past and thereby to reduce its ongoing influence in his or her present life.

More research needs to be done on different helping approaches for traumatized children. For example, when a child has witnessed one or both parents being murdered, it is difficult to conceive of *any* intervention that could help the child to accept this terrible reality. My own belief, based on many years' experience with traumatized children, is that a child's best interests lie in remembering the experience and then placing the memory in the past, so that the child can carry on with his or her life in a way that honors the lost or deceased parent. In this manner the child holds onto the memory while focusing on the present rather than the past. A critical component of this intervention is the assurance of safety in the child's present life. Unfortunately, this guarantee is not possible for immigrants and refugees who may have fled gang warfare and who, in the United States, fear the possibility of arrest and deportation based on their lack of necessary documentation.

TRENDS IN DIRECT PRACTICE WITH CHILDREN

Direct practice with children must adapt to the realities of modern life. Some trends are becoming apparent in the work of practitioners who deal directly with children. These trends include the following:

- Greater awareness of multiple interacting factors in the etiology of childhood problems, including increased emphasis on biological and environmental influences, with special attention to the nature of the child's early attachment experiences, and the impact of these on neurological development.
- Understanding and utilizing concepts of risk and resilience and a strengths perspective in formulating an assessment.
- Utilizing interprofessional collaboration and viewing parents as partners in their children's treatment.
- Practice that is culturally sensitive.
- Practice that integrates child and family therapy.
- Practice that is guided by research and research that utilizes practice experience.
- Practice that employs cognitive and behavioral approaches, where appropriate.
- Practice that utilizes play therapy with children under 12 years of age.

Greater Awareness of Multiple Interacting Factors in the Etiology of Childhood Problems

There are many approaches to the assessment and treatment of childhood disorders, but despite differences in emphasis and methods, most models recognize the role of multiple interactive influences rather than subscribing to unitary causes of behavior (Mash & Barkley, 2003, 2007). The literature increasingly acknowledges the importance of biological factors in shaping behavior (Chess, 1988; Karr-Morse & Wiley, 1997; Perry, 1997; Siegel, 2012). It also recognizes the pivotal role of the environment in either protecting or exposing the child to potentially stressful experiences, such as traumatic events, that can lead to subsequent psychological and somatic disorders in children (Jenkins & Bell, 1997; Garbarino & Kostelny, 1997). The work of Chess and Thomas (1986) on temperament made a significant contribution to our understanding of the innate temperamental characteristics that influence children's and adults' responses to the world. This temperamental disposition, furthermore, may influence the manner in which the child responds to stress and trauma.

In addition to the genetic reality of temperamental characteristics that we all possess, some children's biological inheritance predisposes them to certain conditions, such as schizophrenia, autism, alcoholism, Tourette syndrome, ADHD, and other emotional, learning, and/or behavioral disorders. These conditions are multidetermined, and we do not know the elusive reasons why one child in a family develops a disease or disorder, whereas another child in the same family with the same parents does not. Johnson (1989) states that

> some combination of intrinsic constitutional factors and environmental forces, in continuous interaction with each other, gives rise to conditions classified under disruptive behavior disorder. In some instances, biological factors play the major determining role, in others, environmental factors predominate, and in still others both biology and environment significantly contribute to an outcome identified as a "behavior disorder." (p. 91)

Furthermore, persistent psychosocial adversity, such as poverty, abuse, or neglect, increases the risk of mental illness in children (Institute of Medicine, 1989, cited in Johnson & Friesen, 1993).

Because of the complexity of conditions with both constitutional and environmental components, a multifaceted, multimodal approach to treatment is recommended. The use of psychopharmacology brings dramatic results for some conditions, but ideally this treatment will be combined with simultaneous parent guidance and possible behavioral approaches with the child.

Understanding and Utilizing Concepts of Risk and Resilience and a Strengths Perspective

Because risk and protective factors often occur simultaneously at multiple system levels, assessments must involve the use of multiple sources of information and multiple methods of data collection (Fraser, 1997). As previously discussed, risks can be assessed as they pertain to the child, to the parental/family system, and/or to the social environment (B. Davies, 1999; D. Davies, 2011). Although multiple risk factors may lead to diminished resilience, "*risk factors are not fate*" (Davies, 1999, p. 81; emphasis added), and clinical experience demonstrates that when protective factors are marshaled, the risk may diminish. For example, Alexa's background of repeated experiences of loss and separation might lead one to expect that she could not overcome the impact of her tragic history. However, the timely interventions of the school social worker on multiple levels brought about gradual improvement in the child's behavior, which in turn resulted in more positive interactions with her teacher and her parents.

Saleebey's (1992, 1996) conceptualization of the "strengths perspective" has had a profound impact in directing social workers to focus on the client's positive attributes and to work with the client in a relationship of respect and courtesy (DeJong & Miller, 1995; Nelson, 1997; Ronnau, 2001; Saleebey, 1992, 1996). This applies as much to work with children as with adults.

Interprofessional Collaboration and Parents as Partners in Their Children's Treatment

We have come a long way from the view that parents (especially mothers) cause or substantially contribute to their children's emotional difficulties.

Our enhanced understanding of the biological components of human behavior, together with a broader awareness of the complexity of behavior, leads us to include parents as partners in helping efforts that involve their children. The Amendments to the Education of the Handicapped Act, which passed in 1986, *mandate* a family-centered approach to provision of services to infants and young children with handicaps (Bishop, 1993; Bishop, Rounds, & Weil, 1993; Allen-Meares et al., 2000; Openshaw, 2008). That act, along with programs such as Homebuilders (Kinney et al., 1991) and Family-Centered Services (Wilson & Lipsey, 2001), demonstrate belief in the importance of the parents' role in their children's lives. Studies of early intervention programs for children have shown that the most effective programs actively involve parents along with the children (LeCroy & Ashford, 1992; Groves, 2002).

In addition to the primary role of the parents in helping their own children, many other specialists often participate in the assessment and treatment of some complicated disorders, such as ADHD. For example, special education teachers usually have an essential role in the education of a child with ADHD. In addition, the school nurse may dispense medication to the child during the day; a pediatrician, neurologist, or psychiatrist prescribes the medication; and various other medical and educational personnel may be involved in providing support services to the child and family. Often the social worker functions as case coordinator to ensure that necessary information is transmitted among the different personnel and parents.

Interprofessional collaboration and inclusion of parents as partners result in enriched information about the child, which assists the social worker/counselor while also contributing to a sense of teamwork. The ongoing challenge for the social worker is to keep the members of the "team" working together over the necessary period of time, depending on the child's needs.

Merging Goals of Clinicians and Advocates

Faced with the cruel realities of our changing world, practitioners who work directly with children realize that political and economic remedies are required to reduce poverty and bring about improved living conditions. All citizens who care about children and families must join together to raise the consciousness of the nation, and especially that of its political leaders, who allocate resources for programs and services. When families suffer the combined throes of poverty, racism, unemployment, and lack of opportunity, their children pay the price. All of us must work together to try to correct this social injustice and help families that are too overwhelmed to help themselves.

A philosophy of shared responsibility for the health and well-being of children becomes critical in the face of family breakdown, as I pointed out in Chapter 1. Examples throughout this book have demonstrated the indisputable need for programs and services for children who are homeless, orphaned, maltreated, and disadvantaged. When parents and other family members are absent due to deployment, imprisonment, or abandonment, or when they are addicted, poor, violent, and/or otherwise unable to help their own children, society has a moral responsibility to do so. The slogans "it takes a village to raise a child" and "leave no child behind" deserve to be implemented at every opportunity.

Practice That Is Culturally Sensitive

Implicit (and often explicit) throughout this book is the recognition that social workers and other practitioners with children must be prepared to work with the many different nationalities, races, and ethnic groups that contribute to the diversity of the United States and the world. Children are products of the particular culture in which they grow up, and an understanding of a particular child (and his or her parents and extended family) depends to a great extent on an appreciation and respect for the uniqueness of a culture that may be very different from one's own.

Social work education requires that students examine their own cultural heritage, values, and biases in order to sensitize them to the feelings and beliefs of others who subscribe to different points of view. As I have pointed out in Chapter 2, self-awareness about one's own cultural beliefs and an openness to the beliefs of others form the necessary foundation for the ability to interact effectively with a client from a different culture (Webb, 2001). Because no one person can realistically expect to have knowledge about *every* different culture, the essential attitude for the worker is a willingness to put aside his or her own values and to try to identify the assumptions and values of a different culture. The worker must acknowledge and believe in the concept that there is more than one valid way to raise a child. A reference such as *Culturally Diverse Parent–Child and Family Relationships* (Webb, 2001) can guide practitioners who are working with children and families from a variety of cultural backgrounds.

Practice That Integrates Child and Family Therapy

The tension between the child-centered view of assessment and treatment and one that sees the child's problems as reflecting family dysfunction has a long history. In their enthusiasm for a systems view, the early family therapists, according to LeVine and Sallee (1992, p. 107), believed that

> all children's problems were best dealt with by intervening in the family system. Some still subscribe to this position, but a number now agree that the difficulties of the identified child patient may be so internalized that individual therapy is preferred. In other cases, a family member besides the identified child may be so disturbed that individual therapy with [that family member] must precede effective family intervention.

As an experienced child and family therapist and social work educator, I find that the impact of family factors on the child is uppermost in my mind. I always acknowledge the essential role of the family for the child. However, during my career I have not noted a corresponding recognition among family therapists of the influence of the *child's* problems on the family system. In my opinion, many family therapists fail to recognize that children often have their own intrinsic problems, which do not necessarily emanate from some dysfunction in the family. The essential individuality of the child, unfortunately, is thus diminished by many family systems theories and practitioners.

With this point of view as background, I urge an end to the polarization implicit in either a child-centered or a family-centered approach to helping children. It seems patently obvious that children need their families and that families respond to their children, either by giving them a voice or by expecting them to meld into the larger family gestalt. Children who have special problems and needs cannot conform to their families' expectations. When this is the case, the best skills of both child and family therapists are required to understand each problem situation and devise an intervention that is respectful of both a child's and a family's needs. A systems view recognizes that a child's fundamental problems will affect the family and that effective helping includes *both* child and family approaches.

Practice That Is Guided by Research and Research That Utilizes Practice Experience

Historically, social work researchers and practitioners have tended to pursue their own interests and goals without much interaction. Practitioners strove to understand a case in all its complexity (as in the tripartite assessment), whereas researchers were more likely to focus their attention on a narrow facet of the problem situation in their effort to measure change.

During the second decade of the 21st century, members of each group are realizing that they can learn from one another and even collaborate on projects that simultaneously benefit clients and generate new knowledge (Hess & Mullen, 1995). More social workers are continuing their educations to the doctoral level, and, in completing the required dissertation, they have learned to appreciate both the complexity and the rewards of carrying out a research project whose findings can help practitioners help other clients. Furthermore, as social workers increasingly collaborate with other professionals who routinely employ empirical research and present their findings in interdisciplinary meetings, the social workers need to understand and use this research language in order to be respected. Thus a worker who previously may have had a somewhat limited vision may begin to appreciate how practice wisdom can be translated into a research protocol that, after testing, can result in findings that will apply broadly to many clients and situations.

Both researchers and practitioners have to bend to the effort to develop research that is grounded in practice. Researchers must consult and confer with practitioners in drafting procedures that "make sense" and that will contribute to the client's treatment, even as the research questions are being investigated. Research using child clients needs to follow certain safeguards in order to conform to the child's developmental level, limited ability to conceptualize, and frequent intolerance with demands and expectations. The key to a successful partnership and collaboration is for researchers and practitioners to learn to talk to one another with respect and to come to the conclusion that together they will achieve more than either group can accomplish alone.

Practice That Employs Cognitive and Behavioral Approaches, Where Appropriate

A good example of successful blending of practice and research is in the field of cognitive-behavioral therapy. Interest in this treatment approach has increased in recent years because of the research that attests to its effectiveness. In addition, it satisfies the desire of child practitioners to work with children in a manner that conforms to the children's developmental need for concrete, detailed information, combined with a method for tracking their progress. Cognitive-behavioral methods provide a means of contracting and of monitoring success in regard to a specific problem situation. The specificity of this approach also appeals to managed care companies, which view this method as time limited and easy to monitor. From the child's point of view, a behavioral method that can be followed on a chart offers the empowering opportunity to identify and reward his or her own daily successes. Chapter 6 demonstrated the use of a behavioral method with a boy with ADHD, and Chapter 7 illustrated its use with a girl with a sleep disorder. The fourth edition of Kendall's (2012) edited book on child and adolescent therapy features clinician-researchers who address specific behavioral and emotional problems such as aggression, ADHD, depression, anxiety disorders, and difficulties faced by children with chronic health problems.

Practice That Utilizes Play Therapy with Children Younger Than 12 Years of Age

Social workers subscribe to a principle of "starting where the client is." When applied to working with children, this mandate requires that practitioners understand that children communicate their thoughts, feelings, and worries through their play. This means that practitioners must learn some of the basics of play therapy to be able to engage and treat their child clients effectively. Many schools of social work teach some play therapy methods in clinical practice courses, and some have post-master's-level programs to train practitioners to use a variety of play therapy interventions with children and their parents. A listing of such training programs can be found in Webb (2015).

CONCLUDING COMMENTS

As a clinical practitioner, I know that the various methods demonstrated through the case examples in this book can substantially help children living in stressful family and social environments. We know a great deal about how to treat and support families, school personnel, and children themselves who are in distress. However, no matter how successful the outcome of our therapeutic/helping efforts, as thoughtful practitioners we must reflect seriously about the underlying reasons for the children's difficulties and question whether something might have been done *sooner* to forestall the predictable deterioration of a child's situation in the absence of intervention.

The value of prevention as a worthwhile goal is most appealing. Almost everyone would agree with the wisdom of improving children's lives so that they will not require special remediation services. Over the years since the Community Mental Health Centers Act of 1963, there has been consistent attention to the three levels of prevention—primary, secondary, and tertiary—originally outlined by Caplan (1964).

Social workers have been especially interested in the notion of "primary prevention," which aims to "keep something unwanted from occurring" (Bowker, 1983, p. 2). This proactive approach seeks to build adaptive strengths through education, especially with groups at high risk (LeVine & Sallee, 1992). A philosophy of primary prevention implies intervening *before* a problem becomes visible; implementing a primary prevention program thus requires a leap of faith and a belief that the desired end product of improved well-being will be worth the costs of mounting such a program. Unfortunately, many politicians prefer to deal with the squeaky wheel instead of applying some oil to prevent the squeak. Therefore, the neglect of children's well-being continues; although we know what to do, we don't do it. Bloom (1981, p. 214), with tongue in cheek, says: "It obviously takes a creative practitioner to prevent problems that don't exist, among persons who don't want to be bothered, with methods that haven't been fully demonstrated to be efficacious, with regard to complex situations and powerfully competing forces."

Actually not *all* children's problems lend themselves to primary intervention, valid as that concept may be for many of the social problems arising from poverty, substance abuse/dependence, violence, and lack of good schooling and nutrition. Some conditions of childhood (e.g., ADHD and other emotional, learning, and behavioral disorders with a constitutional component) may require the combined efforts of social workers and other professionals to provide ongoing necessary services to the affected children and their families. Some problems simply do not get better with the methods we have at present, no matter how skilled the worker or how promptly help is made available.

Helping with a problem in its early phases is referred to as "secondary prevention." For example, in the case of a child with suspected ADHD, a secondary prevention approach emphasizes early screening, testing, and goal setting so that the problem situation can be managed effectively before it reaches a dysfunctional level and requires a "tertiary prevention" approach. When disorders such as ADHD are not diagnosed and treated in an early stage, a child may become unmotivated and disruptive in class to the point that he or she begins to engage in antisocial behavior. In later years, such behavior may result in the need to transfer the child to a residential treatment facility. Tertiary prevention such as this should more appropriately be called "remediation," not "prevention" (LeVine & Sallee, 1992).

In addition to innate conditions that require intervention in a timely manner, certain life events, transitions, and crises that may occur in the course of the child's development may create a justifiable need for services. For example, the death of a parent or sibling, parental divorce, and chronic illness in the family all generate stress that may interfere with a child's ability to carry on his or her usual activities. As demonstrated in several chapters in this book, helping interventions focused on either the individual child or the family as a unit can provide a child with the opportunity to express and receive support for his or her feelings. *Timely* interventions in circumstances such as these can prevent the further escalation of the problem.

DISCUSSION QUESTIONS AND ROLE-PLAY EXERCISE

1. Indicate how you might respond to a refugee child like Alexa who refers to a "faraway place" in her drawings. Do you think that it might be too painful for the child to recall these memories, or that this would be beneficial? Give reasons for your opinion.
2. Discuss the role of the social worker as consultant to teachers. Role-play a meeting with a teacher in which the social worker tries to sensitize the teacher to a refugee child's losses as possible determinants of the child's aggressive behavior in school. How is the issue of confidentiality applicable here, and how could this be managed?
3. How can the social worker deal with his or her negative feelings about a client from a culture that puts the parents' needs ahead of those of the child and demands the child's instant obedience to the parents' authority?
4. Identify an issue related to children that you consider as appropriate for uniting child advocates and practitioners around a specific goal or purpose. Outline a plan of action, indicating how this effort would be funded.

APPENDICES

Child-Related Professional Organizations

American Academy of Child and Adolescent Psychiatry
www.aacap.org

American Academy of Experts in Traumatic Stress
www.aaets.org

American Academy of Pediatrics
www.aap.org

American Art Therapy Association
www.arttherapy.org

American Association of Suicidology
www.suicidology.org

American Dance Therapy Association
www.adta.org

American Music Therapy Association
www.musictherapy.org

American Professional Society on the Abuse of Children
www.apsac.org

American Psychiatric Association
www.psych.org

American Psychological Association
www.apa.org

American Red Cross
www.redcross.org

American Society of Group Psychotherapy and Psychodrama
www.asgpp.org

Annie E. Casey Foundation
www.aecf.org

Association for Play Therapy
www.a4pt.org

Association for Traumatic Stress Specialists
www.atss.info

Association of Pediatric Oncology Social Workers
www.aposw.org

Asthma and Allergy Foundation of America
www.aafa.org

Brain Injury Association
www.biausa.org

Child Welfare League of America
www.cwla.org

Child Witness to Violence Project
www.childwitnesstoviolence.org

Council for Exceptional Children
www.cec.sped.org

CureSearch for Children's Cancer
www.curesearch.org

International Expressive Arts Therapy Association
www.ieata.org

International Society for Traumatic Stress Studies
www.istss.org

Juvenile Diabetes Research Foundation International
www.jdrf.org

National Association of Perinatal Social Workers
www.napsw.org

National Association of Social Workers
www.naswdc.org

National Child Traumatic Stress Network
www.nctsn.org

National Coalition of Creative Arts Therapies Associations
www.nccata.org

North American Drama Therapy Association
www.nadta.org

Sandplay Therapists of America
www.sandplay.org

Starlight Children's Foundation
www.starlight.org

Child-Related Professional Journals

The Arts in Psychotherapy
www.elsevier.com

Art Therapy: Journal of the American Art Therapy Association
www.arttherapyjournal.org

Brown University Child and Adolescent Behavioral Letter
www.childadolescentbehavior.com

Child Abuse and Neglect
www.elsevier.com

Child and Adolescent Group Psychotherapy
www.springerlink.com

Child and Adolescent Social Work Journal
www.springerlink.com

Child: Care, Health and Development
www.onlinelibrary.wiley.com

Child Development
www.srcd.org

Child Psychiatry and Human Development
www.springerlink.com

Child Study Journal
https://catalyst.library.jhu.edu/catalog/bib_3471542

Child Welfare (formerly *Child Welfare Quarterly*)
www.cwla.org

Children and Youth Care Forum
www.springerlink.com

Children and Youth Services Review
www.elsevier.com

Children's Health Care
www.tandfonline.com

Drama Therapy Review
www.nadta.org

Early Child Research Quarterly
www.elsevier.com

Gifted Child Quarterly
www.nagc.org

Groupwork
www.whitingbirch.net

Health and Social Work
www.naswpress.org

Infant Mental Health Journal
www.onlinelibrary.wiley.com

International Journal of Group Psychotherapy
www.guilford.com/journals

International Journal of Play Therapy
www.apa.org/journals

Journal of Abnormal Child Psychology
www.springerlink.com

Journal of Adolescence
www.elsevier.com

Journal of the American Academy of Child and Adolescent Psychiatry
www.jaacap.com

Journal of Child and Adolescent Group Therapy
www.springerlink.com

Journal of Child and Adolescent Trauma
www.springerlink.com

Journal of Child and Family Studies
www.springerlink.com

Journal of Child and Youth Care (formerly *Journal of Child Care*)
www.cyc-net.org/journals/jcyc/jcycw.html

Journal of Child Psychology and Psychiatry and Allied Disciplines
www.onlinelibrary.wiley.com

Journal of Clinical Child and Adolescent Psychology
(formerly *Journal of Clinical Child Psychology*)
www.tandfonline.com

Journal of Family Violence
www.springerlink.com

Journal of Music Therapy
www.academic.oup.com/jmt

Journal of Research on Adolescence
www.onlinelibrary.wiley.com

Journal of Traumatic Stress
www.onlinelibrary.wiley.com

Journal of Youth and Adolescence
www.springerlink.com

Play Therapy
www.a4pt.org

Psychoanalytic Study of the Child
www.tandfonline.com

School Psychology International
http://journals.sagepub.com/home/spi

Social Work in Health Care
www.tandfonline.com

Social Work with Groups
www.tandfonline.com

Trauma, Violence and Abuse
http://journals.sagepub.com/home/tva

Training Programs and Certifications

PLAY THERAPY

A comprehensive directory of play therapy training programs may be obtained for a fee from the Center for Play Therapy, Denton, TX 76203. The programs listed here represent a small selection of those available in different parts of the United States.

Boston University School of Social Work
Postgraduate Certificate Program in Assessment and Treatment of Psychological Trauma
Boston, MA 02215
www.bu.edu/ssw/careers/pep

California School of Professional Psychology
Alliant International University
Fresno, CA 93727
www.alliant.edu/cspp

Center for Play Therapy
University of North Texas
Denton, TX 76203
https://cpt.unt.edu

Center for Sandplay Studies
Upper Grandview, NY 10969
www.facebook.com/CenterforSandplayStudies

Chesapeake Beach Professional Seminars
Chesapeake Beach, MD 20732
www.cbpseminars.org

Lesley University
Graduate Certificate in Play Therapy
Cambridge, MA 02138
http://lesley.smartcatalogiq.com/en/2016-2017/Graduate-Catalog/Graduate-School-of-Arts-and-Social-Sciences/Division-of-Expressive-Therapies/Graduate-Certificates/Graduate-Certificate-in-Play-Therapy

Play Therapy Training Institute
Hightstown, NJ 08520
www.ptti.org

Theraplay Institute
Evanston, IL 60201
www.theraplay.org

Vista Del Mar Child and Family Services
Los Angeles, CA 90034
www.vistadelmar.org

CREATIVE ARTS/EXPRESSIVE THERAPY

Creative Arts and Health Certificate
The New School
New York, NY 10011
www.newschool.edu/academics

Dance/Movement Therapy
Drexel University
Philadelphia, PA 19102
www.drexel.edu/cnhp/academics/departments/Creative-Arts-Therapies

Expressive Arts Florida Institute
Sarasota, FL 34236
www.expressiveartsflorida.com/certificate-training-program

Graduate Program in Drama Therapy
Department of Music and Performing Arts Professions
New York University
New York, NY 10012
www.steinhardt.nyu.edu/music/dramatherapy

Lesley University
Certificate of Advanced Graduate Study in Expressive Therapies
Cambridge, MA 02138
www.lesley.edu/academics/graduate/expressive-therapies-0

School of the Art Institute of Chicago
Chicago, IL 60603
www.artic.edu

GRIEF COUNSELING

Association for Death Education and Counseling
Deerfield, IL 60015
www.adec.org

Certificate Program in Thanatology
Graduate School of the College of New Rochelle
New Rochelle, NY 10805
www.cnr.edu/web/graduate-school/thanatology

Children's Hospice International
Alexandria, VA 22314
www.chionline.org

The Dougy Center: The National Center for Grieving Children and Families
Portland, OR 97286
www.dougy.org

Hospice Foundation of America
Washington, DC 20036
www.hospicefoundation.org

Make-A-Wish Foundation of America
Phoenix, AZ 85016
www.wish.org

National Center for Death Education
Newton, MA 02459
www.mountida.edu/academics/continuing-education/ncde

TRAUMA/CRISIS COUNSELING

American Academy of Experts in Traumatic Stress
Ronkonkoma, NY 11779
www.aaets.org

American Association of Suicidology
Washington, DC 20015
www.suicidology.org

Child Trauma Academy
Houston, TX 77056
www.childtrauma.org

Child Trauma Institute
Northampton, MA 01060
www.childtrauma.com

EMDR International Association
Austin, TX 78714
www.emdria.org

National Child Traumatic Stress Network
Los Angeles, CA 90064
www.nctsn.org

National Institute for Trauma and Loss in Children
Albion, MI 49224
www.starr.org/training/tlc

ANIMAL-ASSISTED THERAPY

Mercy College
Dobbs Ferry, NY 10522
www.mercy.edu

Pet Partners (formerly Delta Society)
Bellevue, WA 98005
www.petpartners.org

Suppliers of Play Materials

Child Therapy Toys
www.childtherapytoys.com

Childcraft
www.childcrafteducation.com

Childswork/Childsplay
www.childswork.com

Constructive Playthings
www.constructiveplaythings.com

Magic Cabin
www.magiccabin.com

Play Therapy Supply
www.playtherapysupply.com

School Specialty
www.schoolspecialty.com

Self-Esteem Shop
www.selfesteemshop.com

U.S. Toy Company
www.ustoy.com

Western Psychological Services
www.wpspublish.com

Bereavement Resources

American Hospice Foundation
www.americanhospice.org

Association of Death Education and Counseling
www.adec.org

Children's Hospice International
www.chionline.org

Compassion Books
www.compassionbooks.com

Good Grief Program at Boston Medical Center
www.bmc.org/programs/good-grief-program

National Alliance for Grieving Children
www.nationalallianceforgrievingchildren.org

National Center for Death Education
www.mountida.edu/academics/continuing-education/ncde

Forms for Assessment of the Bereaved Child

FIGURE A1. Individual factors in childhood bereavement. This form is one part of the three-part assessment of the bereaved child, which also includes an assessment of death-related factors (Figure A2) and family/social/religious/cultural factors (Figure A3).

1. Age ________ years ________ months Date of birth ____________________

   Date of assessment ____________________

   a. Developmental stage:

      Freud ____________________

      Erikson ____________________

   b. Cognitive level:

      Piaget ____________________

   c. Temperamental characteristics:

      Thomas and Chess ____________________

2. Past coping/adjustment
   a. Home (as reported by parents): Good _____ Fair _____ Poor _____
   b. School (as reported by parents and teachers): Good _____ Fair _____ Poor _____
   c. Interpersonal/peers: Good _____ Fair _____ Poor _____
   d. Hobbies/interests (list) ____________________

3. Medical history (as reported by parents and pediatrician)—describe serious illnesses, operations, and injuries since birth, with dates and outcome ____________________

   ____

   ____

   ____

4. Past experience with death/loss—give details with dates and outcome *or* complete Wolfelt's Loss Inventory ____________________

   ____

   ____

   ____

From Webb (1993, p. 31). Copyright © 1993 The Guilford Press. Reprinted in *Social Work Practice with Children, Fourth Edition,* by Nancy Boyd Webb (The Guilford Press, 2019). Permission to photocopy this figure is granted to purchasers of this book for personal use or use with clients (see copyright page for details). Purchasers can download enlarged versions of this material (see the box at the end of the table of contents).

FIGURE A2. Death-related factors in childhood bereavement. This form is one part of the three-part assessment of the bereaved child, which also includes an assessment of individual factors (Figure A1) and family/social/religious/cultural factors (Figure A3).

1. Type of death

   Anticipated: Yes ______ No ______ If yes, how long? ______ or sudden ________________

   "Timeliness" of death: Age of the deceased ______________________________________

   Perception of preventability:

   Definitely preventable ______ Maybe ______ Not ____

   Degree of pain associated with death:

   None ______ Some ______ Much ______

   Presence of violence/trauma: Yes ______ No ___________

   If yes, describe, indicating whether the child witnessed, heard about, or was present and experienced the trauma personally. ______________________________________

   ____

   ____

   Element of stigma: Yes ______ No ______

   If yes, describe, indicating nature of death, and degree of openness of family in discussing. ____

   ____

   ____

2. Contact with deceased

   Present at moment of death? Yes ______ No ______

   If yes, describe circumstances, including who else was present and whether the deceased said anything specifically to the child. ____________________________________

   ____

   ____

   Did the child view the dead body? Yes ______ No ______

   If yes, describe circumstances, including reactions of the child and others who were present. ____

   Did the child attend funeral/memorial service/graveside service?

   Yes ______ No ______ Which? ______________________________________

   Child's reactions ____

   ____

   Has the child visited grave/mausoleum since the death? Yes ______ No ___________

   If yes, describe circumstances. ____

   ____

3. Did the child make any expression of "goodbye" to the deceased, either spontaneous or suggested? Yes ______ No ______

   If yes, describe. ____

   ____

   ____

From Webb (1993, p. 35). Copyright © 1993 The Guilford Press. Reprinted in *Social Work Practice with Children, Fourth Edition*, by Nancy Boyd Webb (The Guilford Press, 2019). Permission to photocopy this figure is granted to purchasers of this book for personal use or use with clients (see copyright page for details). Purchasers can download enlarged versions of this material (see the box at the end of the table of contents).

FIGURE A3. Family/social/religious/cultural factors in childhood bereavement. This form is one part of the three-part assessment of the bereaved child, which also includes an assessment of individual factors (Figure A1) and death-related factors (Figure A2).

1. Family influences

   Nuclear family: How responding to death? Describe in terms of relative degree of openness of response.

   Very expressive ______ Moderately expressive ______ Very guarded ______

   To what extent is child included in family discussions/rituals related to the deceased?

   Some ______ A great deal ______ Not at all _

   Extended family: How responding to death? Describe, as above, in terms of relative degree of openness of response.

   Very expressive ______ Moderately expressive ______ Very guarded ______

   To what extent do the views of the extended family differ or agree with those of the nuclear family with regard to the planning of rituals and inclusion of child?

   Very different ______ Very similar __________

   If different, describe the nature of the disagreement ________________________________

   ____

2. School/peer influences

   Child's grade in school ________

   Did any of the child's friends/peers attend the funeral/memorial services?

   Yes ______ No ______

   Was teacher informed of death? Yes ______ No ______

   Did child receive condolence messages from friends/peers? Yes ______ No ______

   Does child know anyone his/her age who has been bereaved? Yes ______ No ______

   If yes, has child spoken to this person since the death? Yes ______ No ______

   Does child express feelings about wanting or not wanting peers/friends to know about the death? Yes ______ No ______

   If yes, what has the child said? ____

3. Religious/cultural influences

   What is the child's religion? ____

   Has he/she been observant? Yes ______ No ______

   What are the beliefs of the child's religion regarding death? ____________________

   ____

   What about life after death? ____

   Has child expressed any thoughts/feelings about this? ____________________

   ____

From Webb (1993, p. 39). Copyright © 1993 The Guilford Press. Reprinted in *Social Work Practice with Children, Fourth Edition*, by Nancy Boyd Webb (The Guilford Press, 2019). Permission to photocopy this figure is granted to purchasers of this book for personal use or use with clients (see copyright page for details). Purchasers can download enlarged versions of this material (see the box at the end of the table of contents).

FIGURE A4. Recording form for childhood grief reactions. This form is an extension of "Death-Related Factors in Childhood Bereavement" (Figure A2), focusing specifically on the nature of the child's grief.

Age of child _____ years _____ months _____ Date of birth ____________________

Date of assessment ____________________

See the form "Individual Factors in Childhood Bereavement" (Figure A1) for recording of personal history factors.

Date of death ____________________

Relationship to deceased ____________________

Favorite activities shared with deceased ____________________

What the child will miss the most ____________________

If the child could see the deceased again for 1 hour, what would he/she like to do or say? ____

____

____

Nature of grief reactions (describe) ____________________

____

Signs of the following feelings? Y = Yes; N = No

Sadness _____ Anger _____ Confusion _____ Guilt _____ Relief _____

Other ____________________

Source of information on which this form has been completed

_____ Parent _____ Observation _____ Other

From Webb (1993, p. 38). Copyright © 1993 The Guilford Press. Reprinted in *Social Work Practice with Children, Fourth Edition,* by Nancy Boyd Webb (The Guilford Press, 2019). Permission to photocopy this figure is granted to purchasers of this book for personal use or use with clients (see copyright page for details). Purchasers can download enlarged versions of this material (see the box at the end of the table of contents).

Forms for Assessment of the Child in Crisis

FIGURE A5. Crisis situation rating form. This form is one part of a three-part crisis assessment, which also includes an assessment of individual factors (Figure A6) and support system factors (Figure A7).

1. Psychosocial and environmental problems:
   List problems = ______________________________
   ____
2. Anticipated or sudden __________ crisis (check where appropriate)
   Amount of preparation ______________________________
3. Single __________ or recurring __________ crisis events (list discrete crisis events)
   a. ______________________ c. ______________________
   b. ______________________ d. ______________________
4. Solitary __________ or shared __________ crisis experience
   Number of other individuals involved __________
5. Presence of loss factor
   a. Separation from family members (list relationship and length of separation) __________
   ____
   ____
   b. Death of family members (list relationship and cause of death) __________
   ____
   ____
   c. Loss of familiar environment (describe) __________
   ____
   ____
   d. Loss of familiar role/status (describe; temporary or permanent) __________
   ____
   ____
   e. Loss of body part or function (describe, with prognosis) __________
   ____
   ____
6. Physical injury or pain (describe, with prognosis) __________
   ____
   ____
7. Presence of violence: verbal and/or physical
   a. Witnessed __________ Verbal __________ Physical __________
   b. Experienced __________ Verbal __________ Physical __________
8. Degree of life threat
   a. Personal (describe) ______________________________
   ____
   ____
   b. To family members (describe, identifying relationship) __________
   ____
   ____
   c. To others (describe) ______________________________
   ____
   ____
9. Other components of the crisis situation ______________________________
   ____
   ____

From Webb (1991, p. 11). Copyright © 1991 The Guilford Press. Reprinted in *Social Work Practice with Children, Fourth Edition*, by Nancy Boyd Webb (The Guilford Press, 2019). Permission to photocopy this figure is granted to purchasers of this book for personal use or use with clients (see copyright page for details). Purchasers can download enlarged versions of this material (see the box at the end of the table of contents).

FIGURE A6. Individual factors in the assessment of the child in crisis. This form is one part of a three-part crisis assessment, which also includes a crisis situation rating form (Figure A5) and support system factors (Figure A7).

1. Age ______ years ______ months ______ Date of birth ____________

   Date of assessment ____________

   a. Developmental stage:
      Freud ___________
      Erikson ___________
   b. Cognitive level:
      Piaget ___________
   c. Moral development:
      Kohlberg ___________
   d. Temperamental characteristics:
      Thomas and Chess ___________

2. Pre-crisis adjustment
   a. Home (as reported by parents): Good ______ Fair ______ Poor ______
   b. School (as reported by parents and teachers): Good ______ Fair ______ Poor ______
   c. Interpersonal/peers: Good ______ Fair ______ Poor ______
   d. Medical (as reported by parents/and pediatrician)—describe serious illnesses, operations, and injuries since birth, with dates and outcome ____________

      ____

      ____

      Past or current use of medications ____________

      ____

3. Coping style/ego assessment (as reported by parents and observed in interviews with child)
   a. Degree of anxiety: High ______ Moderate ______ Low ______
   b. Ability to separate from parent: High anxiety ______ Some anxiety ______ No anxiety ______
   c. Child's ability to discuss "the problem/crisis situation": Good ______ Fair ______ None ______
   d. Presence of symptoms (describe, including the extent to which these bind the anxiety)

      ____

      ____

      ____

   e. Defenses (list, indicating appropriateness) ____________

      ____

4. Child's past experience with crises ____________
   a. Previous losses (list, giving age) ____________

      ____

   b. Major life transitions/adjustments (list, giving age) ____________

      ____

   c. Past experience with violence ____________

      ____

   d. Other (describe) ____________

      ____

5. Specific meaning of crisis to the child: Why is this crisis situation so difficult for *this* child at *this* time? (describe) ____________

   ____

From Webb (1991, p. 14). Copyright © 1991 The Guilford Press. Reprinted in *Social Work Practice with Children, Fourth Edition,* by Nancy Boyd Webb (The Guilford Press, 2019). Permission to photocopy this figure is granted to purchasers of this book for personal use or use with clients (see copyright page for details). Purchasers can download enlarged versions of this material (see the box at the end of the table of contents).

FIGURE A7. Support system factors. This form is one part of a three-part crisis assessment, which also includes a crisis situation rating form (Figure A5) and an assessment of individual factors (Figure A6).

1. Nuclear family members
   a. How responsive are they to the child's needs? Not at all ____ Somewhat ____ Very ______
   b. To what extent is the child included in discussions about "the problem situation"?
      Frequently ____ Never ____ Sometimes ____
   c. Do parents tend to show a judgmental attitude toward the child's behavior?
      Yes ____ No ____
2. Extended family members
   a. How frequently are they in contact with the child?
      Rarely ____ Monthly ____ Weekly ____ Daily ____
   b. Describe nature of the relationships, indicating who is the most supportive relative to the child ______________________________
   c. To what extent do the views of the extended family differ from or agree with those of the nuclear family on matters pertaining to the child? (give details)
      ____
3. School/peers/social network
   a. Child's grade in school ______________
   b. Child's friendship network: How many friends does child have?
      Many ____ "A few" ____ None ____
   c. Would child like to have more friends than he or she has? Yes ____ No ____
   d. How many days after school, on the average, does the child play with another child?
      Most days ____ Once or twice ____ Never ____
4. Religious affiliation
   a. Does the child/family participate in religious services?
      Yes ____ (If yes, give name of religious group:) ______________________
      No ____
   b. If yes, indicate how frequently the child/family participates:
      Weekly ____ Major holiday observances ____ Rarely ____
5. Neighborhood/school activities
   a. Is the family involved with neighborhood/school activities? No ____ Yes ____
   b. If yes, describe ______________________________

From Webb (1991, p. 14). Copyright © 1991 The Guilford Press. Reprinted in *Social Work Practice with Children, Fourth Edition,* by Nancy Boyd Webb (The Guilford Press, 2019). Permission to photocopy this figure is granted to purchasers of this book for personal use or use with clients (see copyright page for details). Purchasers can download enlarged versions of this material (see the box at the end of the table of contents).

References

Achenbach, T. M. (1991). *Integrative guide for the 1991 CBCL/4–18, YSR, and TRF profiles*. Burlington: University of Vermont, Department of Psychiatry.

Achenbach, T. M., & Edelbrock, C. E. (1983). *Manual for the Child Behavior Checklist and Revised Child Behavior Profile*. Burlington: University of Vermont, Department of Psychiatry.

Achenbach, T. M., & Howell, C. T. (1993). Are American children's problems getting worse? A 13-year comparison. *Journal of the American Academy of Child Psychiatry, 32*(6), 1145–1154.

Achenbach, T. M., Howell, C. T., Quay, H. C., & Conners, C. K. (1991). National survey of problems and competencies reported by parents of normal and disturbed children aged four through sixteen. *Monographs of the Society for Research in Child Development, 46*(1, Serial No. 188).

Achenbach, T. M., McConaughy, S. H., & Howell, C. T. (1987). Child/adolescent behavioral and emotional problems: Implications of cross-informant correlations for situational specificity. *Psychological Bulletin, 101*, 213–232.

Administration for Children and Families. (2016). *Child maltreatment*. Washington, DC: Author.

Adoption Assistance and Child Welfare Reform Act, Public Law 96-272, 94 Stat. 500 (1980).

Ainsworth, M. D. S. (1979). Infant–mother attachment. *American Psychologist, 34*, 932–937.

Ainsworth, M. D. S., & Bell, S. M. (1971). Attachment, exploration, and separation: Illustrated by the behavior of one-year-olds in a Strange Situation. In S. Chess & A. Thomas (Eds.), *Annual progress in child psychiatry and child development* (pp. 41–60). New York: Brunner/Mazel.

Ajdukovic, M., & Ajdukovic, D. (1993). Psychological well-being of refugee children. *Child Abuse and Neglect, 17*, 843–854.

Alexander, D. W. (1992). *Something bad happened series: The world I see*. Plainview, NY: Bureau for At-Risk Youth.

Allen, B., Cisneros, E. M., & Tellez, A. (2015). The children left behind: The impact of parental deportation on mental health. *Journal of Child and Family Studies, 24(2)*, 386–392.

Allen-Meares, P. (2007). *Social work services in schools* (5th ed.). Boston: Pearson.

Allen-Meares, P., Washington, R. O., & Welsh, B. L. (2000). *Social work services in schools* (3rd ed.). Boston: Allyn & Bacon.

Amendments to the Education of the Handicapped Act, Public Law 99-457, 100 Stat. 1145-1158 (1986).

Amenta, C. A. (1992). *Russell is extra special: A book about autism for children.* Washington, DC: Magination Press.

American Psychiatric Association. (2013). *Diagnostic and statistical manual of mental disorders* (5th ed.). Arlington, VA: Author.

American Psychological Association. (1993). *Violence and youth: Psychology's response* (Vol. 1). Washington, DC: Author.

American Psychological Association. (2007). *Report of the APA Task Force on Socioeconomic Status.* Washington, DC: Author.

American Psychological Association Ad Hoc Committee on Legal and Ethical Issues in the Treatment of Interpersonal Violence. (1996). *Professional, ethical, and legal issues concerning interpersonal violence, maltreatment, and related trauma.* Washington, DC: American Psychological Association.

Anderson, G. R., & Seita, J. (2006). Family and social factors affecting youth in the child welfare system. In N. B. Webb (Ed.), *Working with traumatized youth in child welfare* (pp. 67–90). New York: Guilford Press.

Angelou, M. (1991). *All God's children need traveling shoes.* New York: Random House. (Original work published 1986)

Annie E. Casey Foundation. (2017). Baltimore: Author.

Anthony, E. J., & Cohler, B. J. (Eds.). (1987). *The invulnerable child.* New York: Guilford Press.

Aponte, H. (1990). *Tres madres* [Videotape]. Kansas City, MO: Golden Triad.

Applegate, J. S., & Shapiro, J. R. (2005). *Neurobiology for clinical social work: Theory and practice.* New York: Norton.

Aries, P. (1962). *Centuries of childhood.* New York: Vintage Books.

Aronson, S. (2017). Origins of group therapy with children and adolescents. In C. Haen & S. Aronson (Eds.), *Handbook of child and adolescent group therapy* (pp. 1–3). New York: Routledge.

Aust, P. H. (1981). Using the life story book to treat children in placement. *Child Welfare, 60,* 535–560.

Axline, V. (1947). *Play therapy.* Boston: Houghton Mifflin.

Axline, V. (1964). *Dibs: In search of self.* New York: Ballantine.

Backhaus, K. (1984). Life books: Tool for working with children in placement. *Social Work, 29*(6), 551–554.

Baggerly, J. (2007). International interventions and challenges following the crisis of natural disasters. In N. B. Webb (Ed.), *Play therapy with children in crisis: Individual, group, and family treatment* (3rd ed., pp. 345–367). New York: Guilford Press.

Baggerly, J., & Bratton, S. (2010). Building a firm foundation in play therapy research: Response to Phillips (2010). *International Journal of Play Therapy, 19*(1), 26–38.

Baggerly, J. N., Ray, D. C., & Bratton, S. C. (Eds.). (2010). *Child-centered play therapy research: The evidence base for effective practice.* Hoboken, NJ: Wiley.

Baggerly, J., & Salloum, A. (2010). Deaths connected to natural disasters. In N. B. Webb (Ed.), *Helping bereaved children: A handbook for practitioners* (3rd ed., pp. 240–260). New York: Guilford Press.

Ballan, M. S., & Hoban, K. S. (2006). Effective interventions for students with autism and Asperger's syndrome. In C. Franklin, M. B. Harris, & P. Allen-Meares (Eds.), *The school services sourcebook: A guide for school-based professionals* (pp. 147–163). New York: Oxford University Press.

Bank, S. P., & Kahn, M. (1982). *The sibling bond.* New York: Basic Books.

Banks, R. (1997). *Bullying in school.* Retrieved from *www.ericdigests.org/1997-4/bullying.htm.*

Barker, P. (1995). *Basic child psychiatry* (6th ed.). Oxford, UK: Blackwell Scientific.

Barkley, R. A. (2006). *Attention-deficit hyperactivity disorder. A handbook for diagnosis and treatment* (3rd ed.). New York: Guilford Press.

Barkley, R. A. (2013). *Taking charge of ADHD: The complete, authoritative guide for parents* (3rd ed.). New York: Guilford Press.

Barkley, R. A., Robin, A. R., & Benton, C. (2014). *Your defiant teen: 10 steps to resolve conflict and rebuild your relationship* (2nd ed.). New York: Guilford Press.

Barnard, M., & McKeganey, N. (2004). The impact of parental problem drug use on children: What is the problem and what can be done to help? *Addictions, 95*(5), 552–559.

Barth, R., Courtney, M., Berrick, J., & Albert, V. (1994). *From child abuse to permanency planning: Child welfare services, pathways, and placements.* New York: Aldine de Gruyter.

Bassuk, E. L. (1993). Social and economic hardships of homeless and other poor women. *American Journal of Orthopsychiatry, 63*(3), 340–347.

Bassuk, E. L., & Rubin, L. (1986). Homeless children: A neglected population. *American Journal of Orthopsychiatry, 57*(2), 279–286.

Bean, N., McAllister, E., & Hudgins, L. (2001). Cross-cultural lessons and inspirations from grandparents and great-grandparents raising grandchildren. *Reflections, 7*(2), 40–51.

Beauchaine, T. P., & Hinshaw, S. P. (2008). *Child and adolescent psychopathology.* Hoboken, NJ: Wiley.

Beck, A. T., Rush, A. J., Shaw, B. F., & Emery, G. (1979). *Cognitive therapy of depression.* New York: Guilford Press.

Begleiter, H. (1988). Advances in alcoholism and chemical dependence [Editorial]. *American Journal of Medicine, 85*, 465.

Belsky, J. (1993). Etiology of child maltreatment: A developmental–ecological analysis. *Psychological Bulletin, 114*, 413–434.

Bernier, J. C., & Siegel, D. H. (1994). Attention-deficit hyperactivity disorder: A family and ecological systems perspective. *Families in Society, 75*(3), 142–151.

Berrick, J. D., Needell, B., Barth, R. P., & Jonson-Reid, M. (1998). *The tender years: Toward developmentally sensitive child welfare services for very young children.* New York: Oxford University Press.

Besharov, D. J. (1989). The children of crack: Will we protect them? *Public Welfare, 46*(4), 7–11.

Bevin, T. (1999). Multiple traumas of refugees—near drowning and witnessing of maternal rape: Case of Sergio, age 9, and follow-up at age 16. In N. B. Webb (Ed.), *Play therapy with children in crisis: Individual, group, and family treatment* (2nd ed., pp. 164–182). New York: Guilford Press.

Bing, N. M., Nelson, W. M., III, & Wesolowski, K. L. (2009). Comparing the effects of conflict on children's adjustment following parental divorce. *Journal of Divorce and Remarriage, 50*, 159–171.

Bishop, K. K. (1993). P.L. 99-457: A family-centered continuing education curriculum for social workers. *Journal of Teaching in Social Work, 7*(2), 47–61.

Bishop, K. K., Rounds, K. A., & Weil, M. (1993). P.L. 97–457: Preparation for social work practice with infants and toddlers with disabilities and their families. *Journal of Social Work Education, 29*(1), 36–45.

Black, R., & Mayer, J. (1980). Parents with special problems: Alcoholism and opiate addictions. In C. H. Kempe & R. Helfer (Eds.), *The battered child* (pp. 104–113). Chicago: University of Chicago Press.

Blaustein, M. E., & Kinniburgh, K. M. (2019). *Treating traumatic stress in children and adolescents: How to foster resilience through attachment, self-regulation, and competency* (2nd ed.). New York: Guilford Press.

Block, J., & Margolis, J. (1986). Feelings of shame: Siblings of handicapped children. In A. Gitterman & L. Shulman (Eds.), *Mutual aid groups and the life cycle* (pp. 91–108). Itasca, IL: Peacock.

Bloom, M. (1981). *Primary prevention: The possible science.* Englewood Cliffs, NJ: Prentice-Hall.

Bloomquist, M. L. (1996). *Skills training for children with behavior disorders: A parent and therapist guidebook.* New York: Guilford Press.

Boulanger, M. D., & Langevin, C. (1992). Direct observation of play group therapy for social skills deficits. *Journal of Child and Adolescent Group Therapy, 2*(4), 227–236.

Bowker, J. P. (1983). Overview. In J. P. Bowker (Ed.), *Education for primary prevention in social work* (pp. 1–6). New York: Council on Social Work Education.

Bowlby, J. (1969). *Attachment and loss: Vol. 1. Attachment.* New York: Basic Books.

Bowlby, J. (1973). *Attachment and loss: Vol. 2. Separation: Anxiety and anger.* New York: Basic Books.

Bowlby, J. (1977). The making and breaking of affectional bonds. *British Journal of Psychiatry, 130*, 201–210, 421–431.

Bowlby, J. (1979). *The making and breaking of affectional bonds.* London: Tavistock.

Bowlby, J. (1980). *Attachment and loss: Vol. 3. Loss: Sadness and depression.* New York: Basic Books.

Bowlby, J. (1988). *A secure base: Parent–child attachment and healthy human development.* New York: Basic Books.

Boyle, M. H., Offord, D. R., Hoffman, H. G., Catlin, G. P., Byles, J. A., Cadman, D. T., et al. (1987). Ontario Child Health Study: I. Methodology. *Archives of General Psychiatry, 44*, 826–831.

Brandell, J. (2002). The marginalization of psychoanalysis in social work. *Psychoanalysis in Social Work, 9*(2), 41.

Brandenburg, N. A., Friedman, R. M., & Silver, S. E. (1990). The epidemiology of childhood psychiatric disorders: Prevalence findings from recent studies. *Journal of the American Academy of Child and Adolescent Psychiatry, 29*, 76–83.

Brandler, S., & Roman, C. P. (1991). *Group work skills and strategies for effective intervention.* New York: Haworth Press.

Brané, M., & Wang, L. (2013, September). Women: The invisible detainees. *Forced Migration Review, 44*, 37–39.

Brendler, J. (2006). A model for disrupting cycles of violence in families with young children. In L. Combrinck-Graham (Ed.), *Children in family contexts: Perspectives on treatment* (pp. 433–455). New York: Guilford Press.

Breslau, N. (2001). The epidemiology of posttraumatic stress disorder: What is the extent of the problem? *Journal of Clinical Psychiatry, 62*(17, Suppl.), 16–22.

Brieland, D., Costin, L. B., & Atherton, C. R. (1985). *Contemporary social work: An introduction to social work and social welfare* (3rd ed.). New York: McGraw-Hill.

Briggs, H. E., & Rzepnicki, T. L. (2004). *Using evidence in social work practice: Behavioral perspectives.* Chicago: Lyceum Books.

Bronfenbrenner, U. (1979). *The ecology of human development.* Cambridge, MA: Harvard University Press.

Bronstein, I. R. (2003). A model for interdisciplinary collaboration. *Social Work, 48*(3), 297–307.

Brooks-Gunn, J., & Duncan, G. J. (1997). The effects of poverty on children. *Future of Children, 7,* 55–71.

Brown, T. (1999, January 18). *The bullying reference, 1*(4). Zanesville, OH: Broken Toy Project. Retrieved February 6, 1999, from *members.tripod.com/-Ghoul2x/Bully1.html.*

Browne, A. (1993). Family violence and homelessness: The relevance of trauma histories in the lives of homeless women. *American Journal of Orthopsychiatry, 63*(3), 370–384.

Bruni, F. (1995, November 24). The case of Elisa: A child dies, and the questions abound. *New York Times,* p. B-1.

Bruning, P. S. (2007). The crisis of adoption disruption and dissolution. In N. B. Webb (Ed.), *Play therapy with children in crisis. Individual, group, and family treatment* (3rd ed., pp. 152–172). New York: Guilford Press.

Bullock, R. B. (2007). The crisis of deaths in schools: Interventions with students, parents, and teachers. In N. B. Webb (Ed.), *Play therapy with children in crisis: Individual, group, and family treatment* (3rd ed., pp. 270–293). New York: Guilford Press.

Bullock, R. B. (2009). Medical conditions that appear during early childhood. In N. B. Webb (Ed.), *Helping children and adolescents with chronic and serious medical conditions* (pp. 205–224). Hoboken, NJ: Wiley.

Burns, R. C., & Kaufman, S. H. (1970). *Kinetic Family Drawing (K-F-D): Research and application.* New York: Brunner/Mazel.

Burns, R. C., & Kaufman, S. H. (1972). *Actions, styles and symbols in Kinetic Family Drawings (K-F-D): An interpretive manual.* New York: Brunner/Mazel.

Caldwell, B., & Bradley, R. (1979). *Home observation for measurement of the environment.* Little Rock: University of Arkansas Center for Child Development and Education.

Call, D. A. (1990). School-based groups: A valuable support for children of cancer patients. *Journal of Psychosocial Oncology, 8*(1), 97–118.

Calohan, C. J., & Peeler, C. M. (2007). Autistic disorder. In B. A. Thyer & J. S. Wodarski (Eds.), *Social work in mental health. An evidence-based approach* (pp. 53–73). Hoboken, NJ: Wiley.

Cancino, A. (2016, February). More grandparents raising their grandchildren. Retrieved from *www.pbs.org/newshour/nation/more-grandparents-raising-their-grandchildren.*

Caplan, G. (1964). *Principles of preventive psychiatry.* New York: Basic Books.

Capps, R., Casteñeda, R. M., Chaudry, A., & Santos, R. (2007). *Paying the price: The impact of immigration raids on America's children.* Washington, DC: Urban Institute for National Council of La Raza.

Carlson, B. E. (1984). Children's observations of interpersonal violence. In A. R. Roberts (Ed.), *Battered women and their families* (pp. 147–167). New York: Springer.

Carrillo, D. F., Holzhalb, C. M., & Thyer, B. A. (1993). Assessing social work students' attitudes related to cultural diversity: A review of selected measures. *Journal of Social Work Education, 29*(3), 263–268.

Casper, L. M., & Bryson, K. R. (1998). *Co-resident grandparents and their grandchildren: Grandparent-maintained families* (Population Division Technical Working Paper 26). Washington, DC: U.S. Bureau of the Census.

Ceballo, R. (2000). The neighborhood club: A supportive intervention group for children exposed to urban violence. *American Journal of Orthopsychiatry, 70*(3), 401–407.

Centers for Disease Control and Prevention. (2018, May). *About autism spectrum disorder.* Retrieved June 29, 2018 from *www.cdc.gov/ncbddd/autism.*

Chadiha, L., Miller-Cribbs, J., & Wilson-Klar, D. (1997). Course syllabus on human diversity. In George Warren Brown School of Social Work (Ed.), *Human diversity content in social work education: A collection of course outlines with content on racial, ethnic, and cultural diversity* (pp. 103–129). Alexandria, VA: Council on Social Work Education.

Chasin, R., & White, T. B. (1989). The child in family therapy: Guidelines for active engagement across the age span. In L. Combrinck-Graham (Ed.), *Children in family contexts: Perspectives on treatment* (pp. 5–25). New York: Guilford Press.

Chess, S. (1988). Child and adolescent psychiatry come of age: A fifty-year perspective. *Journal of the American Academy of Child and Adolescent Psychiatry, 27*(1), 1–7.

Chess, S., & Thomas, A. (1986). *Temperament in clinical practice.* New York: Guilford Press.

Chethik, M. (2000). *Techniques of child therapy: Psychodynamic strategies* (2nd ed.). New York: Guilford Press.

Child Abuse: Part III. (1993). *Harvard Mental Health Letter, 10*(1), 1–5.

Child Abuse Prevention and Treatment Act, Public Law 93-247, 88 Stat. 119 (1974).

Child Welfare Information Gateway. (2017). *Foster care statistics 2015.* Washington, DC: U.S. Department of Health and Human Services, Children's Bureau.

Children's Bureau. (2014). *Trends in foster care and adoption.* Washington, DC: Author.

Children's Bureau. (2016, May). *Kinship caregivers and the child welfare system: Factsheet for families.* Washington, DC: Author.

Children's Defense Fund. (2000). *State of America's children.* Washington, DC. Author.

Children's Defense Fund. (2005, August). *Child abuse and neglect fact sheet.* Washington, DC: Author.

Children's Defense Fund. (2008a). Children in kinship care: 2000 and 2007. In *State of America's children* (p. 43). Washington, DC: Author. Retrieved January 20, 2010, from *www.childrensdefense.org/child-research-data-publication/data/state of Americas-children.*

Children's Defense Fund. (2008b). *State of America's children.* Washington, DC: Author. Retrieved January 20, 2010, from *www.childrensdefense.org/child-research-data-publication/data/state of Americas-children.*

Children's Defense Fund. (2012). *Child abuse and neglect fact sheet.* Washington, DC: Author.

Children's Defense Fund. (2016). *Child poverty in American 2015: National analysis.* Washington, DC: Author.

Choi, N. G., & Snyder, N. G. (1999). *Homeless families with children: A subjective experience of homelessness.* New York: Springer.

Cicchetti, D. (2008). A multiple-levels-of-analysis perspective on research in development and psychopathology. In T. P. Beauchaine & S. P. Hinshaw (Eds.), *Child and adolescent psychopathology* (pp. 27–57). Hoboken, NJ: Wiley.

Cicchetti, D., & Blender, J. A. (2004). A multiple-levels-of-analysis approach to the study of developmental processes in maltreated children. *Proceedings of the National Academy of Sciences of the USA, 101*(50), 17325–17326.

Clinton, B. (2004). *My life.* New York: Random House.

Cohen, J. A., Mannarino, A. P., & Deblinger, E. (2012). *Trauma-focused CBT for children and adolescents: Treatment applications.* New York: Guilford Press.

Cohen, J. A., Mannarino, A. P., & Deblinger, E. (2017). Trauma-focused cognitive-behavioral therapy for traumatized children. In J. R. Weisz & A. E. Kazdin (Eds.), *Evidence-based psychotherapies for children and adolescents* (3rd ed., pp. 253–271). New York: Guilford Press.

Cohn, D. (2016, June 23). *It's official: Minority babies are the majority among the nation's infants, but only just.* Washington, DC: Pew Research Center.

Cohn, D., & Caumont, A. (2016, March 31). *10 demographic trends that are shaping the U.S. and the world.* Washington, DC: Pew Research Center.

Combrinck-Graham, L. (Ed.). (1989). *Children in family contexts: Perspectives on treatment.* New York: Guilford Press.

Combrinck-Graham, L. (Ed.). (2006). *Children in family contexts: Perspectives on treatment* (2nd ed.). New York: Guilford Press.

Committee for Children. (2011). Steps to Respect: A bullying prevention program. Retrieved from *http://cfchildren.org/steps-to-respect.*

Community Mental Health Centers Act, Public Law 88-164, 77 Stat. 290–294 (1963).

Congress, E. P. (1994). The use of culturagrams to assess and empower culturally diverse families. *Families in Society, 75*(9), 531–539.

Congress, E. P. (Ed.). (1997). *Multicultural perspectives in working with families.* New York: Springer.

Congress, E. P. (1999). *Social work values and ethics: Identifying and resolving professional dilemmas.* New York: Wadsworth.

Congress, E. P. (2008). The culturagram. In A. Roberts (Ed.), *Social work desk reference* (2nd ed., pp. 969–975). New York: Oxford University Press.

Conners, C. K. (1969). A teacher rating scale for use in drug studies with children. *American Journal of Psychiatry, 126*, 884–888.

Conners, C. K. (1970). Symptom patterns in hyperkinetic, neurotic, and normal children. *Child Development, 41*, 667–682.

Connors, K., Schamess, G., & Strieder, F. (1997). Children's treatment groups: General principles and their application to group treatment with cumulatively traumatized children. In J. Brandell (Ed.), *Theory and practice in clinical social work* (pp. 288–314). New York: Free Press.

Copans, S. A. (1989). The invisible family member: Children in families with alcohol abuse. In L. Combrinck-Graham (Ed.), *Children in family contexts: Perspectives on treatment* (pp. 277–298). New York: Guilford Press.

Copans, S. A. (2006). The invisible illness: Children in alcoholic families. In L. Combrinck-Graham (Ed.), *Children in family contexts: Perspectives on treatment* (pp. 292–311). New York: Guilford Press.

Corr, C. A., Nabe, C. M., & Corr, D. M. (2000). *Death and dying: Life and living.* Belmont, CA: Wadsworth.

Costin, L. B. (1969). A historical review of school social work. *Social Casework, 50*(10), 439–453.

Costin, L. B. (1987). School social work. In A. Minahan (Ed.), *Encyclopedia of social work* (18th ed., pp. 538–545). Silver Spring, MD: National Association of Social Workers.

Council on Social Work Education. (1984). *Handbook of accreditation standards and procedures* (rev. ed.). New York: Author.

Council on Social Work Education. (1992a). *Curriculum policy statement for baccalaureate degree programs in social work education.* Alexandria, VA: Author.

Council on Social Work Education. (1992b). *Curriculum policy statement for master's degree programs in social work education.* Alexandria, VA: Author.

Council on Social Work Education. (2002). *Education policy and accreditation standards.* New York: Author.

Council on Social Work Education. (2008). *Education policy and accreditation standards.* Alexandria, VA: Author.

Council on Social Work Education. (2015). *Educational policy and accreditation standards.* Alexandria, VA: Author.

Cournoyer, B. (1991). *The social work skills workbook.* Belmont, CA: Wadsworth.

Courtois, C. A., & Ford, J. D. (2009). Defining and understanding complex trauma and complex stress disorders. In C. A. Courtois & J. D. Ford (Eds.), *Treating complex stress disorders: An evidence-based guide* (pp. 13–30). New York: Guilford Press.

Crawford-Brown, C., & Rattray, M. (2001). Parent–child relationships in Caribbean families. In N. B. Webb (Ed.), *Culturally diverse parent–child and family relationships: A guide for social workers and other practitioners* (pp. 107–130). New York: Columbia University Press.

Creeden, K., & Haen, C. (2017). Groups in residential settings. In C. Haen & S. Aronson (Eds.), *Handbook of child and adolescent group therapy* (pp. 229–239). New York: Routledge.

Crenshaw, D. A. (2014). Play therapy approaches to attachment issues. In C. A. Malchiodi & D. A. Crenshaw (Eds.), *Creative arts and play therapy for attachment problems* (pp. 19–32). New York: Guilford Press.

Crick, N. R., & Dodge, K. A. (1996). Social information-processing mechanisms in reactive and proactive aggression. *Child Development, 67*, 993–1002.

D'Andrea, W., Ford, J., Stolbach, B., Spinazzola, J., & van der Kolk, B. A. (2012). Understanding interpersonal trauma in children: Why we need a developmentally appropriate trauma diagnosis. *American Journal of Orthopsychiatry, 82*(2), 187–200.

Dane, B. O. (2002). Bereavement groups for children: Families with HIV/AIDS. In N. B. Webb (Ed.), *Helping bereaved children: A handbook for practitioners* (2nd ed., pp. 265–298). New York: Guilford Press.

Dane, E. (1990). *Painful passages: Working with children with learning disabilities.* Silver Springs, MD: National Association of Social Workers.

Daro, D., & McCurdy, K. L. (1991). *Current trends in child abuse reporting and fatalities: The results of the 1989 annual fifty-state survey.* Chicago: National Center on Child Abuse Prevention Research, National Committee for Prevention of Child Abuse.

Davenport, B. R., & Bourgeois, N. M. (2008). Play, aggression, and the pre-school child, and the family: A review of literature to guide empirically informed play therapy with aggressive preschool children. *International Journal of Play Therapy, 17,* 2–23.

Davies, B. (1988). The family environment in bereaved families and its relationship to surviving sibling behavior. *Children's Health Care, 17,* 22–31.

Davies, B. (1995). Sibling bereavement research: State of the art. In I. Corless, B. Germino, & M. Pittman (Eds.), *A challenge for living: Death, dying, and bereavement* (Vol. 2, pp. 173–202). Boston: Jones & Bartlett.

Davies, B. (1999). *Shadows in the sun: The experiences of sibling bereavement in childhood.* Philadelphia: Brunner/Mazel.

Davies, B., & Limbo, R. (2010). The grief of siblings. In N. B. Webb (Ed.), *Helping bereaved children: A handbook for practitioners* (3rd ed., pp. 69–90). New York: Guilford Press.

Davies, D. (2011). *Child development: A practitioner's guide* (3rd ed.). New York: Guilford Press.

Dawkins, J. L. (1996). Bullying, physical disability and the paediatric patient. *Developmental Medicine and Child Neurology, 38,* 603–612.

Dean, M., & Landis, H. (2017). Creative arts-based approaches with adolescent groups. In C. Haen & S. Aronson (Eds.), *Handbook of child and adolescent group therapy: A practitioner's reference* (pp. 124–136). New York: Routledge.

DeJong, P., & Miller, S. D. (1995). How to interview for client strengths. *Social Work, 40*(6), 729–736.

Dempsey, J. P., Fireman, G. D., & Wang, E. M. (2006). Transitioning out of peer victimization in school children: Gender and behavior characteristics. *Journal of Psychopathology and Behavioral Assessment, 28*(4), 271–280.

deRidder, N. F. (1999). HIV/AIDS in the family: Group treatment for latency-age children affected by the illness of a family member. In N. B. Webb (Ed.), *Play therapy with children in crisis: Individual, group, and family treatment* (2nd ed., pp. 341–355). New York: Guilford Press.

Deutsch, C. (1982). *Broken bottles, broken dreams.* New York: Teachers College Press.

Devore, W., & Schlesinger, E. (1987). *Ethnic-sensitive social work practice* (2nd ed.). Columbus, OH: Merrill.

Devore, W., & Schlesinger, E. (1996). *Ethnic-sensitive social work practice* (4th ed.). Boston: Allyn & Bacon.

Di Leo, J. H. (1973). *Children's drawings as diagnostic aids.* New York: Brunner/Mazel.

Diamond, E., Gans, D., & Mortola, P. (2017). Groups in schools. In C. Haen & S. Aronson (Eds.), *Handbook of child and adolescent group therapy* (pp. 205–213). New York: Routledge.

Dillard, H. K., Donenberg, B., & Glickman, H. (1986). A support system for parents with learning disabled children. In M. T. Hawkins (Ed.), *Achieving educational excellence for children at risk* (pp. 50–55). Silver Spring, MD: National Association of Social Workers.

Docker-Drysdale, B. (1993). *Therapy and consultation in child care.* London: Free Association Books.

Doka, K. J. (Ed.). (1989). *Disenfranchised grief: Recognizing hidden sorrow.* Lexington, MA: Lexington Books.

Doka, K. J. (Ed.). (2002). *Disenfranchised grief: New directions, challenges, and strategies for practice.* Champaign, IL: Research Press.

Dore, M. M. (1993). Family preservation and poor families: When homebuilding is not enough. *Families in Society, 74*(9), 545–556.

Doster, G., & McElroy, C. Q. (1993). Sudden death of a teacher: Multilevel intervention in an elementary school. In N. B. Webb (Ed.), *Helping bereaved children: A handbook for practitioners* (pp. 212–238). New York: Guilford Press.

Doyle, J. S., & Bauer, S. K. (1989). Post-traumatic stress disorder in children: Its identification and treatment in a residential setting for emotionally disturbed youths. *Journal of Traumatic Stress, 2*(3), 275–288.

Doyle, J. S., & Stoop, D. (1991). Witness and victim of multiple abuses: Collaborative treatment of 10-year-old Randy in a residential treatment center. In N. B. Webb (Ed.), *Play therapy with children in crisis: A casebook for practitioners* (pp. 111–140). New York: Guilford Press.

Doyle, J. S., & Stoop, D. (1999). Witness and victim of multiple abuses: Case of Randy, age 10, in a residential treatment center, and follow-up at age 19 in prison. In N. B. Webb (Ed.), *Play therapy with children in crisis: Individual, group, and family treatment* (2nd ed., pp. 131–163). New York: Guilford Press.

Dreby, J. (2012). The burden of deportation on children in Mexican immigrant families. *Journal of Marriage and the Family, 74*, 829–845.

Drewes, A. A., Bratton, S. C., & Schaefer, C. E. (2011). *Integrative play therapy*. Hoboken, NJ: Wiley.

Duenwald, M. (2002, March 26). Two portraits of children of divorce: Rosy and dark. *New York Times*, p. D6.

Dupper, D. R., & Halter, A. P. (1994). Barriers in educating children from homeless shelters: Perspectives of school and shelter staff. *Social Work in Education, 16*(1), 39–45.

Dyson, P. (2015). The traumatic aftermath of parental abandonment, separation, and divorce: Play and family therapy to deal with ongoing crises. In N. B. Webb (Ed.), *Play therapy with children and adolescents in crisis* (4th ed., pp. 179–195). New York: Guilford Press.

Edelman, M. W. (1998). *Stand for children*. Washington, DC: Children's Defense Fund.

Edelstein, S. B., Burge, D., & Waterman, J. (2002). Older children in preadoptive homes: Issues before termination of parental rights. *Child Welfare, 81*(2), 101–121.

Edleson, J. L. (1999). Children's witnessing of adult domestic violence. *Journal of Interpersonal Violence, 14*, 839–870.

Education for All Handicapped Children Act, Public Law 94-142, 89 Stat. 77 (1975).

Eiden, R. D., Edwards, E. P., & Leonard, K. E. (2007). A conceptual model for the development of externalizing behavior problems among kindergarten children of alcoholic families: Role of parenting and children's self-regulation. *Developmental Psychology, 43*(5), 1187–1201.

Ellis, D. A., Zucker, R. A., & Fitzgerald, H. E. (1997). The role of family influences in development and risk. *Alcohol Health and Research World, 21*(3), 218–226.

Englander, E. K., & Lawson, C. (2007). New approaches to preventing peer abuse among children. In N. B. Webb (Ed.), *Play therapy with children in crisis: Individual, group, and family treatment* (3rd ed., pp. 251–269). New York: Guilford Press.

English, A. (1990). Prenatal drug exposure: Grounds for mandatory child abuse reports? *Youth Law News, 11*(1), 3–8.

Enzer, N. B. (1988). *Overview of play therapy.* Paper presented at the annual meeting of the American Academy of Child and Adolescent Psychiatry, Seattle, WA.

Erikson, E. H. (1963). *Childhood and society* (rev. ed.). New York: Norton.

Erikson, E. H. (1968). *Identity: Youth and crisis.* New York: Norton.

Espelage, D. L., Swearer, S. M. (Eds.). (2011). *Bullying in North American schools* (2nd ed.). New York: Routledge.

Eth, S., & Pynoos, R. S. (Eds.). (1985). *Post-traumatic stress disorder in children.* Washington, DC: American Psychiatric Press.

Evans, M. D. (1986). *This is me and my two families: An awareness scrapbook/journal for children living in stepfamilies.* New York: Magination Press.

Evans, S. E., Davies, C., & DiLillo, D. (2008). Exposure to domestic violence: A meta-analysis of child and adolescent outcomes. *Aggression and Violent Behavior, 13,* 131–140.

Every Child Matters Education Fund. (2010). We can do better: Child abuse and neglect deaths in America. Retrieved from *www.everychildmatters.org/storage/documents/pdf/reports/wcdbv2.pdf.*

Ewing, C. P. (1990). *Kids who kill.* Lexington, MA: Lexington Books.

Family Educational Rights and Privacy Act, Public Law 93-380, 88 Stat. 571, 20 (1974).

Family Educational Rights and Privacy Act (FERPA), 20 U.S.C. § 1232g. 34CFR Part 99 (1974).

Federal Emergency Management Agency. (1991). *Children and trauma* [Videotape]. Washington, DC: Author.

Feig, L. (1990). *Drug-exposed infants and children: Service needs and policy questions.* Washington, DC: U.S. Department of Health and Human Services.

Feigelman, B., & Feigelman, W. (1993). Treating the adolescent substance abuser. In L. S. L. Straussner (Ed.), *Clinical work with substance-abusing clients* (pp. 233–250). New York: Guilford Press.

Feinberg, F. (1995). Substance-abusing mothers and their children: Treatment for the family. In L. Combrinck-Graham (Ed.), *Children in families at risk: Maintaining the connections* (pp. 228–247). New York: Guilford Press.

Ficaro, R. (1999). The many losses of children in substance-disordered families: Individual and group interventions. In N. B. Webb (Ed.), *Play therapy with children in crisis: Individual, group, and family treatment* (2nd ed., pp. 294–317). New York: Guilford Press.

Fineran, K. R., Nitza, A., & Patterson, K. W. (2017). Planning for groups. In C. Haen & S. Aronson (Eds.), *Handbook of child and adolescent group therapy* (pp. 9–19). New York: Routledge.

Finkelhor, D., & Berliner, L. (1995). Research on the treatment of sexually abused children: A review and recommendations. *Journal of the American Academy of Child and Adolescent Psychiatry, 34,* 1408–1423.

Fitzgerald, M. M., Schneider, R. A., Salstrom, S., Zinzow, H. M., Jackson, J., & Fosel, R. V. (2008). Child sexual abuse, early family risk, and childhood parentification: Pathways to current psychosocial adjustment. *Journal of Family Psychology, 22*(2), 320–324.

Foa, E. B., Johnson, K. M., Feeny, N. C., & Treadwell, K. R. H. (2001). The Child PTSD Symptom Scale: A preliminary examination of its psychometric properties. *Journal of Clinical Child and Adolescent Psychology, 30,* 376–384.

Foa, E. B., Keane, T. M., Friedman, M. J., & Cohen, J. A. (Eds.). (2009). *Effective treatments for PTSD: Practice guidelines from the International Society for Traumatic Stress Studies.* New York: Guilford Press.

Fong, R. (2001). Cultural competency in providing family-centered services. In E. Walton, P. Sandau-Beckler, & M. Mannes (Eds.), *Balancing family-centered services and child well-being: Exploring issues in policy, practice, theory, and research* (pp. 55–68). New York: Columbia University Press.

Fong, R. (2004). *Culturally competent practice with immigrant and refugee children and families.* New York: Guilford Press.

Fong, R., & Earner, I. (2015). Multiple traumas of undocumented immigrants: Crisis reenactment play therapy. In N. B. Webb (Ed.), *Play therapy with children and adolescents in crisis* (pp. 372–392). New York: Guilford Press.

Fox, J. A., Elliott, D. S., Kerlikowske, R. G., Newman, S. A., & Christeson, W. (2003). *Bullying prevention is crime prevention.* Washington, DC: Fight Crime: Invest in Kids.

Fox, R. (2001). *Elements of the helping process: A guide for clinicians* (2nd ed.). New York: Haworth Press.

Franklin, C. (2000). The delivery of school social work services. In P. Allen-Meares, R. O. Washington, & B. L. Welsh (Eds.), *Social work services in schools* (3rd ed., pp. 273–298). Boston: Allyn & Bacon.

Fraser, M. W. (Ed.). (1997). *Risk and resilience in childhood: An ecological perspective.* Washington, DC: National Association of Social Workers Press.

Freud, A. (1937). *The ego and the mechanisms of defense.* London: Hogarth Press.

Freud, A. (1968). *The psychoanalytic treatment of children: Technical lectures and essays.* New York: International Universities Press. (Original work published 1946)

Freud, A. (1970). The concept of the rejecting mother. In E. J. Anthony & T. Benedek (Eds.), *Parenthood: Its psychology and psychopathology* (pp. 376–386). Boston: Little, Brown.

Friedberg, R. D., Berlyant, M., Mulalti, S., Birt, M., Brehm, L., & Trafalis, S. (2017). Anxious children and adolescents. In C. Haen & S. Aronson (Eds.), *Handbook of child and adolescent group therapy* (pp. 299–310). New York: Routledge.

Friedberg, R. D., McClure, J. M., & Garcia, J. H. (2014). *Cognitive therapy techniques for children and adolescents: Tools for enhancing practice.* New York: Guilford Press.

Fuchs, D., Mock, D., Morgan, P. L., & Young, C. L. (2003). Responsiveness-to-intervention: Definitions, evidence, and implications for the learning disabilities construct. *Learning Disabilities Research and Practice, 18*(3), 157–171.

Furman, E. (1974). *A child's parent dies.* New Haven, CT: Yale University Press.

Gallo-Lopez, L. (2006). A creative play therapy approach to the group treatment of young sexually abused children. In H. G. Kaduson & C. E. Schaefer (Eds.), *Short-term play therapy for children* (2nd ed., pp. 245–272). New York: Guilford Press.

Garbarino, J. (1992). Developmental consequences of living in dangerous and unstable environments: The situation of refugee children. In M. McCallin (Ed.), *The psychological well-being of refugee children* (pp. 1–23). Geneva, Switzerland: International Catholic Child Bureau.

Garbarino, J., & deLara, E. (2002). *And words can hurt forever: How to protect adolescents from bullying, harassment, and emotional violence.* New York: Free Press.

Garbarino, J., Dubrow, N., Kostelny, K., & Pardo, C. (1992). *Children in danger: Coping with the consequences of community violence.* San Francisco: Jossey-Bass.

Garbarino, J., & Kostelny, K. (1997). What children can tell us about living in a war zone. In J. D. Osofsky (Ed.), *Children in a violent society* (pp. 32–41). New York: Guilford Press.

Garbarino, J., Stott, F. M., & Associates. (1989). *What children can tell us.* San Francisco: Jossey-Bass.

Gardner, R. A. (1983). Children's reactions to parental death. In J. E. Schowalter, P. E. Patterson, M. Tallmer, A. H. Kutscher, S. W. Gullo, & D. Peretz (Eds.), *The child and death* (pp. 104–124). New York: Columbia University Press.

Garmezy, N. (1985). Stress-resistant children: The search for protective factors. In J. E. Stevenson (Ed.), *Recent research in developmental psychopathology* (pp. 213–233). Tarrytown, NY: Pergamon Press.

Garrett, K. J. (1994). Caught in a bind: Ethical decision making in schools. *Social Work in Education, 16*(2), 97–105.

Garrity, C. B., & Baris, M. A. (1994). *Caught in the middle: Protecting children of high-conflict divorce.* New York: Free Press.

Gelles, R. J. (1979). *Family violence.* Beverly Hills, CA: SAGE.

Gentry, D. B., & Beneson, W. A. (1993). School-to-home transfer of conflict management skills among school-age children. *Families in Society, 74*(2), 67–73.

George, H. (1988). Child therapy and animals. In C. E. Schaefer (Ed.), *Innovative interventions in child and adolescent therapy* (pp. 400–418). New York: Wiley.

Germain, C. B. (1973). An ecological perspective in casework practice. *Social Casework, 54*, 323–330.

Germain, C. B., & Gitterman, A. (1987). Ecological perspective. In A. Minahan (Ed.), *Encyclopedia of social work* (18th ed., pp. 488–499). Silver Spring, MD: National Association of Social Workers.

Gibbs, J. T., Huang, L. N., & Associates (Eds.). (1989). *Children of color: Psychological interventions with minority youth.* San Francisco: Jossey-Bass.

Gibelman, M., & Schervish, P. (1997). *Who we are: A second look.* Washington, DC: National Association of Social Workers Press.

Gil, E. (1994). *Play in family therapy.* New York: Guilford Press.

Gil, E. (2017). *Posttraumatic play in children. What clinicians need to know.* New York: Guilford Press.

Gil, E., & Selekman, M. D. (Eds.). (2015). *Play in family therapy* (2nd ed.). New York: Guilford Press.

Gilliland, B. E., & James, R. K. (2001). *Crisis intervention strategies* (4th ed.). Pacific Grove, CA: Brooks/Cole.

Ginott, H. G. (1961). *Group psychotherapies with children.* New York: McGraw-Hill.

Ginsburg, E. H. (1989). *School social work: A practitioner's guidebook.* Springfield, IL: Charles C Thomas.

Ginsburg, G. S., Silverman, W. K., & Kurtines, W. S. (1995). Cognitive-behavioral group therapy. In A. R. Eisen, C. A. Kearney, & C. E. Schaefer (Eds.), *Clinical handbook of anxiety disorders in children and adolescents* (pp. 521–549). Northvale, NJ: Jason Aronson.

Gitterman, A. (Ed.). (2001). *Handbook of social work practice with vulnerable and resilient populations* (2nd ed.). New York: Columbia University Press.

Gitterman, A., & Germain, C. B. (2008). *The life model of social work practice: Advances in theory and practice.* New York: Columbia University Press.

Gitterman, A., & Shulman, L. (Eds.). (1986). *Mutual aid groups and the life cycle.* Itasca, IL: Peacock.

Gittler, J., & McPherson, M. (1990). Prenatal substance abuse: An overview of the problem. *Children Today, 19*(4), 3–7.

Gladstone, R. (2016, September 7). Nearly 50 million children are refugees, report finds. *New York Times*, p. 9.

Goldberg, M. E. (1995). Substance-abusing women: False stereotypes and real needs. *Social Work, 40*(6), 789–798.

Goldberg, S. B. (1973). Family tasks and reactions in the crisis of death. *Social Casework, 54*, 398–405.

Goldman, J., Stein, C. L'E., & Guerry, S. (1983). *Psychological methods of child assessment.* New York: Brunner/Mazel.

Goldman, L. (2008). *Coming out, coming in: Nurturing the well-being and inclusion of gay youth in mainstream society.* New York: Routledge.

Goleman, D. (1993, December 8). New study portrays the young as more and more troubled. *New York Times*, p. C16.

Gonzales-Ramos, G., & Goldstein, E. (1989). Child maltreatment: An overview. In S. Ehrenkrantz, E. G. Goldstein, L. Goodman, & J. Seinfeld (Eds.), *Clinical social work with maltreated children and their families* (pp. 3–20). New York: New York University Press.

Goodman, R. F. (2007). Living beyond the crisis of childhood cancer. In N. B. Webb (Ed.), *Play therapy with children in crisis: Individual, group, and family treatment* (3rd ed., pp. 197–227). New York: Guilford Press.

Goodwin, D. W., Schulsinger, F., Hermansen, S. B., Guze, S. B., & Winokur, G. (1973). Alcohol problems in adoptees raised apart from biological parents. *Archives of General Psychiatry, 28*, 238–243.

Green, E. J., & Myrick, A. C. (2015). *Play therapy with vulnerable populations: No child forgotten.* Lanham, MD: Rowman & Littlefield.

Green, J. W. (1999). *Cultural awareness in the human services: A multi-ethnic approach* (3rd ed.). Boston: Allyn & Bacon.

Gregory, P. (1990). *Body map of feelings.* Lethbridge, Alberta, Canada: Family and Community Development Program.

Griffin, R. (2010). Play, create, express, understand: Bereavement groups in schools. In A. Drewes & C. E. Schaefer (Eds.), *School-based play therapy* (2nd ed., pp. 379–405). Hoboken, NJ: Wiley.

Grollman, E. (1967). *Explaining death to children.* Boston: Beacon Press.

Groves, B. M. (2002). *Children who see too much: Lessons from the Child Witness to Violence Project.* Boston: Beacon Press.

Guidubaldi, J. (1989). The poor achievement of children of divorce. *Children and Teens Today, 9*(5), 5–6.

Gustafsson, P. E., Larson, I. B., Nelson, N., & Gustafsson, P. A. (2009). Sociocultural disadvantage, traumatic life events, and psychiatric symptoms in preadolescent children. *American Journal of Orthopsychiatry, 79*(3), 387–397.

Guterman, N., & Cameron, M. (1997). Assessing the impact of community violence on children and youths. *Social Work, 42*(5), 495–505.

Haen, C. (2017). An integrative perspective on group therapy. In C. Haen & S. Aronson (Eds.), *Handbook of child and adolescent group therapy* (pp. 193–202). New York: Routledge.

Haen, C., & Aronson, S. (2017). *Handbook of child and adolescent group therapy: A practitioner's reference.* New York: Routledge.

Hall, K. B. (Ed.). (1992). *Orphan train riders.* Springdale, AR: Springdale Public Library.
Hallowell, E. M., & Ratey, J. J. (1994). *Driven to distraction.* New York: Pantheon Books.
Hancock, B. L. (1982). *School social work.* Englewood Cliffs, NJ: Prentice-Hall.
Harachi, T. W., Fleming, C. B., White, H. R., Ensminger, M. E., Abbott, R. D., Catalano, R. E., et al. (2006). Aggressive behavior among girls and boys during middle childhood: Predictors and sequelae of trajectory group membership. *Aggressive Behavior, 32,* 279–293.
Harader, D., & Fullwood, H. (2010). Overview of the implications of response to intervention with students with SLD. *Dasman Model School Special Needs Education Journal, 1*(1), 4.
Hariton, J. (2017). Social skills groups for children and adolescents. In C. Haen & S. Aronson (Eds.), *Handbook of child and adolescent group therapy* (pp. 357–367). New York: Routledge.
Hartley, B. (2004). Bereavement groups soon after traumatic death. In N. B. Webb (Ed.), *Mass trauma and violence: Helping families and children cope* (pp. 167–190). New York: Guilford Press.
Hartman, A. (1978). Diagrammatic assessment of family relationships. *Social Casework, 59,* 465–476.
Hazelden Foundation. (2002). *Children Are People: Circle of prevention (facilitator's manual).* Center City, MN: Author.
Heath, S. (2004). *Parent's guide to No Child Left Behind.* Deltaville, VA: Harbor House Law Press. Retrieved from *www.wrightslaw.com/nclb.parent.guide.heath.pdf.*
Heegaard, M. (1991). *When something terrible happens: Children can learn to cope with grief.* Minneapolis, MN: Woodland Press.
Heide, K. M. (1999). *Young killers: The challenge of juvenile homicide.* Thousand Oaks, CA: SAGE.
Hennessy-Fiske, M. (2015, August 31). Immigration: Are male detainees treated differently than women? *Los Angeles Times.* Retrieved from *www.latimes.com/nation/la-na-family-detention-fathers-20150829-story.html.*
Hepworth, D. H., & Larsen, J. A. (1982). *Direct social work practice: Theory and skills.* Homewood, IL: Dorsey Press.
Hepworth, D. H., & Larsen, J. A. (1993). *Direct social work practice: Theory and skills* (4th ed.). Pacific Grove, CA: Brooks/Cole.
Hepworth, D. H., Rooney, R. H., & Larsen, J. A. (2002). *Direct social work practice: Theory and skills* (6th ed.). Pacific Grove, CA: Brooks/Cole.
Herman, J. L. (1992). *Trauma and recovery.* New York: Basic Books.
Hershorn, M., & Rosenbaum, A. (1985). Children of marital violence: A close look at the unintended victims. *American Journal of Orthopsychiatry, 55*(2), 260–266.
Hess, P. M., & Mullen, E. J. (1995). *Practitioner–researcher partnerships: Building knowledge from, in, and for practice.* Washington, DC: National Association of Social Workers Press.
Hetherington, E. M., & Kelly, J. (2002). *For better or for worse: Divorce reconsidered.* New York: Norton.
Hickey, L. O. (1993). Death of a counselor: A bereavement group for junior high school students. In N. B. Webb (Ed.), *Helping bereaved children: A handbook for practitioners* (pp. 239–266). New York: Guilford Press.
Hinshaw, S. P. (2008). Developmental psychopathology as a scientific discipline:

Relevance to behavioral and emotional disorder of childhood and adolescence. In T. P. Beauchaine & S. P. Hinshaw (Eds.), *Child and adolescent psychopathology* (pp. 3–26). Hoboken, NJ: Wiley.

Ho, M. K. (1992). *Minority children and adolescents in therapy*. Newbury Park, CA: SAGE.

Hodges, V. G., Morgan, L. J., & Johnston, B. (1993). Educating for excellence in child welfare practice: A model for graduate training in intensive family preservation. *Journal of Teaching in Social Work, 7*(1), 31–48.

Hoefer, M., Rytina, N., & Baker, B. C. (2011). *Estimates of the unauthorized immigrant population residing in the United States: January 2010*. Washington, DC: U.S. Department of Homeland Security, Policy Directorate, Office of Immigration Statistics.

Hoffman, J., & Rogers, P. (1991). A crisis play group in a shelter following the Santa Cruz earthquake. In N. B. Webb (Ed.), *Play therapy with children in crisis: A casebook for practitioners* (pp. 379–395). New York: Guilford Press.

Hooker, C. E. (1976). Learned helplessness. *Social Work, 21*(3), 194–198.

Horne, A. M., Bartolomucci, C. L., & Newman-Carlson, D. (2003). *Bully Busters: A teacher's manual for helping bullies, victims, and bystanders, grades K–5*. Champaign, IL: Research Press.

Huang, L. N. (1989). Southeast Asian refugee children and adolescents. In J. T. Gibbs, L. N. Huang, & Associates (Eds.), *Children of color: Psychological interventions with minority youth* (pp. 278–321). San Francisco: Jossey-Bass.

Hunt, K. (Director & Producer). (1992). *No place like home* [Videotape]. Berkeley: University of California Extension Center for Media and Independent Learning. (Available from 2000 Center St., Fourth Floor, Berkeley, CA 94704)

Hylton, W. S. (2015, February 4). American nightmare: The shame of family detention camps. *New York Times*, pp. 26–49.

Immigration report hits home. (2017, January 27). *Tampa Times*, p. 3A.

Individuals with Disabilities Education Improvement Act of 2004, Public Law 108-446 (2004).

Institute of Medicine. (1989). *Research on children and adolescents with mental, behavioral, and developmental disorders: Mobilizing a national initiative*. Washington, DC: Author.

Jackson, K. (2000). *Family homelessness: More than a lack of housing*. New York: Garland.

Jaeger, E., Hahn, N. B., & Weinraub, M. (2000). Attachment in adult daughters of alcoholic fathers. *Addiction, 95*(2), 267–276.

James, B. (1989). *Treating traumatized children: New insights and creative interventions*. Lexington, MA: Lexington Books.

James, B. (1994). *Handbook for treatment of attachment-trauma problems in children*. New York: Free Press.

James, B. (2009). *Treating traumatized children: New insights and creative innovations*. New York: Free Press.

Jenkins, E. J., & Bell, C. C. (1997). Exposure and response to community violence among children and adolescents. In J. D. Osofsky (Ed.), *Children in a violent society* (pp. 9–31). New York: Guilford Press.

Johnson, H. C. (1989). Behavior disorders. In F. J. Turner (Ed.), *Child psychopathology: A social work perspective* (pp. 73–140). New York: Free Press.

Johnson, H. C. (1993a). The disruptive child: Problems of definition. In J. B. Rauch

(Ed.), *Assessment: A source book for social work practice* (pp. 144–157). Milwaukee, WI: Families International.
Johnson, H. C. (1993b). Family issues and interventions. In H. C. Johnson (Ed.), *Child mental health in the 1990s: Curricula for graduate and undergraduate professional education* (pp. 86–105). Rockville, MD: U.S. Department of Health and Human Services.
Johnson, H. C. (1994). [Review of *Child psychopathology: Diagnostic criteria and clinical assessment* (Vols. 1–2)]. *Families and Society, 39*(5), 613–614.
Johnson, H. C., & Friesen, B. J. (1993). Etiologies of mental and emotional disorders in children and adolescents. In H. C. Johnson (Ed.), *Child mental health in the 1990s: Curricula for graduate and undergraduate professional education* (pp. 27–46). Rockville, MD: U.S. Department of Health and Human Services.
Johnson, J. H., Rasbury, W. C., & Siegel, L. J. (1986). *Approaches to child treatment: Introduction to theory, research, and practice.* Elmsford, NY: Pergamon Press.
Johnson, M. E. (1991). Multiple losses in children of chemically dependent families: Case of RJ, age 7. In N. B. Webb (Ed.), *Play therapy with children in crisis: A casebook for practitioners* (pp. 276–292). New York: Guilford Press.
Jones, T. (2017, January 28). How my mom learned to love her son. *New York Times*, p. 9.
Jordan, J. V. (1991). Empathy and the mother–daughter relationship. In J. V. Jordan, A. G. Kaplan, J. B. Miller, I. P. Stiver, & J. L. Surrey (Eds.), *Women's growth in connection: Writings from the Stone Center* (pp. 28–34). New York: Guilford Press.
Kadushin, A. (1987). Child welfare services. In A. Minahan (Ed.), *Encyclopedia of social work* (18th ed., pp. 265–275). Silver Spring, MD: National Association of Social Workers.
Kadushin, G. (1995). Review of *Assessment: A sourcebook for social work practice. Families in Society, 76*(1), 62–63.
Kalter, N., & Schreier, S. (1994). Developmental facilitation groups for children of divorce: The elementary school model. In C. W. LeCroy (Ed.), *Handbook of child and adolescent treatment manuals* (pp. 307–342). New York: Lexington.
Kamen, B., & Gewirtz, B. (1989). Child maltreatment and the court. In S. Ehrenkrantz, E. G. Goldstein, L. Goodman, & J. Seinfeld (Eds.), *Clinical social work with maltreated children and their families* (pp. 178–201). New York: New York University Press.
Kaplan, C. P., & Joslin, H. (1993). Accidental sibling death. In N. B. Webb (Ed.), *Helping bereaved children: A handbook for practitioners* (pp. 118–136). New York: Guilford Press.
Karr-Morse, R., & Wiley, M. S. (1997). *Ghosts from the nursery: Tracing the roots of violence.* New York: Atlantic Monthly Press.
Kastenbaum, R. J. (2001). *Death, society, and human experience* (7th ed.). Boston: Allyn & Bacon.
Kastenbaum, R. J. (2006). *Death, society and human experience* (9th ed.). Boston: Allyn & Bacon.
Kazdin, A. E. (1988). *Child psychotherapy: Developing and identifying effective treatments.* New York: Pergamon Press.
Kazdin, A. E., & Weisz, J. R. (Eds.). (2003). *Evidence-based psychotherapies for children and adolescents.* New York: Guilford Press.

Kelly, J. (2014, March 3). Focus on the figures: Reasons for removal from home. *Chronicle of Social Change.*

Kendall, P. C. (Ed.). (2000). *Child and adolescent therapy: Cognitive-behavioral procedures* (2nd ed.). New York: Guilford Press.

Kendall, P. C. (Ed.). (2006). *Child and adolescent therapy: Cognitive-behavioral procedures* (3rd ed.). New York: Guilford Press.

Kendall, P. C. (Ed.). (2012). *Child and adolescent therapy: Cognitive-behavioral procedures* (4th ed.). New York: Guilford Press.

Kendall, P. C. (Ed.). (2018). *Cognitive therapy with children and adolescents: A casebook for clinical practice* (3rd ed.). New York: Guilford Press.

Kestly, T. (2010). Group sandplay in elementary schools. In A. Drewes & C. E. Schaefer (Eds.), *School-based play therapy* (2nd ed., pp. 257–281). Hoboken, NJ: Wiley.

Kight, M. (1998). *Forever changed: Remembering Okahoma City, April 19, 1995.* Amherst, NY: Prometheus Books.

Kinney, J. M., Haapala, D. A., & Booth, C. (1991). *Keeping families together: The Homebuilders model.* New York: Aldine de Gruyter.

Kirby, J. (n.d.). Single-parent families in poverty. Retrieved from *www3vakron.edu/schulze/401/readings/singleparfam.htm.*

Kirby, L. D., & Fraser, M. W. (1997). Risk and resilience in childhood. In M. Fraser (Ed.), *Risk and resilience in childhood: An ecological perspective* (pp. 2–33). Washington, DC: National Association of Social Workers Press.

Klein, M. (1937). *The psychoanalysis of children* (2nd ed.). London: Hogarth Press.

Kliman, G. (1989). Facilitation of mourning during childhood. In S. C. Klagsbrun, G. W. Kliman, E. J. Clark, A. H. Kutscher, R. DeBellis, & C. A. Lambert (Eds.), *Preventive psychiatry: Early intervention and situational crisis management* (pp. 59–82). Philadelphia: Charles Press.

Kochanek, K. D., & Hudson, B. L. (1995). Advance report of final mortality statistics, 1992. *Monthly Vital Statistics Report, 43*(Suppl. 6).

Kochenderfer, B. J., & Ladd, G. W. (1996). Peer victimization: Manifestations and relations to social adjustment in kindergarten. *Journal of School Psychology, 34,* 267–283.

Kolodny, R. L., & Garland, J. A. (1984). Guest editorial. *Social Work with Groups,* 7(4), 3–5.

Koocher, C., & Keith-Spiegel, P. (1990). *Children, ethics and the law.* Lincoln: University of Nebraska Press.

Kotani, H., Nakamura, Y., Hashimoto, M., & Hanai, T. (2017). Post-traumatic stress disorder in children and adolescents in the aftermath of disaster. In C. Haen & S. Aronson (Eds.), *Handbook of child and adolescent group therapy* (pp. 415–426). New York: Routledge.

Kovacs, M. (1978). *The Children's Depression Inventory: A self-rated depression scale.* Unpublished manuscript, University of Pittsburgh School of Medicine.

Kovaleski, J. F. (2003). *The three tier model for identifying learning disabilities: Critical program features and system issues.* Paper presented at the NRCLD Responsiveness-to-Intervention Symposium, Kansas City, MO.

Krestan, J., & Bepko, C. (1989). Alcohol problems and the family life cycle. In B. Carter & M. McGoldrick (Eds.), *The changing family life cycle* (2nd ed., pp. 483–511). Boston: Allyn & Bacon.

La Greca, A. M. (2008). Interventions for posttraumatic stress disorders in children and adolescents following natural disasters and acts of terrorism. In R. G. Steele,

T. D. Elkin, & M. C. Roberts (Eds.), *Handbook of evidence-based therapies for children and adolescents: Bridging science and practice* (pp. 121–141). New York: Springer Science.

Lander, L., Howsare, J., & Byrne, M. (2013). The impact of substance use disorders on families and children: From theory to practice. *Social Work Public Health, 28*, 194–205.

Landreth, G. L. (2002a). *Child-centered play therapy. The art of the relationship* (2nd ed.). New York: Brunner-Routledge.

Landreth, G. L. (2002b). *Play therapy: The art of the relationship* (2nd ed.). Independence, KY: Brunner-Routledge.

Landreth, G. L. (2012). *Play therapy: The art of the relationship* (3rd ed.). New York: Routledge.

Landreth, G. L., & Bratton, S. C. (2006). *Child parent relationship therapy (CPRT): A 10-session filial therapy model.* New York: Taylor & Francis.

Lavin, C. (2002). Disenfranchised grief and individuals with developmental disabilities. In K. J. Doka (Ed.), *Disenfranchised grief: New directions, challenges, and strategies for practice* (pp. 307–322). Champaign, IL: Research Press.

LeCroy, C. W., & Ashford, J. B. (1992). Children's mental health: Current findings and research directions. In S. M. Buttrick (Ed.), *Research on children* (pp. 14–24). Washington, DC: National Association of Social Workers Press.

LeProhn, N. S., Wetherbee, K. M., Lamont, E. R., Achenbach, T. M., & Pecora, P. J. (Eds.). (2002). *Assessing youth behavior using the Child Behavior Checklist in family and children's services.* Washington, DC: Child Welfare League of America Press.

LeVine, E. S., & Sallee, A. L. (1992). *Listen to our children: Clinical theory and practice* (2nd ed.). Dubuque, IA: Kendall/Hunt.

Levinson, B. M. (1962). The dog as "co-therapist." *Mental Hygiene, 46*, 59–65.

Levinson, B. M. (1969). *Pet-oriented child psychotherapy.* Springfield, IL: Charles C Thomas.

Levinson, B. M. (1978). Pets and personality development. *Psychological Reports, 42*, 1031–1038.

Li, H. C., Lopez, V., & Lee, T. L. (2007). Effects of preoperative therapeutic play on outcomes of school-age children undergoing day surgery. *Research in Nursing and Health, 30*(3), 320–332.

Lidz, T. (1963). *The family and human development.* New York: International Universities Press.

Lieberman, A. F. (1990). Culturally sensitive intervention with children and families. *Child and Adolescent Social Work, 7*(2), 101–120.

Lieberman, A. F. (2004). Traumatic stress and quality of attachment; Reality and internalization in disorders of infant mental health. *Journal of Infant Mental Health, 25*(4), 336–351.

Lieberman, F. (1987). Mental health and illness in children. In A. Minahan (Ed.), *Encyclopedia of social work* (18th ed., pp. 111–125). Silver Spring, MD: National Association of Social Workers.

Lindy, J. (1986). An outline for the psychoanalytic psychotherapy of post-traumatic stress disorder. In C. Figley (Ed.), *Trauma and its wake: Vol. 2. Traumatic stress theory, research, and interventions* (pp. 195–212). New York: Brunner/Mazel.

Lorion, R., & Saltzman, W. (1993). Children's exposure to community violence following a path from concern to research to action. In D. Reiss, J. Richters, M.

Radke-Yarrow, & D. Scharff (Eds.), *Children and violence* (pp. 55–65). New York: Guilford Press.

Lourie, I. S., & Katz-Leavy, J. (1991). New directions for mental health services for families and children. *Families in Society, 72*(5), 277–285.

Lowenberg, F. M., & Dolgoff, R. (1996). *Ethical decisions for social work practice* (5th ed.). Itasca, IL: Peacock.

Lowinson, J. H., Ruiz, P., Millman, R. B., & Langrod, J. G. (Eds.). (1997). *Substance abuse: A comprehensive textbook*. Baltimore: Williams & Wilkins.

Lukas, S. (1993). *Where to start and what to ask: An assessment handbook*. New York: Norton.

Lum, D. (1996). *Social work practice with people of color: A process-stage approach* (3rd ed.). Belmont, CA: Wadsworth.

Lum, D. (1999). *Culturally competent practice: A framework for growth and action*. Pacific Grove, CA: Brooks/Cole.

Lum, D. (Ed.). (2003). *Culturally competent practice: A framework for understanding diverse groups and social justice*. Pacific Grove, CA: Brooks/Cole.

Mahler, M., Pine, F., & Bergman, A. (1975). *The psychological birth of the human infant: Symbiosis and individuation*. New York: Basic Books.

Main, M., & Solomon, J. (1990). Procedures for identifying infants as disorganized/disoriented during the Ainsworth Strange Situation. In M. T. Greenberg, D. Cicchetti, & E. M. Cummings (Eds.), *Attachment in the preschool years: Theory, research, and intervention* (pp. 121–160). Chicago: University of Chicago Press.

Makin, C. (2014, July 26). More granparents raising their grandkids. *USA Today*.

Malchiodi, C. A. (1998). *Understanding children's drawings*. New York: Guilford Press.

Malchiodi, C. A. (2006). *Art therapy sourcebook* (2nd ed.). New York: McGraw Hill.

Malchiodi, C. A. (2011). *Handbook of art therapy* (2nd ed.). New York: Guilford Press.

Malchiodi, C. A. (2014a). Creative arts therapy approaches to attachment issues. In C. A. Malchiodi & D. A. Crenshaw (Eds.), *Creative arts and play therapy for attachment problems* (pp. 3–18). New York: Guilford Press.

Malchiodi, C. A. (2014b). Art therapy, attachment, and parent–child dyads. In C. A. Malchiodi & D. A. Crenshaw (Eds.), *Creative arts and play therapy for attachment problems* (pp. 52–66). New York: Guilford Press.

Malchiodi, C. A., & Crenshaw, D. A. (Eds.). (2014). *Creative arts and play therapy for attachment problems*. New York: Guilford Press.

Malekoff, A. (2002). Malekoff responds to debriefing article. *Social Work with Groups Newsletter, 17*(3), 11.

Maluccio, A. N. (1985). Education and training for child welfare practice. In J. Laird & A. Hartman (Eds.), *Handbook of child welfare* (pp. 741–759). New York: Free Press.

Maluccio, A. N. (2006). The nature and scope of the problem. In N. B. Webb (Ed.), *Working with traumatized youth in child welfare* (pp. 3–12). New York: Guilford Press.

Mannes, M. (2001). Reclaiming a family-centered services reform agenda. In E. Walton, P. Sandau-Beckler, & M. Mannes (Eds.), *Balancing family-centered services and child well-being: Exploring issues in policy, practice, theory, and research* (pp. 336–358). New York: Columbia University Press.

Marans, S., & Cohen, D. (1993). Children and inner-city violence: Strategies for intervention. In L. Leavitt & N. Fox (Eds.), *Psychological effects of war and violence on children* (pp. 281–302). Hillsdale, NJ: Erlbaum.

Margolin, G. (1979). *Conjoint marital therapy to enhance anger management and reduce spouse abuse.* Los Angeles: University of Southern California Psychological Research and Service Center.

Markowitz, R. (2014). Dynamics and treatment issues with children of individuals with substance use disorders. In S. L. A. Straussner (Ed.), *Clinical work with substance-abusing clients* (3rd ed., pp. 348–368). New York: Guilford Press.

Marquart, E. (2006). *Between two worlds: The inner life of children of divorce.* New York: Harmony.

Maschi, T. (2015). Professonal self-care and the prevention of secondary trauma among play therapists working with traumatized youth. In N. B. Webb (Ed.), *Play therapy with children and adolescents in crisis* (4th ed., pp. 373–414). New York: Guilford Press.

Mash, E. J., & Barkley, R. A. (Eds.). (2003). *Child psychopathology* (2nd ed.). New York: Guilford Press.

Mash, E. J., & Barkley, R. A. (Eds.). (2007). *Assessment of childhood disorders* (4th ed.). New York: Guilford Press.

Mash, E. J., & Barkley, R. A. (2014). *Child psychopathology* (3rd ed.). New York: Guilford Press.

Mash, E. J., & Dozois, D. J. (1996). Child psychopathology: A developmental–systems perspective. In E. J. Mash & R. A. Barkley (Eds.), *Child psychopathology* (pp. 3–60). New York: Guilford Press.

Mash, E. J., & Dozois, D. J. (2003). Child psychopathology: A developmental–systems perspective. In E. J. Mash & R. A. Barkley (Eds.), *Child psychopathology* (2nd ed., pp. 3–71). New York: Guilford Press.

Mash, E. J., & Hunsley, J. (Eds.). (2007). *Assessment of childhood disorders* (4th ed.). New York: Guilford Press.

Mash, E. J., & Terdal, L. G. (1997). *Assessment of childhood disorders* (3rd ed.). New York: Guilford Press.

Maslow, A. (1970). *Motivation and personality* (2nd ed.). New York: Harper & Row.

Mason, S., & Linsk, N. (2002). Relative foster parents of HIV-affected children. *Child Welfare, 81*(4), 541–569.

May, P. A., Gossage, J. P., Kalberg, W. O., Robinson, L. K., Buckley, D., Manning, M., et al. (2009). Prevalence and epidemiologic characteristics of FASD from various research methods with an emphasis on recent in-school studies. *Developmental Disabilities Research Reviews, 15*(3), 176–192.

McFarlane, A. C. (1990). Post-traumatic stress syndrome revisited. In H. J. Parad & L. G. Parad (Eds.), *Crisis intervention book 2* (pp. 69–92). Milwaukee, WI: Family Service America.

McGoldrick, M., Carter, B., & Garcia-Preto, N. (2010). *The expanded family life cycle* (4th ed.). New York: Pearson.

McGoldrick, M., & Gerson, R. (1985). *Genograms in family assessment.* New York: Norton.

McGoldrick, M., Gerson, R., & Petry, S. (2008). *Genograms: Assessment and intervention* (3rd ed.). New York: Norton.

McGoldrick, M., & Walsh, F. (Eds.). (1991). *Living beyond loss: Death in the family.* New York: Norton.

McGonagle, E. (1989). *Banana Splits: A school/parent support program for children of divorce.* Carlsbad, CA: Interaction. (Original work published 1978)

Mellard, D. (2005). Basic principles of the responsiveness-to-intervention approach. Retrieved from *www.schwablearning.org/articles.asp?r=1056.*

Meyer, C. H. (Ed.). (1983). *Clinical social work in an eco-systems perspective.* New York: Columbia University Press.

Meyer, C. H. (1993). *Assessment in social work practice.* New York: Columbia University Press.

Michaels, D., & Levine, C. (1992). Estimates of the number of motherless youth orphaned by AIDS in the United States. *Journal of the American Medical Association, 268*(24), 3456–3460.

Millay, E. St. V. (1969). Childhood is the kingdom where nobody dies. In *Edna St. Vincent Millay collected lyrics* (p. 203). New York: Harper & Row. (Original work published 1934)

Miller, D. (1989). Family violence and the helping system. In L. Combrinck-Graham (Ed.), *Children in family contexts: Perspectives on treatment* (pp. 413–434). New York: Guilford Press.

Miller, J. (2003). Critical incident stress debriefing and social work: Expanding the frame. *Journal of Social Service Research, 30*(2), 7–25.

Miller, J. (2012). *Psychosocial capacity building in response to disasters.* New York: Columbia University Press.

Miller, W. M. (1994). Family play therapy: History, theory, and convergence. In C. E. Schaefer & L. J. Carey (Eds.), *Family play therapy* (pp. 3–19). Northvale, NJ: Jason Aronson.

Minuchin, P. (1995). Foster and natural families: Forming a cooperative network. In L. Combrinck-Graham (Ed.), *Children in families at risk: Maintaining the connections* (pp. 251–274). New York: Guilford Press.

Minuchin, S. (1974). *Family and family therapy.* Cambridge, MA: Harvard University Press.

Minuchin, S., & Fishman, H. C. (1981). *Family therapy techniques.* Cambridge, MA: Harvard University Press.

Mishne, J. M. (1983). *Clinical work with children.* New York: Free Press.

Moe, J. (1989). *Kids' power: Healing games for children of alcoholics.* Tucson, AZ: Imagine Works.

Moe, J. (1993). *Discovery: Finding the buried treasure: A prevention/intervention program for youths from high-stress families.* Tucson, AZ: Stem.

Moustakas, C. (1959). *Psychotherapy with children.* New York: Harper & Row.

Murphy, L., Pynoos, R. S., & James, C. B. (1997). The trauma/grief-focused group psychotherapy module of an elementary school-based violence prevention/intervention program. In J. Osofsky (Ed.), *Children in a violent society* (pp. 223–255). New York: Guilford Press.

Nadel, M., & Straussner, S. L. A. (1997). Children in substance-abusing families. In N. K. Phillips & S. L. A. Straussner (Eds.), *Children in the urban environment* (pp. 154–174). Springfield, IL: Charles C Thomas.

Nader, K. (2008). *Understanding and assessing trauma in children and adolescents: Measures, methods, and youth in context.* New York: Routledge.

Nader, K. (2010). Children's and adolescents' exposure to the mass violence of war and terrorism. In N. B. Webb (Ed.), *Helping bereaved children: A handbook for practitioners* (3rd ed., pp. 215–239). New York: Guilford Press.

Nader, K., & Fletcher, K. E. (2014). *The child trauma reaction inventories.* Austin, TX: Two Suns.

Nader, K., & Fletcher, K. E. (2014). Childhood posttraumatic stress disorder. In E. J. Mash & R. A. Barkley (Eds.), *Child psychopathology* (3rd ed., pp. 476–528). New York: Guilford Press.

Nagin, D. S., & Tremblay, R. E. (2001). Parental and early childhood predictors of persistent physical aggression in boys from kindergarten to high school. *Archives of General Psychiatry, 58*(4), 389–394.

Nansel, T. R., Overpeck, M., Pilla, R. S., Ruan, W. J., Simons-Morton, B., & Scheidt, P. (2001). Bullying behaviors among U.S. youth: Prevalence and association with psychosocial adjustment. *Journal of the American Medical Association, 285*, 2094–2100.

National Association of Social Workers. (1993, July). Foster care up despite “permanency” efforts. *NASW News*, p. 9.

National Association of Social Workers. (1994, September 8). Simpson case: Confidences survive clients. *NASW News*, p. 8.

National Association of Social Workers. (1996, August). *NASW code of ethics* (approved ed.). Washington, DC: Author.

National Association of Social Workers. (2002). *NASW standards for school social work services.* Washington, DC: Author.

National Association of Social Workers. (2008). *NASW code of ethics* (approved ed.). Washington, DC: Author.

National Association of Social Workers. (2010). *Legal rights of children.* Washington, DC: Author.

National Association of Social Workers. (2012). *NASW standards for school social workers.* Washington, DC: Author.

National Association of Social Workers. (2015). *Standards and indicators for cultural competence in social work practice.* Washington, DC: Author.

National Association of Social Workers. (2016). *Code of ethics.* Alexandria, VA: Author.

National Center for PTSD. (2005). Psychological first aid: Field operations guide. Retrieved from *www.nctsnet.org/nccts/nav.do?pid=typ_terrresources_pfa.*

National Dissemination Center for Children with Disabilities. (2010). IDEA 2004 definitions and terms. Retrieved June 23, 2010, from *www.nichcy.org/SchoolsAndAdministrators/Pages/KeyTerms.aspx#point.*

National Geographic. (2017, January). The shifting landscape of gender revolution [Special issue]. *National Geographic, 231*(1).

National Institute for Dispute Resolution. (1999). *Conflict resolution: Education facts.* Retrieved from *www.CRFnet.org.*

National Organization on Fetal Alcohol Syndrome. (2010). FASD: What everyone should know. Retrieved from *www.nofas.org/MediaFiles/PDFs/factsheets/everyone.pdf.*

National Research Center on Learning Disabilities. (2006). *RTI manual.* Lawrence, KS: Author.

Nelson, K. E. (1997). Family preservation: What is it? *Children and Youth Services Review, 19*(1, 2), 101–118.

New York State Department of Education. (2009, July). *Special education in New York State for children ages 3–21: A parent's guide.* Albany: Author.

New York State Department of Education/University of the State of New York.

(2002a, May). *Special education in New York State for children ages 3–21: A parent's guide*. Albany: Author.

New York State Department of Education/University of the State of New York. (2002b, June). *Regulations of the Commissioner of Education: Part 200. Students with disabilities*. Albany: Author.

Newton-Logston, G., & Armstrong, M. I. (1993). School-based mental health services. *Social Work in Education, 15*(3), 187–191.

Nigg, J., & Nikolas, M. (2008). Attention-deficit/hyperactivity disorder. In T. Beauchaine & S. P. Hinshaw (Eds.), *Child and adolescent psychopathology* (pp. 301–334). Hoboken, NJ: Wiley.

Nisivoccia, D., & Lynn, M. (1999). Helping forgotten victims: Using activity groups with children who witness violence. In N. B. Webb (Ed.), *Play therapy with children in crisis: Individual, group, and family treatment* (2nd ed., pp. 74–103). New York: Guilford Press.

Nisivoccia, D., & Lynn, M. (2007). Helping forgotten victims: Using activity groups with children who witness violence. In N. B. Webb (Ed.), *Play therapy with children in crisis: Individual, group, and family treatment* (3rd ed., pp. 294–321). New York: Guilford Press.

Norman, E. (Ed.). (2000). *Resiliency enhancement: Putting the strengths perspective into social work practice*. New York: Columbia University Press.

Northen, H. (1987). Assessment in direct practice. In A. Minahan (Ed.), *Encyclopedia of social work* (18th ed., pp. 171–183). Silver Spring, MD: National Association of Social Workers.

Nuñez, R. D. C. (1994). Access to success: Meeting the educational needs of homeless children and families. *Social Work in Education, 16*(1), 21–30.

O'Hara, M. E. (2017, April 11). Domestic violence: Nearly three U.S. women killed every day by intimate partners. Available at *www.nbcnews.com/news/us-news/domestic-violence-nearly-three-u-s-women-killed-every-day-n745166*.

O'Malley, B. (2006). *My foster care journey*. Winthrop, MA: Adoption Works.

Oaklander, V. (1988). *Windows to our children*. Highland, NY: Center for Gestalt Development.

Office for Civil Rights. (2009). Protecting students with disabilities. Retrieved June 23, 2010, from *ed.gov/about/offices/list/ocr/504faq.html*.

Olshansky, S. (1962). Chronic sorrow: A response to having a mentally defective child. *Social Casework, 43*, 190–193.

Olweus, D. (1993). *Bullying at school: What we know and what we can do*. Cambridge, MA: Blackwell.

Olweus, D., & Limber, S. P. (2002). *The bullying prevention program: Blueprints for violence prevention*. Boulder, CO: Center for the Study and Prevention of Violence.

Olweus, D., Limber, S., & Mihalic, S. (1999). *Blueprints for violence prevention: The Bullying prevention program*. Boulder, CO: Center for the Study and Prevention of Violence.

Openshaw, L. (2008). *Social work in schools: Principles and practice*. New York: Guilford Press.

Oppenheim, D., & Goldsmith, D. F. (Eds.). (2007). *Attachment theory in clinical work with children: Bridging the gap between research and practice*. New York: Guilford Press.

Osofsky, J. D. (Ed.). (1997). *Children in a violent society*. New York: Guilford Press.

Osofsky, J. D., Wewers, S., Hann, D. M., & Fick, A. C. (1993). Chronic community violence: What is happening to our children? *Psychiatry: Interpersonal and Biological Processes, 56*, 36–45.

Oster, G. D., & Gould, P. (1987). *Using drawings in assessment and therapy: A guide for mental health professionals.* New York: Brunner/Mazel.

Otis, J. (2017, January 17). Dangers behind and uncertainties ahead, but together at last. *New York Times*, p. 19.

Ozonoff, S., Dawson, G., & McPartland, J. (2002). *A parent's guide to Asperger syndrome and high-functioning autism.* New York: Guilford Press.

Pace, P. (2010, July). Lawmakers briefed on abuse. *NASW News*, p. 6.

Pahl, K. M., & Barrett, P. M. (2010). Interventions for anxiety disorders in children using group cognitive-behavioral therapy with family involvement. In J. R. Weisz & A. E. Kazdin (Eds.), *Evidence-based psychotherapies for children and adolescents* (2nd ed., pp. 61–79). New York: Guilford Press.

Palombo, J. (1985). Self-psychology and countertransference in the treatment of children. *Child and Adolescent Social Work, 2*(1), 36–48.

Palombo, J. (2002). The therapeutic process with children with learning disorders. In J. R. Brandell (Ed.), *Psychoanalytic approaches to the treatment of children and adolescents: Tradition and transformation* (pp. 143–168). New York: Haworth Press.

Paniagua, F. A. (1998). *Assessing and treating culturally diverse clients: A practical guide* (2nd ed.). Thousand Oaks, CA: SAGE.

Papell, C. P., & Rothman, B. (1966). Social work group models: Possession and heritage. *Journal of Education for Social Work, 11*(2), 66–77.

Parnell, M., & Vanderkloot, J. (1989). Ghetto children growing up in poverty. In L. Combrinck-Graham (Ed.), *Children in family contexts: Perspectives on treatment* (pp. 437–462). New York: Guilford Press.

Patterson, S. L., & Marsiglia, F. F. (2000). "Mi casa es su casa": Beginning exploration of Mexican Americans' natural helping. *Families in Society, 81*(1), 22–31.

Peachman, R. R. (2017). Raising a transgender child. *New York Times*, p. D4.

Pecora, P. J., Reed-Ashcraft, K., & Kirk, R. S. (2001). Family-centered services. In E. Walton, P. Sandau-Beckler, & M. Mannes (Eds.), *Balancing family-centered services and child well-being: Exploring issues in policy, practice, theory, and research* (pp. 1–33). New York: Columbia University Press.

Pegasus Therapeutic Riding. (2001). *Riding a dream.* Darien. CT: Author.

Pelcovitz, D. (1999). Betrayed by a trusted adult: Structured time-limited group therapy with elementary school children abused by a school employee. In N. B. Webb (Ed.), *Play therapy with children in crisis: Individual, group, and family treatment* (2nd ed., pp. 183–199). New York: Guilford Press.

Pelham, W. E., & Fabiano, G. H. (2008). Evidence-based psychosocial treatments for ADHD: An update. *Journal of Clinical Child and Adolescent Psychology, 17*(1), 185–214.

Pelham, W. E., Guaggy, E. M., Greiner, A. R., Fabiano, G. A., Waschbusch, D. A., & Coles, E. K. (2017). Summer treatment programs for attention-deficit/hyperactivity disorder. In J. R. Weisz & A. E. Kazdin (Eds.), *Evidence-based psychotherapies for children and adolescents* (3rd ed., pp. 215–232). New York: Guilford Press.

Pelzer, D. (1995). *A child called it.* Deerfield Beach, FL: Health Communications.

Pelzer, D. (1997). *The lost boy.* Deerfield Beach, FL: Health Communications.

Pelzer, D. (2000). *A man named Dave: A story of triumph and forgiveness.* New York: Plume/Penguin Putnam.
Perlman, H. H. (1979). *Relationship: The heart of helping.* Chicago: University of Chicago Press.
Perry, B. D. (1996). Neurodevelopmental adaptations to violence: How children survive the intergenerational vortex of violence. In *Violence and childhood trauma. Understanding and responding to the effects of violence on young children* (pp. 66–80). Cleveland, OH: Gund Foundation.
Perry, B. D. (1997). Incubated in terror: Neurodevelopmental factors in the cycle of violence. In J. D. Osofsky (Ed.), *Children in a violent society* (pp. 124–149). New York: Guilford Press.
Perry, B. D. (1999). Memories of fear: How the brain stores and retrieves physiologic states, feelings, behaviors and thoughts from traumatic events. In J. Goodwin & R. Attias (Eds.), *Splintered reflections: Images of the body in trauma* (pp. 9–38). New York: Basic Books.
Perry, B. D. (2006). Applying principles of neurodevelopment to clinical work with maltreated and traumatized children. The neurosequential model of therapeutics. In N. B. Webb (Ed.), *Working with traumatized youth in child welfare* (pp. 27–52). New York: Guilford Press.
Perry, B. D., & Szalavitz, M. (2006). *The boy who was raised as a dog and other stories from a child psychiatrist's notebook.* New York: Basic Books.
Petitti, D. B., & Coleman, C. (1990). Cocaine and the risk of low birth weight. *American Journal of Public Health, 80*, 25–28.
Petyr, C. (1992). Adultcentrism to practice with children. *Families in Society, 73*(7), 408–416.
Pew Research Center. (2015, December 17). The American family today. Retrieved from *www.pewsocialtrends.org/2015/12/17/1.the-american-family-today.*
Pfeffer, C. R. (1986). *The suicidal child.* New York: Guilford Press.
Phillips, M. H., DeChillo, N., Kronenfeld, D., & Middleton-Jeter, V. (1988). Homeless families: Services make a difference. *Social Casework, 69*(1), 48–49.
Phillips, R. D. (2010). How firm is our foundation?: Current play therapy research. *International Journal of Play Therapy, 19*(1), 13–25.
Phippen, J. W. (2016, May 6). Is it an immigration detention facility or a child-care center? *Atlantic.*
Piaget, J. (1955). *The child's construction of reality.* New York: Basic Books.
Piaget, J. (1968). *Six psychological studies.* New York: Vintage Books.
Piaget, J. (1972). Intellectual evolution from childhood to adolescence. *Human Development, 115*, 1–12.
Piaget, J., & Inhelder, B. (1969). *The psychology of the child.* New York: Basic Books.
Post-Traumatic Stress: Part II. (1991). *Harvard Mental Health Letter, 7*(9), 1–4.
Price, J. O., & Webb, N. B. (1999). A suicide threat uncovers multiple family problems: Case of Philip, age 8, evaluated in a psychiatric emergency room. In N. B. Webb (Ed.), *Play therapy with children in crisis: Individual, group, and family treatment* (2nd ed., pp. 252–271). New York: Guilford Press.
Pynoos, R. S., & Eth, S. (1985). Children traumatized by witnessing acts of personal violence: Homicide, rape, or suicidal behavior. In S. Eth & R. S. Pynoos (Eds.), *Post-traumatic stress disorder in children* (pp. 19–40). Washington, DC: American Psychiatric Press.
Pynoos, R. S., & Eth, S. (1986). Witness to violence: The child interview. *Journal of the American Academy of Child Psychiatry, 25*, 306–319.

Pynoos, R. S., & Nader, K. (1988). Children who witness the sexual assaults of their mothers. *Journal of the American Academy of Child and Adolescent Psychiatry, 27*, 567–572.

Pynoos, R. S., & Nader, K. (1993). Issues in the treatment of post-traumatic stress in children and adolescents. In J. P. Wilson & B. Raphael (Eds.), *The international handbook of traumatic stress syndromes* (pp. 535–549). New York: Plenum Press.

Rando, T. A. (1991). *How to go on living when someone you love dies.* New York: Bantam.

Rando, T. A. (1993). *Treatment of complicated mourning.* Champaign, IL: Research Press.

Raphael, B. (1983). *The anatomy of bereavement.* New York: Basic Books.

Rapoport, J. L., & Ismond, D. R. (1990). *DSM-III-R training guide for diagnosis of childhood disorders.* New York: Brunner/Mazel.

Reamer, F. G. (2006). *Social work values and ethics* (3rd ed.). New York: Columbia University Press.

Reamer, F. G. (2013). *Social work values and ethics* (4th ed.). New York: Columbia University Press.

Reddy, L. (2010). Group play interventions for children with attention-deficit/hyperactivity disorder. In A. Drewes & C. E. Schaefer (Eds.), *School-based play therapy* (2nd ed., pp. 307–329). Hoboken, NJ: Wiley.

Reddy, L. A., & Alperin, A. (2017). Children with attention-deficit disorder. In C. Haen & S. Aronson (Eds.), *Handbook of child and adolescent group therapy* (pp. 322–334). New York: Routledge.

Reddy, L. A., Files-Hall, T. M., & Schaefer, C. E. (Eds.). (2005). *Empirically based play interventions for children.* Washington, DC: American Psychological Association.

Redl, F. (1944). Diagnostic group work. *American Journal of Orthopsychiatry, 14*, 53–67.

Rehabilitation Act of 1973. Public Law 93-112.

Remkus, J. (1991). Repeated foster placements and attachment failure: Case of Joseph, age 3. In N. B. Webb (Ed.), *Play therapy with children in crisis: A casebook for practitioners* (pp. 143–161). New York: Guilford Press.

Rhodes, J. E. (1994). Older and wiser: Mentoring relationships in childhood and adolescence. *Journal of Primary Prevention, 14*(3), 187–196.

Rice, J. K., & Rice, D. G. (1986). *Living through divorce: A developmental approach to divorce therapy.* New York: Guilford Press.

Richmond, M. (1917). *Social diagnosis.* New York: Russell Sage Foundation.

Robbins, L. (2017, January 19). A passport stamp gives young immigrants hope for the future. *New York Times*, p. 20.

Robert Wood Johnson Foundation. (2001). *Substance abuse: The nation's number one health problem.* Princeton, NJ: Author.

Robert Wood Johnson Foundation. (2010). *FASD: What everyone should know.* Washington, DC: Author.

Roberts, A. R., & Roberts, B. S. (1990). A comprehensive model for crisis intervention with battered women and their children. In A. R. Roberts (Ed.), *Crisis intervention handbook: Assessment, treatment, and research* (pp. 105–123). Belmont, CA: Wadsworth.

Rogers, C. (1951). *Client-centered therapy.* Boston: Houghton Mifflin.

Ronnau, J. P. (2001). Values and ethics for family-centered practice. In E. Walton,

P. Sandau-Beckler, & M. Mannes (Eds.), *Balancing family-centered services and child well-being: Exploring issues in policy, practice, theory, and research* (pp. 34–54). New York: Columbia University Press.

Rooney, R. H. (1988). Socialization strategies for involuntary clients. *Social Casework, 69*(3), 131–140.

Rose, R., & Philpot, T. (2005). *The child's own story: Life story work with traumatized children*. Philadelphia: Jessica Kingsley.

Rose, S. D. (1967). A behavioral approach to group treatment of children. In E. J. Thomas (Ed.), *The sociobehavioral approach and applications to social work* (pp. 39–58). New York: Council on Social Work Education.

Rose, S. D. (1972). *Treating children in groups: A behavioral approach*. San Francisco: Jossey-Bass.

Rose, S. R. (1998). *Group work with children and adolescents: Prevention and intervention in school and community systems*. Thousand Oaks, CA: SAGE.

Rosen, H. (1986). *Unspoken grief: Coping with childhood sibling loss*. Lexington, MA: Lexington Books.

Rosen, H. (1991). Child and adolescent bereavement. *Child and Adolescent Social Work, 8*(1), 5–16.

Rosenbaum, A., & O'Leary, K. (1981). Children: The unintended victims of marital violence. *American Journal of Orthopsychiatry, 51*(4), 692–699.

Rosenberg, E. (1988). Stepsiblings in therapy. In M. D. Kahn & K. G. Lewis (Eds.), *Siblings in therapy: Life span and clinical issues* (pp. 209–227). New York: Norton.

Rothschild, M. (1986). Chronic sorrow: Plight of parents of special children. In M. T. Hawkins (Ed.), *Achieving educational excellence for children at risk* (pp. 41–49). Silver Spring, MD: National Association of Social Workers.

Rounds, K. A., Weil, M., & Bishop, K. K. (1994). Practice with culturally diverse families of young children with disabilities. *Families in Society, 75*(1), 3–14.

Rubin, J. A. (1984). *Child art therapy* (2nd ed.). New York: Van Nostrand Reinhold.

Ruffin, P. A., & Zimmerman, S. A. (2010). Bereavement groups and camps for children: An interdisciplinary approach. In N. B. Webb (Ed.), *Helping bereaved children: A handbook for practitioners* (3rd ed., pp. 296–317). New York: Guilford Press.

Russell, J. (2010, November 28). A world of misery left by bullying. *Boston Globe*.

Russell, M. (1990). Prevalence of alcoholism among children of alcoholics. In M. Windle & J. Searles (Eds.), *Children of alcoholics: Critical perspectives* (pp. 9–38). New York: Guilford Press.

Rutter, M. (1979). Protective factors in children's responses to stress and disadvantage. In M. W. Kent & J. E. Rolf (Eds.), *Primary prevention of psychopathology: Vol. 3. Social competence in children* (pp. 49–74). Hanover, NH: University Press of New England.

Rutter, M. (1987). Psychosocial resilience and protective mechanisms. *American Journal of Orthopsychiatry, 57*, 57–72.

Rynearson, E. (1987). Psychological adjustment to unnatural dying. In S. Zisook (Ed.), *Biopsychosocial aspects of bereavement* (pp. 75–93). Washington, DC: American Psychiatric Press.

Saleebey, D. (Ed.). (1992). *The strengths perspective in social work practice*. New York: Longman.

Saleebey, D. (1996). The strengths perspective in social work practice: Extensions and cautions. *Social Work, 41*(3), 296–304.

Sanchez, E., Robertson, T. R., Lewis, C. M., Rosenbluth, B., Bohman, T., & Casey, D. M. (2001). Preventing bullying and sexual harassment in elementary schools: The expect respect model. In R. A. Geffner, M. Loring, & C. Young (Eds.), *Bullying behavior: Current issues, research, and interventions* (pp. 157–180). New York: Haworth Press.

Sarnoff, C. A. (1976). *Latency.* Northvale, NJ: Jason Aronson.

Sarton, M. (1973). A letter to James Stephens. In *Collected poems, 1930–1973* (pp. 42–43). New York: Norton. (Original work, Inner Landscapes, published 1936–1938)

Satir, V. (1983). *Conjoint family therapy* (3rd ed., rev.). Palo Alto, CA: Science and Behavior Books.

Saunders, C. (1997). When push comes to shove: Dealing with bullies requires adult supervision. *Our Children, 22*(4), 34–35.

Schaefer, C. E., & Carey, L. J. (Eds.). (1994). *Family play therapy.* Northvale, NJ: Jason Aronson.

Schaefer, C. E., Jacobsen, H. E., & Ghahramanlou, M. (2000). Play group therapy for social skills deficits in children. In H. G. Kaduson & C. E. Schaefer (Eds.), *Short-term play therapy for children* (pp. 296–341). New York: Guilford Press.

Schaefer, C. E., & Reid, S. E. (Eds.). (1986). *Game play.* New York: Wiley.

Schaefer, C., & Reid, S. (Eds.). (2001). *Game play: Therapeutic use of childhood games* (2nd ed.). New York: Wiley.

Scheeringa, M. S., & Zeanah, C. H. (1995). Symptom expression and trauma variables in children under 48 months of age. *Infant Mental Health Journal, 16*(4), 259–270.

Schiffer, M. (1984). *Children's group therapy: Methods and case histories.* New York: Free Press.

Schlosberg, S. B., & Kagan, R. M. (1988). Practice strategies for engaging chronic, multiproblem families. *Social Casework, 69*(1), 3–9.

Schore, A. N. (2001). The effects of early relational trauma on right brain development, affect regulation, and infant mental health. *Infant Mental Health Journal, 22*(1–2), 201–269.

Schowalter, J. E., Patterson, P. E., Tallmer, M., Kutscher, A. H., Gullo, S. W., & Peretz, D. (Eds.). (1983). *The child and death.* New York: Columbia University Press.

Schore, A. N. (2012). *The science of the art of psychotherapy.* New York: Norton.

Schteingart, J. S., Molnar, J., Klein, T. P., Lowe, C. B., & Hartmann, A. H. (1995). Homelessness and child functioning in the context of risk and protective factors moderating child outcomes. *Journal of Clinical Child Psychology, 24*, 320–331.

Schuckit, M. A. (1985). Genetics and the role of alcoholism. *Journal of the American Medical Association, 25*(18), 2614–2617.

Schuckit, M. A. (1994). A clinical model of genetic influences in alcohol dependence. *Journal of Studies on Alcohol, 55*, 5–17.

Schuurman, D. L. (2008). Grief groups for children and adolescents. In K. Doka & A. S. Tucci (Eds.), *Living with grief: Children and adolescents* (pp. 255–268). Washington, DC: Hospice Foundation of America.

Schuurman, D. L., & DeCristofaro, J. (2007). After a parent's death: Group, family, and individual therapy to help children. In N. B. Webb (Ed.), *Play therapy with children in crisis: Individual, group, and family treatment* (3rd ed., pp. 173–196). New York: Guilford Press.

Schuurman, D. L., & DeCristofaro, J. (2015). After a parent's death. Group, family and individual therapy to help children and adolescents. In N. B. Webb (Ed.), *Play therapy with children and adolescents in crisis* (4th ed., pp. 196–217). New York: Guilford Press.

Schwab, F. (1986). *Just tell the truth.* Charlotte, NC: Kidsrights.

Schwartz, W. (1977). Social group work: The interactionist approach. In J. B. Turner (Ed.), *Encyclopedia of social work* (17th ed., pp. 1328–1338). Washington, DC: National Association of Social Workers.

Schwartz, W., & Zalba, S. (Eds.). (1971). *The practice of group work.* New York: Columbia University Press.

Sedlak, A. J., & Broadhurst, D. D. (1996). *Third national incidence study of child abuse and neglect: Final report.* Washington, DC: National Center on Child Abuse and Neglect.

Sedlak, A. J., Doueck, B., & Gragg, F. (2005). Child maltreatment and the justice system: Predictors of court involvement. *Research on Social Work Practice, 15*(5), 389–403.

Shahinfar, A., Fox, N. A., & Leavitt, L. A. (2000). Preschool children's exposure to violence: Relation of behavior problems to parent and child reports. *American Journal of Orthopsychiatry, 70*(1), 115–125.

Shapiro, V. B., Shapiro, J. R., & Paret, I. H. (2001a). *Complex adoption and assisted reproductive technology: A developmental approach to clinical practice.* New York: Guilford Press.

Shapiro, V. B., Shapiro, J. R., & Paret, I. H. (2001b). Skipped-generation kinship care: Grandparents and their grandchildren. In V. B. Shapiro, J. R. Shapiro, & I. H. Paret (Eds.), *Complex adoption and assisted reproductive technology: A developmental approach to clinical practice* (pp. 125–147). New York: Guilford Press.

Sheafor, B. W., & Landon, P. S. (1987). Generalist perspective. In A. Minahan (Ed.), *Encyclopedia of social work* (18th ed., pp. 660–669). Silver Spring, MD: National Association of Social Workers.

Shear, M. D., & Yee, V. (2017, June). "Dreamers" to stay in U.S. for now, but their long-term fate is unclear. *New York Times*, p. A17.

Shinagawa, L. H., & Jang, M. (1998). *Atlas of American diversity.* Walnut Creek, CA: AltaMira Press.

Shulman, L. (1984). *The skills of helping individuals and groups* (2nd ed.). Itasca, IL: Peacock.

Shulman, L. (1999). *The skills of helping individuals, families, and groups* (3rd ed.). Itasca, IL: Peacock.

Shulman, L. (2006). *The skills of helping individuals, families, groups, and communities* (6th ed.). Pacific Grove, CA: Brooks/Cole.

Siegel, D. (2012). *The developing mind: How relationships and the brain interact to shape who we are* (2nd ed.). New York: Guilford Press.

Siegel, J. P. (2007). The enduring crisis of divorce for children and their parents. In N. B. Webb (Ed.), *Play therapy with children in crisis: Individual, group, and family treatment* (3rd ed., pp. 133–151). New York: Guilford Press.

Silverman, P., & Worden, J. W. (1992). Children's reactions in the early months after the death of a parent. *American Journal of Orthopsychiatry, 62*(1), 93–104.

Slavson, S. R. (1943). *An introduction to group therapy.* New York: Commonwealth Fund.

Slavson, S. R., & Schiffer, M. (1975). *Group psychotherapies for children.* New York: International Universities Press.

Smith, I. E. (2011). Prevention and intervention programs for pregnant women who abuse substances. In S. L. A. Straussner & C. H. Fewell (Eds.), *Children of substance abusing parents: Dynamics and treatment* (pp. 161–184). New York: Springer.

Snyder, S., Bell, H., & Busch-Armendariz, N. (2015, April). Immigrant detention and faith-based organizations. *Social Work, 60*(2), 165–173.

Spielberger, C. D. (1973). *Preliminary manual for the State–Trait Anxiety Inventory for Children.* Palo Alto, CA: Consulting Psychologists Press.

Sroufe, L. A. (1979a). The coherence of individual development: Early care, attachment, and subsequent developmental issues. *American Psychologist, 34*, 834–841.

Sroufe, L. A. (1979b). Socioemotional development. In J. Osofsky (Ed.), *Handbook of infant development* (pp. 462–516). New York: Wiley.

Sroufe, L. A., & Waters, E. (1977). Attachment as an organizational construct. *Child Development, 48*, 1184–1199.

Stahlman, S. D. (1996). Children and the death of a sibling. In C. A. Corr & D. M. Corr (Eds.), *Handbook of childhood death and bereavement* (pp. 149–164). New York: Springer.

Stark, K. D., Rafaelle, L., & Reysa, A. (1994). The treatment of depressed children: A skills training approach to working with children and families. In C. W. LeCroy (Ed.), *Handbook of child and adolescent treatment manuals* (pp. 343–397). New York: Lexington Books.

Steele, W. (1998). *Children of trauma: Tools to help the helper* [Video]. Grosse Pointe Woods, MI: Institute for Trauma and Loss in Children.

Stein, N. (1996). *Bullyproof: A teacher's guide on teasing and bullying for use with fourth and fifth grade students.* Wellesley, MA: Wellesley College Center for Research on Women.

Stern, D. (1985). *The interpersonal world of the infant.* New York: Basic Books.

Strand, V. C. (1999). The assessment and treatment of family sexual abuse: Case of Rosa, age 6. In N. B. Webb (Ed.), *Play therapy with children in crisis: Individual, group, and family treatment* (2nd ed., pp. 104–130). New York: Guilford Press.

Straussner, S. L. A. (1989). Intervention with maltreating parents who are drug and alcohol abusers. In S. Ehrenkrantz (Ed.), *Clinical social work with maltreated children and their families* (pp. 149–177). New York: New York University Press.

Straussner, S. L. A. (Ed.). (1993). *Clinical work with substance-abusing clients.* New York: Guilford Press.

Straussner, S. L. A. (Ed.). (2004). *Clinical work with substance-abusing clients* (2nd ed.). New York: Guilford Press.

Straussner, S. L. A. (Ed.). (2014). *Clinical work with substance-abusing clients* (3rd ed.). New York: Guilford Press.

Straussner, S. L. A., & Donath, R. (2015). Children and teens with substance-abusing parents. In N. B. Webb (Ed.), *Play therapy with children and adolescents in crisis* (4th ed., pp. 79–98). New York: Guilford Press.

Sullivan, D. F. (1952). *Readings in group work.* New York: Association Press.

Swearer, S. M., & Espelage, D. L. (2004). Introduction: A social–ecological framework of bullying among youth. In D. L. Espelage & S. W. Swearer (Eds.), *Bullying in American schools: A social–ecological perspective on prevention and intervention* (pp. 1–12). Mahwah, NJ: Erlbaum.

Swearer, S. M., Espelage, D. L., & Napolitano, S. A. (Eds.). (2009). *Bullying: Prevention and intervention.* New York: Guilford Press.

Swearer, S. M., & Givens, J. E. (2006, March). *Designing an alternative to suspension for middle school bullies.* Paper presented at the annual convention of the National Association of School Psychologists, Anaheim, CA.

Swearer, S. M., Limber, S. P., & Alley, R. (2009). Developing and implementing an effective anti-bullying policy. In S. M. Swearer, D. L. Espelage, & S. A. Napolitano (Eds.), *Bullying: Prevention and intervention* (pp. 39–52). New York: Guilford Press.

Swearer, S. M., Schwartz, H., & Garcia, A. (2015). Bullying. Interpersonal trauma among children and adolescents. In N. B. Webb (Ed.), *Play therapy with children and adolescents in crisis* (4th ed., pp. 259–276). New York: Guilford Press.

Sweeney, D. S., & Homeyer, L. E. (Eds.). (2000). *Group play therapy.* San Francisco: Jossey-Bass.

Tait, D. C., & Depta, J. L. (1993). Play therapy group for bereaved children. In N. B. Webb (Ed.), *Helping bereaved children: A handbook for practitioners* (pp. 169–185). New York: Guilford Press.

Temkin, D. (2015, January 27). All 50 states now have a bullying law: Now what? *The Blog.* Huffington Post.

Terr, L. C. (1983). Play therapy and psychic trauma: A preliminary report. In C. E. Schaefer & K. O'Connor (Eds.), *Handbook of play therapy* (pp. 308–319). New York: Wiley.

Terr, L. C. (1988). What happens to early memories of trauma?: A study of twenty children under age 5 at the time of documented traumatic events. *Journal of the American Academy of Child and Adolescent Psychiatry, 27*(1), 96–104.

Terr, L. C. (1989). Treating psychic trauma in children: A preliminary discussion. *Journal of Traumatic Stress, 2,* 3–20.

Theresa's Fund. (2018). Arizona 501(c)3. When children witness violence.

Thomas, A., Chess, S., & Birch, H. G. (1968). *Temperament and behavior disorders in children.* New York: New York University Press.

Thompson, C. L., & Rudolph, L. B. (1992). *Counseling children* (3rd ed.). Pacific Grove, CA: Brooks/Cole.

Timberlake, E. M., & Sabatino, C. A. (1994). Homeless children: Impact of school attendance on self-esteem and loneliness. *Social Work in Education, 16*(1), 9–20.

Tonning, L. M. (1999). Persistent and chronic neglect in the context of poverty: When parents can't parent. In N. B. Webb (Ed.), *Play therapy with children in crisis: Individual, group, and family treatment* (pp. 203–224). New York: Guilford Press.

Tracy, E. M. (1994). Maternal substance abuse: Protecting the child, preserving the family. *Social Work, 39*(5), 534–540.

Tracy, E. M. (1999). Review of the family at risk: Issues and trends in family preservation services. *Social Services Review, 73,* 262–263.

Tracy, E. M. (2001). Interventions: Hard and soft services. In E. Walton, P. Sandau-Beckler, & M. Mannes (Eds.), *Balancing family-centered services and child well-being: Exploring issues in policy, practice, theory, and research* (pp. 155–178). New York: Columbia University Press.

Twemlow, S. W., Biggs, B. K., Nelson, T. D., Vernberge, E. M., Fonagy, P., & Twemlow, S. (2009). Effects of participation in a martial arts-based antibullying program on children's aggression in elementary schools. *Psychology in the Schools, 45*, 947–959.

Tyson, K. (1995, March). *Empowering children and their caregivers: Beyond adult-centrism.* Paper presented at the annual meeting of the Council on Social Work Education, San Diego, CA.

Understood Team, The. (2017). The difference between the Every Student Succeeds Act and No Child Left Behind. Retrieved August 7, 2017, from *www.understood.org/en/school-learning/your-childs-rights/basics-about-the-childs-rights/the-difference-between-the-every-student-succeds-act-and-no-child-left-behind.*

University of Kentucky College of Social Work. (1989). *Collaboration for competency: Examining social work curriculum in the perspective of current practice with children and families.* Lexington, KY: Author.

U.S. Bureau of the Census. (2011, June 29). Census bureau reports 64 percent increase in number of children living with a grandparent over last two decades. Retreved from *www.census.gov/newsroom/releases/archives/children/cb11-117.html.*

U.S. Bureau of the Census. (2016, November 17). *The majority of children live with two parents, Census Bureau reports.* Washington, DC: Public Information Office.

U.S. Citizenship and Immigration Services. (2011). Green card eligibility. Retrieved from *www.uscis.gov/greencard/eligibility/-categories.*

U.S. Department of Health and Human Services. (2003). *Child abuse and neglect data.* Washington, DC: U.S. Government Printing Office.

U.S. Department of Health and Human Services. (1993). *Eighth special report to the U.S. Congress on alcohol and health.* Rockville, MD: National Institute on Alcohol Abuse and Alcoholism.

U.S. Department of Health and Human Services. (1999). *Mental health. A report of the Surgeon General.* Rockville, MD: National Institutes of Health, National Institute of Mental Health.

U.S. Department of Health and Human Services, Children's Bureau. (1978). *Substance abuse and child abuse and neglect.* Washington, DC: U.S. Government Printing Office.

U.S. Department of Justice. (2009). A guide to disability rights laws. Retrieved August 7, 2017, from *www.ada.gov/cguide.htm.*

U.S. Immigration & Customs Enforcement. (2016). *FY 2016 ICE immigration removals.* Washington, DC: Office of the Department of Homeland Security.

Vail, P. L. (1989). The gifted learning disabled child. In L. B. Silver (Ed.), *The assessment of learning disabilities: Preschool through adulthood* (pp. 135–159). New York: Little, Brown.

Vaillant, G. (1983). *The natural history of alcoholism: Causes, patterns, and paths to recovery.* Cambridge, MA: Harvard University Press.

van der Kolk, B. A. (Ed.). (1987). *Psychological trauma.* Washington, DC: American Psychiatric Press.

van der Kolk, B. A. (1989). The compulsion to repeat the trauma: Re-enactment, re-victimization, and masochism. *Psychiatric Clinics of North America, 12*(2), 389–406.

van der Kolk, B. A. (2005). Developmental trauma disorder: Toward a rational diagnosis for children with complex trauma histories. *Psychiatric Annals, 35*, 401–408.

Vernberg, E. M., La Greca, A. M., Silverman, W. K., & Prinstein, M. J. (1996).

Prediction of posttraumatic stress symptoms after Hurricane Andrew. *Journal of Abnormal Psychology, 105*(2), 237–248.

Vinter, R. (1959). Group work: Perspective and prospects. In *Social work with groups*. New York: National Association of Social Workers.

Vogel, J., & Vernberg, E. M. (1993). Children's psychological response to disaster. *Journal of Clinical Child Psychology, 22*, 470–484.

Vostanis, P., & Cumella, S. (Eds.). (1999). *Homeless children: Problems and needs*. London: Jessica Kingsley.

Wachtel, E. F. (1994). *Treating troubled children and their families*. New York: Guilford Press.

Wallerstein, J. (1983). Children of divorce: The psychological tasks of the child. *American Journal of Orthopsychiatry, 53*, 230–243.

Wallerstein, J., & Blakeslee, S. (1989). *Second chances*. New York: Ticknor & Fields.

Wallerstein, J., & Kelly, J. (1980). *Surviving the breakup: How children and parents cope with divorce*. New York: Basic Books.

Wallerstein, J., Lewis, J. M., & Blakeslee, S. (2000). *The unexpected legacy of divorce: A 25-year landmark study*. New York: Hyperion.

Walsh, F. (Ed.). (2012). *Normal family processes: Growing diversity and complexity* (4th ed.). New York: Guilford Press.

Walton, E., Sandau-Beckler, P., & Mannes, M. (Eds.). (2001). *Balancing family-centered services and child well-being: Exploring issues in policy, practice, theory, and research*. New York: Columbia University Press.

Webb, N. B. (1983). Developing competent clinical practitioners: A model for supervisors. *The Clinical Supervisor, 1*(4), 41–51.

Webb, N. B. (1989). Supervision of child therapy: Analyzing therapeutic impasses and monitoring countertransference. *The Clinical Supervisor, 73*, 51–76.

Webb, N. B. (1994a). Assessment and intervention with kindergarten children following the New York World Trade Center disaster. *Crisis Intervention and Time-Limited Treatment, 1*(1), 47–59.

Webb, N. B. (1994b). *Techniques of play therapy: A clinical demonstration* [Videotape]. New York: Guilford Press.

Webb, N. B. (1995). *Survey of Westchester County child welfare administrators*. Unpublished data.

Webb, N. B. (1996). *Social work practice with children*. New York: Guilford Press.

Webb, N. B. (Ed.). (1991). *Play therapy with children in crisis: A casebook for practitioners*. New York: Guilford Press.

Webb, N. B. (Ed.). (1993). *Helping bereaved children: A handbook for practitioners*. New York: Guilford Press.

Webb, N. B. (Ed.). (1999). *Play therapy with children in crisis: Individual, group, and family treatment* (2nd ed.). New York: Guilford Press.

Webb, N. B. (Ed.). (2001). *Culturally diverse parent–child and family relationships: A guide for social workers and other practitioners*. New York: Columbia University Press.

Webb, N. B. (Ed.). (2002a). *Helping bereaved children: A handbook for practitioners* (2nd ed.). New York: Guilford Press.

Webb, N. B. (2002b). September 11, 2001. In N. B. Webb (Ed.), *Helping bereaved children: A handbook for practitioners* (2nd ed., pp. 365–384). New York: Guilford Press.

Webb, N. B. (2003). *Social work practice with children* (2nd ed.). New York: Guilford Press.
Webb, N. B. (Ed.). (2004). *Mass trauma and violence: Helping families and children cope.* New York: Guilford Press.
Webb, N. B. (2006a). *Techniques of play therapy: A clinical demonstration* [DVD]. New York: Guilford Press.
Webb, N. B. (Ed.). (2006b). *Working with traumatized youth in child welfare.* New York: Guilford Press.
Webb, N. B. (Ed.). (2007). *Play therapy with children in crisis: Individual, group, and family treatment* (3rd ed.). New York: Guilford Press.
Webb, N. B. (Ed.). (2010). *Helping bereaved children: A handbook for practitioners* (3rd ed.). New York: Guilford Press.
Webb, N. B. (Ed.). (2011). *Social work practice with children and adolescents* (4th ed.). New York: Guilford Press.
Webb, N. B. (Ed.). (2015). *Play therapy with children and adolescents in crisis* (4th ed.). New York: Guilford Press.
Wegscheider, S. (1981). *Another chance: Hope and health for the alcoholic family.* Palo Alto, CA: Science & Behavior Books.
Weick, A., & Pope, L. (1988). Knowing what's best: A new look at self-determination. *Social Casework, 69*(1), 10–16.
Weinhold, B. K. (2003). Uncovering the hidden causes of bullying and school violence. In J. Miller, I. R. Martin, & G. Schamess (Eds.), *School violence and children in crisis: Community and school interventions for social workers and counselors* (pp. 103–134). Denver, CO: Love.
Weisz, J. R., & Kazdin, A. E. (Eds.). (2010). *Evidence-based psychotherapies for children and adolescents* (2nd ed.). New York: Guilford Press.
Weisz, J. R., & Kazdin, A. E. (Eds.). (2017). *Evidence-based psychotherapies for children and adolescents* (3rd ed.). New York: Guilford Press.
Werner, E. E., & Smith, R. S. (1982). *Vulnerable but invincible: A study of resilient children.* New York: McGraw-Hill.
Wertz, R. (1986, November–December). Children of alcoholics. *Chemical People Newsletter*, p. 9.
Wessler, S. (2011). *Shattered families: The perilous intersection between immigration enforcement and the child welfare system.* New York: Applied Research Center.
Whittaker, J. K. (1987). Group care for children. In A. Minahan (Ed.), *Encyclopedia of social work* (18th ed., pp. 672–682). Silver Spring, MD: National Association of Social Workers.
Whittaker, J. K. (1991). The leadership challenge in family-based services: Policy, practice and research. *Families in Society, 72*(5), 294–300.
Wilkerson, I. (1994, May 16). Two boys, a debt, a gun, a victim: The face of violence. *New York Times*, pp. A-1, A-14.
Wilson, D. B., & Lipsey, M. W. (2001). The role of method in treatment effectiveness research: Evidence from meta-analysis. *Psychological Methods, 6*(4), 413–429.
Wilson, J. P., & Keane, T. M. (Eds.). (2004). *Assessing psychological trauma and PTSD* (2nd ed.). New York: Guilford Press.
Winnicott, D. W. (1971a). *Playing and reality.* New York: Basic Books.
Winnicott, D. W. (1971b). *Therapeutic consultations in child psychiatry.* New York: Basic Books.

Wolfenstein, M. (1966). How is mourning possible? *Psychoanalytic Study of the Child, 21*, 432–460.

Wolin, S., & Wolin, S. (1995). Resilience among youth growing up in substance-abusing families. *Pediatric Clinics of North America, 42*, 415–429.

Woltmann, A. G. (1964). The use of puppetry as a projective method in therapy. In M. R. Haworth (Ed.), *Child psychotherapy* (pp. 395–399). New York: Basic Books. (Original work published 1951)

Wu, S. J. (2001). Parenting in Chinese American families. In N. B. Webb (Ed.), *Culturally diverse parent–child and family relationships: A guide for social workers and other practitioners* (pp. 235–260). New York: Columbia University Press.

Yalom, I. (1985). *The theory and practice of group psychotherapy* (3rd ed.). New York: Basic Books.

Ybarra, M. L., & Mitchell, K. J. (2004). Youth engaging in online harassment: Associations with caregiver–child relationships, Internet use, and personal characteristics. *Journal of Adolescence, 27*, 319–336.

Youngstrom, N. (1991, October). Drug exposure in home elicits worst behavior. *Monitor*, p. 3.

Zayas, L. H. (2015). *Forgotten citizens: Deportation, children, and the making of American exiles and orphans*. New York: Oxford University Press.

Zayas, L. H., Aguilar-Gaxiola, S., Yoon, H., & Rey, G. N. (2015). The distress of citizen-children with detained and deported parents. *Journal of Child and Family Studies, 24*(11), 3213–3223.

Zayas, L. H., Canino, I., & Suarez, Z. E. (2001). Parenting in Mainland Puerto Rican families. In N. B. Webb (Ed.), *Culturally diverse parent–child and family relationships* (pp. 133–156). New York: Columbia University Press.

Zevon, M. (1990, September 10). Archway program group therapy. *Mount Vernon Journal*, p. 10.

Zins, J. E., Elias, M. J., & Maher, C. A. (2007). *Bullying, victimization, and peer-harassment: A handbook of prevention intervention*. New York: Routledge.

Zirkel, P. A. (2017). RTI and other approaches to SLD identification under the IDEA: A legal update. *Learning Disability Quarterly, 40*(3), 165–171.

Author Index

B

H

I

M

N

O

P

Q

R

S

T

V

Subject Index

Note. f or *t* after a page number indicates a figure or a table.

B

D

G

S

T

U

V

W